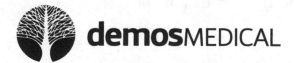 **demos**MEDICAL

Acquisitions Editor: R. Craig Percy
Cover Design: Steve Pisano
Compositor: The Manila Typesetting Company
Printer: Victor Graphics

Visit our website at www.demosmedpub.com

Medicine is an ever-changing science. Research and clinical experience are continually expanding our knowledge, in particular our understanding of proper treatment and drug therapy. The authors, editors, and publisher have made every effort to ensure that all information in this book is in accordance with the state of knowledge at the time of production of the book. Nevertheless, the authors, editors, and publisher are not responsible for errors or omissions or for any consequences from application of the information in this book and make no warranty, express or implied, with respect to the contents of the publication. Every reader should examine carefully the package inserts accompanying each drug and should carefully check whether the dosage schedules mentioned therein or the contraindications stated by the manufacturer differ from the statements made in this book. Such examination is particularly important with drugs that are either rarely used or have been newly released on the market.

Library of Congress Cataloging-in-Publication Data
Medical management of adults with neurologic disabilities / edited by Adrian Cristian.
    p. ; cm.
  Includes bibliographical references and index.
  ISBN-13: 978-1-933864-45-7 (hardcover : alk. paper)
  ISBN-10: 1-933864-45-1 (hardcover : alk. paper)
  1. Nervous system--Diseases--Complications. 2. Nervous system—Diseases—Patients—Medical care. I. Cristian, Adrian, 1964-
  [DNLM: 1. Nervous System Diseases—complications. 2. Primary Health Care—methods.
3. Adult. 4. Disabled Persons—rehabilitation. WL 140 M266 2009]
  RC346.M266 2009
  616.8'043—dc22

                                                                      2008040668

Special discounts on bulk quantities of Demos Medical Publishing books are available to corporations, professional associations, pharmaceutical companies, health care organizations, and other qualifying groups. For details, please contact:
Special Sales Department
Demos Medical Publishing
386 Park Avenue South, Suite 301
New York, NY 10016
Phone: 800–532–8663 or 212–683–0072
Fax: 212–683–0118
Email: orderdept@demosmedpub.com

Printed in the United States of America
08 09 10 11   5 4 3 2 1

This book is dedicated to my wife and children whose love
support and understanding helped make it possible.
To my father, Cali Cristian, a man of wisdom and integrity
who taught by example. To my mother, Stella Cristian,
who embodies caring and compassion.
To the memory of Harriet and Norman Zuller,
Rasela Cru, and Camille Katz.

.

Contents

Preface

As a result of advances in modern medicine and public health measures, adults with neurologic disabilities such as spinal cord injury, traumatic brain injury, stroke, multiple sclerosis, and cerebral palsy are living longer and often very productive lives. The increased longevity, however, subjects them to challenges imposed by the aging process itself as well as the late effects of their neurologic diagnosis.

The goal of this book is to provide a reference that busy clinicians can refer to in the daily management of the medical problems faced by this population with the hope that this will ultimately result in improved health for their patients.

The chapters have been selected based on common medical problems and health care issues that clinicians face daily. Each chapter attempts to cover basic information about pertinent anatomy, physiology, pathophysiology, patient assessment, and practical treatment advice. Chapters have been organized alphabetically by topic to facilitate quick reference in the clinical setting. The index will also facilitate quick data location.

A unique feature of the book is that the topics of patient safety and patient education are an integral part of most chapters. These sections were incorporated out of concern that this population is vulnerable and at a high risk for adverse events given that many have cognitive and communication impairments as well as often severe manifestations of their neurologic disease. It is felt that the likelihood of an adverse event will be reduced by bringing to the attention of health care providers key areas of patient safety as well as important information to educate patients and their caregivers.

The contributing authors represent a wide spectrum of medical, surgical, and rehabilitative expertise and have experience in caring for this population in a variety of settings across the United States.

This book is meant to be used as a general guide and reference for clinicians in the management of their patients; however, individualized care with appropriate local expertise is advised given the complexities of the medical problems that these patients face.

Adrian Cristian, MD

Contributors

Uri S. Adler, MD
Director, Stroke Rehabilitation
Department of Physiatry and Rehabilitation Medicine
Kessler Institute for Rehabilitation
Saddle Brook, New Jersey

Mohamed S. Ahmed, MD
Assistant Professor and Assistant Chief
Department of Rehabilitation Medicine
Mount Sinai School of Medicine
Director Inpatient Rehabilitation Unit
Department of Rehabilitation Medicine
James J. Peters Veterans Affairs Medical Center
New York, New York

Mindy Aisen, MD
Director and Chief Executive Officer
Global Research for Development Brain Disorders
Cerebral Palsy International Research Foundation
Washington, DC

Alan Anschel, MD
Spinal Cord Injury Medicine Fellow
Department of Physical Medicine and Rehabilitation
Rehabilitation Institute of Chicago
Chicago, Illinois

Naomi Betesh, DO
Chief Resident
Department of Rehabilitation Medicine
Mount Sinai School of Medicine
New York, New York

Carol Braunschweig, PhD, RD
Associate Professor
Department of Kinesiology and Nutrition
University of Illinois at Chicago
Chicago, Illinois

Kenneth J. Ciuffreda, OD, PhD
Professor
Department of Vision Sciences
State University of New York College of Optometry
New York, New York

Adrian Cristian, MD
Associate Professor
Department of Rehabilitation Medicine
Mount Sinai School of Medicine
New York, New York
Chief
Rehabilitation Medicine
James J. Peters Veterans Affairs Medical Center
Bronx, New York

George A. Deitrick, MD
Assistant Professor
Department of Surgery
Mount Sinai School of Medicine
New York, New York

Amit Dholakia, DO
Resident
Department of Rehabilitation Medicine
Mount Sinai School of Medicine
New York, New York

Gregory A. Elder, MD
Physician
Department of Rehabilitation Medicine
James J. Peters Veterans Affairs Medical Center
Bronx, New York

Steven R. Flanagan, MD
Professor and Chairman
Department of Rehabilitation Medicine
New York University School of Medicine
New York, New York

Marinella DeFre Galea, MD
Assistant Professor
Department of Physical Medicine and Rehabilitation
Mount Sinai School of Medicine
New York, New York

Clinic Director, Spinal Cord Injury
James J. Peters Veterans Affairs Medical Center
Bronx, New York

Shai Gavi, DO, MPH
Assistant Professor
Department of Clinical Medicine
Stony Brook University School of Medicine
Chief, Section of Hospital Medicine
Department of Medicine
Stony Brook University Medical Center
Stony Brook, New York

Brian D. Greenwald, MD
Assistant Professor
Department of Rehabilitation Medicine
Mount Sinai Medical Center
New York, New York

Neera Kapoor, OD, MS
Associate Clinical Professor
Director, Raymond J. Greenwald Rehabilitation Center
Department of Clinical Sciences
State University of New York College of Optometry
New York, New York

Danielle M. Kerkovich, PhD
Associate Director for Research
Sensory Motor Performance Program
Rehabilitation Institute of Chicago
Chicago, Illinois

Avniel Shetreat-Klein, MD, PhD
Instructor
Department of Rehabilitation Medicine
Mount Sinai Medical Center
New York, New York

Mark A. Korstein, MD
Professor and Chief
Department of Gastroenterology
James J. Peters Veterans Affairs Medical Center
Mount Sinai Medical Center
New York, New York

Michael La Fountaine, EdD
Health Science Specialist
Center of Excellence for the Medical Consequences of Spinal Cord Injury
James J. Peters Veterans Affairs Medical Center
Bronx, New York

Susan A. Laskoski, BA, MA
Clinical Manager
Department of Speech Language Pathology
Kessler Institute for Rehabilitation
Saddle Brook, New Jersey

Marvin Lesser, MD
Pulmonary Consultant
Center of Excellence for the Medical Consequences of Spinal Cord Injury
James J. Peters Veterans Affairs Medical Center
Bronx, New York

HuiFang Liang, MD, PhD
Pharmacoepidemiology Data Analyst
Department of Pharmacoepidemiology Data Analysis
Takeda Global Research and Development Center, Inc.
Lake Forest, Illinois

Julie T. Lin, MD
Assistant Attending Physiatrist
Department of Physiatry and Rehabilitation Medicine
Hospital for Special Surgery
Assistant Professor
Department of Physiatry and Rehabilitation Medicine
Weill Medical College of Cornell University
New York, New York

Kimberly Beckwith McGuire, PhD
Psychologist
Department of Psychology and Neuropsychology
Kessler Institute for Rehabilitation
West Orange, New Jersey

Maria D. McNish, MS CCC-SLP
Clinical Manager
Department of Speech Language Pathology
Kessler Institute for Rehabilitation
West Orange, New Jersey

Jeffrey I. Mechanick, MD, FACP, FACE, FACN
Clinical Professor of Medicine and Director of Metabolic Support
Department of Endocrinology, Diabetes and Bone Disease
Mount Sinai School of Medicine
New York, New York

Dorothy A. Miller, MD
Attending Physician
Spinal Cord Injury Patient Care Center
James J. Peters Veterans Affairs Medical Center
Bronx, New York

Steven Nussbaum, MD
Assistant Professor
Department of Physical Medicine and Rehabilitation
Rehabilitation Institute of Chicago
Northwestern University
Chicago, Illinois

Norma Parets, BA, MS, OTR/L
Admissions Coordinator
Mount Sinai Rehabilitation Center
Mount Sinai Medical Center
New York, New York

Miroslav Radulovic, MD
Staff Physician
Department of Medicine
Associate Investigator
Center of Excellence for the Medical Consequences of Spinal Cord Injury
James J. Peters Veterans Affairs Medical Center
Bronx, New York

John L. Rigg, MD
Traumatic Brain Injury Program Director
Department of Behavioral Health
Dwight D. Eisenhower Army Medical Center
Augusta, Georgia

James H. Rimmer, PhD
Professor
Department of Disability and Human Development
University of Illinois at Chicago
Chicago, Illinois

David L. Ripley, MD, MS
Medical Director of Brain Injury Research
CNS Medical Group
Craig Hospital
Englewood, Colorado

Rosanna C. Sabini, BA
Resident Physician
Department of Rehabilitation Medicine
Mount Sinai Medical Center
New York, New York

Gregory Schilero, MD
Staff Physician
Department of Pulmonary and Critical Care Medicine
James J. Peters Veterans Affairs Medical Center
Bronx, New York
Assistant Professor
Department of Medicine
The Mount Sinai School of Medicine
New York, New York

Audrey J. Schmerzler, RN, MSN, CRRN, NE-BC
Director of Nursing
Mount Sinai Rehabilitation Center
Mount Sinai Medical Center
New York, New York

Hyon Schneider, MD
Chief Resident
Department of Physical Medicine and Rehabilitation
Mount Sinai School of Medicine
New York, New York

Adam Silver
Student
Bronx Science High School
Bronx, New York

Ashwani K. Singal, MD
GI Fellow
Department of Internal Medicine
University of Texas Medical Branch
Galveston, TX

Daniela Spector, DDS
Signature Smiles
Great Neck, New York

Yuval Spector, DDS
Signature Smiles
Great Neck, New York
Fellowship in Implant Dentistry
North Shore University Hospital
Manhasset, New York

Kevin Sperber, MD
Assistant Clinical Professor
Department of Physical Medicine and Rehabilitation
Columbia University College of Physicians and Surgeons
New York, New York

Adam Stein, MD
Chairman
Department of Physical Medicine and Rehabilitation
North Shore-Long Island Jewish Health System
Great Neck, New York

Michelle Stern, MD
Assistant Clinical Professor
Department of Physical Medicine and Rehabilitation
Columbia University College of Physicians and Surgeons
New York, New York

Gene Tekmyster, DO
Resident
Department of Physical Medicine and Rehabilitation
Saint Vincent Catholic Medical Centers
New York, New York

Kristen Tomey, PhD
Assistant Research Scientist
Department of Epidemiology
University of Michigan
Ann Arbor, Michigan

Monique J. Tremaine, PhD
Senior Neuropsychologist
Psychology/Cognitive Rehabilitation Program
Kessler Institute for Rehabilitation
West Orange, New Jersey

Michael A. Via, MD
Clinical Instructor
Department of Endocrinology and Metabolism
Beth Israel Medical Center
New York, New York

Loran C. Vocaturo, EdD, ABPP
Director
Department of Psychology and Neuropsychology
Kessler Institute for Rehabilitation
West Orange, New Jersey

1

Aging with a Neurologic Disability

Adrian Cristian
Adam Silver

According to the 2006 American Community Survey, 13% of Americans between the ages of 21 and 64 have a disability. This number increases dramatically for those over the age of 65 to 41%. Those with a physical disability have less education and lower median earnings and are less likely to be employed in comparison to nondisabled Americans (1).

Respondents to the survey between the ages of 25 and 64 reported: 1) severe difficulties walking and using stairs (6.5%), 2) limitation in a basic activity of daily living (ADL) (2.5%), 3) limitation in an instrumental activity of daily living (IADL) (4.0%), 4) need for personal assistance (2.9%), 5) need of assistance for one or more ADLs or IADLs (3.1%), 6) symptoms of depression or anxiety (3.1%), 7) trouble coping with stress (2.4%), and 8) perceived health status as fair or poor (25.4% for nonseverely disabled and 63.1% for severely disabled). According to the U.S. Census Americans with Disability report, there are 4,174,000 people living with a severe disability and in poverty (1).

Whereas these statistics are not specific for adults aging with a neurologic disability, they underscore the larger problems faced by all adults living with a disability. The goal of this chapter is to provide an overview of the challenges faced by adults aging with spinal cord injury (SCI), traumatic brain injury (TBI), stroke (CVA), and cerebral palsy (CP). The assessment and treatment of physical and mental ailments commonly seen in these diseases are discussed separately in greater detail elsewhere in this book.

PREMATURE AGING

As life expectancy for all Americans has increased, so has that for adults with neurologic disabilities. Advances in public health, better primary and preventive care, and better medical and surgical treatments have all contributed to this increase. Many adults with these disabilities can expect a life span that is comparable to able-bodied individuals. However, as these adults age, they face health challenges similar to their nondisabled counterparts

1

(i.e., coronary artery disease, hypertension, obesity, diabetes, cancer, and osteoarthritic conditions) as well as some that are more specific to their disability (i.e., repetitive use syndrome of the upper extremities in wheelchair users).

The concept of "premature aging" has been described with respect to adults aging with a neurologic disease. Premature aging is believed to be due to the extra functional demands placed on organ systems. The extra demands over time lead to wear and tear on that organ system at a younger age than in able-bodied individuals.

The age of onset of disability is important. If the injury occurred before the maturation of the organ system, then the organs in that system would not function at an optimal level and would break down earlier than in a fully mature organ system. Conversely, if the injury occurred after the maturation of the organ system, but organs in that system are subjected to increased workload or repetitive trauma, then their functional life span would also be shortened (2).

The aging rate for an organ has been estimated to be about 1% per year, whereas in adults with disabilities, this rate can vary between 1.5 and 5%. This accelerated aging rate can also depend on the types of treatments that the person received during his or her life for problems of that organ system. Lack of appropriate treatments at key points in the person's life can contribute to an accelerated aging rate (2).

Changes in various organ systems eventually have an impact on the individual's functional level. The onset of functional issues has been reported as the "20/40" rule. This refers to 20 years of living with the injury or 40 years of age, whichever come first (3). A unique "functional impairment syndrome" has also been reported in adults with severe disabilities. This consists of weakness, fatigue, and pain (2).

Adults with neurologic disabilities face additional challenges such as loss of significant social support systems as their caregivers age as well as loss of income if they had previously been working. Health and social challenges commonly encountered by adults with neurologic disabilities are listed in Table 1.1.

AGING WITH SCI

There are an estimated 253,000 people living with SCI in the United States and 11,000 newly diagnosed each year. The average age at diagnosis is 38, and injuries occur more commonly in men. The most common causes are motor vehicle accidents, falls, gunshot wounds, and recreational activities (4).

Life expectancy for a paraplegic injury at age 20 is 46.3 years and for a low tetraplegic injury (C5–8) is 41.7 years (4). Forty percent of people living with SCI are over the age of 45, and 25% of adults with SCI have lived with the injury for 20 or more years (5).

Whereas the leading cause of death in the past was kidney disease, recently respiratory complications (pneumonia, pulmonary emboli) and septicemia have been reported as more common (4). As people with SCI live longer, they

Table 1.1

Problems Affecting Adults Aging with a Neurologic Disability

- Cognitive impairments
  - o Impaired memory
  - o Impaired concentration
  - o Slowed speed of mental processing
- Communication
- Swallowing
- Dental-caries, periodontal disease
- Seizures
- Hearing and visual problems
- Obesity
- Diabetes
- Hypertension
- Coronary artery disease
- Respiratory-aspiration pneumonia
- Neurogenic bowel and bladder
- Spasticity

- Contractures
- Psychiatric
  - o Depression
  - o Anxiety
  - o PTSD symptoms
  - o Substance abuse
  - o Irritability, anger, poor impulse control
- Weakness
- Fatigue
- Pain syndromes
  - o Musculoskeletal (repetitive use, osteoarthritis)
  - o Neuropathic-entrapment neuropathies, radiculopathy
- Functional decline for ADLs and IADLs
- Aging caregivers
- Limited social support systems and income

are also subject to diseases that are prevalent in the nondisabled population, such as heart disease and cancer (5).

AGING WITH A TRAUMATIC BRAIN INJURY

It has been reported that 1.4 million Americans are evaluated and treated for a TBI each year, 235,000 of which require hospitalization. The leading causes of TBI are falls, motor vehicle accidents, and blows to the head. The direct and indirect costs of TBI have been estimated to be $60 billion (6).

Two percent of Americans (5.3 million) are living with the effects of a traumatic brain injury, with the vast majority being mild injuries. Forty percent of those hospitalized with a TBI have at least one unmet need for services one year after injury (6). The most common unmet needs include: 1) impaired memory, 2) impaired problem solving, 3) stress and emotional upset, 4) temper control, and 5) job-related skills (6).

Additional challenges faced by adults with TBI include the psychosocial impact of lifelong cognitive impairments. Psychiatric symptoms such as depression, anxiety, posttraumatic stress disorder (PTSD), agitation, aggression and impulsivity have been well documented as have challenges to community reintegration (7). Sleep problems are also a common occurrence in adults with TBI.

Elderly adults who sustain a TBI often have a more complicated and lengthier hospitalization with poorer reported rehabilitation outcomes and more severe disabilities at time of discharge. Nevertheless, the benefit of rehab in this population has been reported.

AGING WITH MULTIPLE SCLEROSIS

There are 250,000–350,000 persons living with multiple sclerosis (MS) in the United States, with approximately 10,000 newly diagnosed each year. Women with MS outnumber men, and the highest incidence is in the fourth decade of life. Fifty percent of people with MS survive for 30 years following disease onset (8). Issues commonly affecting adults with MS include pain, weakness, fatigue, heat intolerance, cognitive dysfunction (impaired memory and problem solving and slowed speed of mental processing), depression, and suicide.

AGING WITH CEREBRAL PALSY

It has been estimated that there are approximately 400,000 adults with cerebral palsy (CP), with 8000 babies diagnosed each year. The number of adults with CP will increase due to the increased survival of low-birthweight babies.

The major issues facing adults with CP are communication, swallowing function, musculoskeletal pain, seizures, scoliosis, falls and fractures, visual deficits, hearing impairment, dental caries, and periodontal disease (9).

AGING WITH A STROKE

Each year 780,000 people in the United States have a stroke. Of these, approximately 600,000 have their first stroke and 180,000 have a recurrent stroke. Twenty-five percent of all stroke survivors will have another stroke within 5 years, and 28% of all strokes occur in people under the age of 65. There are 5.8 million stroke survivors in the United States, and stroke is the most common disability. Forty percent of all stroke survivors have moderate to severe impairments that will require specialized care. The risk of stroke is increased significantly in adults with hypertension and diabetes (10,11).

These are sobering statistics with profound implications for those affected. Adults living with a stroke face challenges similar to those described for other neurologic diseases. They include: 1) communication and swallowing problems, 2) weakness, 3) fatigue, 4) neurogenic bowel and bladder, 5) functional losses and need for personal assistance with ADLs and IADLs, 6) limited ambulation, and 7) cognitive impairments.

REFERENCES

1. www.census.gov
2. Kemp BJ. What the rehabilitation professional and the consumer need to know. Phys Med Rehabil Clin N Am 2005; 16:1–18.
3. Gerhart KA, Bergstrom E, Charilifue SW, Menter RR, Whiteneck GG. Longterm spinal cord injury: functional changes over time. Arch Phys Med Rehabil 1993; 74:1030–1034.
4. www.spinalcord.uab.edu
5. Capoor J, Stein AB. Aging with spinal cord injury. Phys Med Rehabil Clin N Am 2005; 16:129–162.
6. www.cdc.gov

7. Flanagan SR, Hibbard MR, Gordon WA. The impact of age on traumatic brain injury. Phys Med Rehabil Clin N Am 2005; 16:163–178.
8. Stern M. Aging with Multiple Sclerosis. Phys Med Rehabil Clin N Am 2005; 16:219–234.
9. Zaffuto-Sforza C. Aging with cerebral Palsy. Phys Med Rehabil Clin N Am 2005; 16:235–251
10. www.americanheart.org
11. www.theuniversityhospital.com

2 | Autonomic Dysreflexia

Steven Nussbaum

Autonomic dysreflexia, a syndrome characterized by an elevation of the systolic and diastolic blood pressures in response to a noxious stimulus below the level of injury, is a serious cause of morbidity in spinal cord injury.

In general, autonomic dysreflexia occurs in individuals with spinal cord injuries above the T6 level. Other names for autonomic dysreflexia include autonomic hyperreflexia, paroxysmal hypertension, paroxysmal neurogenic hypertension, autonomic spasticity, and sympathetic hyperreflexia.

ANATOMY AND PHYSIOLOGY

Autonomic dysreflexia cannot occur until after spinal shock has resolved and reflexes return. Noxious stimuli transmit impulses that ascend via sensory nerves in the spinal cord and stimulate sympathetic neurons below the injury level. Norepinephrine and dopamine are subsequently released, causing vasoconstriction of the arterial vasculature, thus resulting in a sudden elevation in blood pressure. The carotid and aortic baroreceptors detect the elevated blood pressure and stimulate two brainstem reflexes. First, the heart rate slows via parasympathetic stimulation via the vagus nerve, which is not affected by the spinal cord injury. Second, sympathetic inhibitory impulses are stimulated above the injury level. These impulses, however, are blocked by the spinal cord injury and are unable to cause vasodilatation of the arterial vasculature below the injury level. Therefore, despite the lowered heart rate, sympathetic stimuli are relatively unopposed in autonomic dysreflexia.

Autonomic dysreflexia has numerous potential etiologies. The most common etiologies are secondary to bowel, bladder, and skin problems (Table 2.1). Urinary system etiologies include bladder distention, a blocked urinary catheter, bladder or kidney stones, a urinary tract infection, and bladder spasms. Gastrointestinal system etiologies include bowel impaction, bowel distention, gallstones, hemorrhoids, gastritis or gastric ulcers, and an acute abdomen. Integumentary system etiologies include constrictive clothing or shoes, constrictive catheters, blisters, sunburn, burns, insect bites, pressure sores, and ingrown toenails. Reproductive system etiologies in men include sexual intercourse, sexually transmitted diseases, ejaculation, epididymitis, and scrotal compression. Reproductive system etiologies in women include sexual intercourse, sexually transmitted diseases, menstruation, vaginitis, and pregnancy. Skeletal and circulatory system etiologies include fractures, muscle strains, heterotopic ossification, deep vein thrombosis, pulmonary emboli, myocardial infarction, pneumonia, and asthma.

Table 2.1

Etiologies of Autonomic Dysreflexia

Bladder etiologies
    Bladder distension
    Urinary tract infection
    Bladder spasms
    Bladder/kidney stones
Gastrointestinal etiologies
    Constipation/impaction
    Gallstones
    Hemorrhoids
    Gastritis/ulcer
    Acute abdomen
Integument etiologies
    Sunburn
    Burns
    Insect bites
    Pressure sores
    Ingrown toenails
    Constrictive clothing
Reproductive etiologies
    Sexual intercourse
    Sexually transmitted diseases
    Menstruation
    Pregnancy
    Vaginitis
    Scrotal constriction
Skeletal/cardiovascular etiologies
    Fractures
    Muscle strains
    Heterotopic ossification
    Deep vein thrombosis
    Pulmonary embolism
    Myocardial infarction
    Asthma
    Pneumonia

PATIENT ASSESSMENT

Numerous signs and symptoms characteristically occur with autonomic dysreflexia. Table 2.2 outlines some common clinical questions to ask patients with suspected autonomic dysreflexia.

The most common sign of autonomic dysreflexia (Table 2.3) is a sudden increase in both the systolic and diastolic blood pressures of 20–40 mmHg above baseline. It is important to note that a blood pressure of 130/80 may be secondary to autonomic dysreflexia if the individual's baseline blood pressure is 90/50. The most common symptom of autonomic dysreflexia is a pounding headache that corresponds to the heart beat. Bradycardia is often seen in response to the elevated BP. Cardiac arrhythmias such as atrial fibrillation or PVCs are less common but can also occur. An individual may have feelings of apprehension or anxiety during a dysreflexic event. Profuse sweating, piloerection, and flushing of the skin above the injury level are other common symptoms of autonomic dysreflexia. Nasal congestion, blurred vision, and the

Table 2.2

Key Clinical Questions to Ask Patient
Do you have a headache?
What is the character of the headache—pounding, steady, etc?
Are you anxious?
When was your Foley catheter last changed?
Do you have a history of kidney/bladder stones?
How long has it been since you were catheterized?
What do you do for your bowel program? Are you getting good results?
Do you have any pressure sores?
Do you have any ingrown toenails?

Table 2.3

Signs and Symptoms of Autonomic Dysreflexia
Pounding headache
Increase in SBP/DBO >20–40 mmHg
Bradycardia
Cardiac arrhythmias
Anxiety
Diaphoresis
Piloerection
Flushing of skin
Nasal congestion
Blurred vision
Blind spots in VF
Asymptomatic

appearance of blind spots in the visual fields can also occur. It is also possible that no symptoms may occur during autonomic dysreflexia despite a significantly elevated BP.

A complete blood count, basic chemistry panel, liver function tests, and urinalysis should be obtained once initial treatment has begun (Table 2.4). Lowered hemoglobin may indicate an ulcer or another bleeding source. An elevated creatinine may indicate renal failure. Elevated liver function tests may indicate hepatitis or liver failure. A chest x-ray can assess for pneumonia or

---

Table 2.4

Treatment Summary of Autonomic Dysreflexia

---

1. Check blood pressure: if 20 mmHg or more above baseline with symptoms, probable dysreflexia
2. Sit patient up and loosen tight clothing

If indwelling catheter is not present:

3. Instill 2% lidocaine into urethra, wait 2–5 minutes
4. Catheterize 500 cc
5. Clamp catheter for 5 minutes
6. Repeat steps 4 and 5 until bladder empty
7. Check blood pressure
8. Skip to step 13

If indwelling catheter is present:

9. Check catheter for kinks or constrictions and correct
10. If no improvement in urine flow, irrigate with 10–15 cc of saline at body temperature
11. If still no improvement in urine flow, remove catheter and replace with new catheter
12. Check blood pressure
13. Place lidocaine jelly liberally on ingrown toenails and pressure sores
14. Wait 2–3 minutes and check blood pressure
15. Place lidocaine jelly liberally on hemorrhoids and anus
16. Wait 2–3 minutes and check blood pressure
17. Insert gloved and lubricated finger into anus and disimpact
18. Check blood pressure
19. Give Mylanta 15–30 cc
20. Check blood pressure
21. If no sildenafil use in last 24 hours, place 2" of nitropaste 1"above level of injury
22. If sildenafil use in last 24 hours, give prazosin or captopril
23. Check blood pressure
24. If blood pressure at safe level, may send for testing
25. Obtain CBC, chemistry panel, liver function tests, urinalysis, CXR, abdominal x-ray, skeletal x-rays as appropriate, EKG, pulse oximetry, renal/bladder/gall bladder ultrasounds, chest/abdominal/pelvic CT as appropriate
26. Treat findings in #25 as appropriate

pleural effusion, and an abdominal film can assess for an impaction or an ileus. A renal/bladder ultrasound can assess for a kidney or bladder stone, a gallbladder ultrasound can assess for a gallstone, an electrocardiogram (EKG) can assess for cardiac pathology, and skeletal x-rays can assess for broken bones or heterotopic ossification. A pelvic, abdominal, and chest computed tomography (CT) may be necessary if no etiology is found during the extensive workup.

TREATMENT

The first step to treating autonomic dysreflexia is to check the individual's blood pressure. It is important that during the treatment of autonomic dysreflexia, the blood pressure be checked every 2–5 minutes until the blood pressure stabilizes.

If the blood pressure is elevated, sitting the individual up and lowering the legs may cause pooling of blood in the lower extremities, thus lowering the blood pressure. Loosening tight clothing may cause pooling of blood in the abdomen and lower extremities, thus also lowering blood pressure.

Since the most common etiology of autonomic dysreflexia is bladder distention, the *urinary tract* as an etiology should be investigated first. If no indwelling catheter is present, the individual should be catheterized. Prior to catheterization, however, 2% lidocaine jelly should be inserted into the urethra since catheterization may exacerbate dysreflexia. Catheterization should commence 2–5 minutes after the lidocaine jelly is inserted since the peak action of lidocaine jelly occurs between 2 and 5 minutes. No more than 500 cc of urine should be catheterized initially as catheterizing a large amount of urine quickly could cause worsening dysreflexia. The catheter should be clamped after 500 cc is drained, and no more urine should be drained for 5 minutes. The process should be repeated until the bladder is fully drained of urine. If an indwelling catheter is present, the catheter should be checked for kinks or constrictions that could be causing blockage of urinary flow. If the catheter is blocked and correcting any kinks or constrictions does not improve the urinary flow, the catheter should be irrigated with 10–15 cc of saline that is at body temperature. If the catheter continues to be blocked, the indwelling urinary catheter should be changed after inserting 2% lidocaine jelly and waiting 2–5 minutes.

Since the next most common etiology of autonomic dysreflexia is a *pressure ulcer* or ingrown toenail, the individual should be examined closely for any pressure ulcers or ingrown toenails. Lidocaine jelly should be placed on any pressure ulcers or ingrown toenails, and the blood pressure should be rechecked in 2–3 minutes. Autonomic dysreflexia secondary to pressure ulcers occurs more frequently with stage II pressure sores compared to stage III or IV sores since the pain receptors are often not present in deeper pressure sores.

If the blood pressure remains elevated, *gastrointestinal* etiologies such as fecal impactions or hemorrhoids should be investigated. Lidocaine jelly should be placed on the anus and inserted into the rectum. If any hemorrhoids are present, lidocaine jelly should be liberally applied to the hemorrhoid. After waiting 2 minutes to allow the lidocaine jelly to take effect, a lubricated finger should be inserted into the rectum to remove any stool present. Another gastrointestinal inciter of dysreflexia can be gastritis. Mylanta 15–30 cc can be given to relieve any gastric upset, thus lowering blood pressure.

If the blood pressure remains elevated despite the previous treatments, a further workup is required to identify the etiology of the autonomic dysreflexia. Because the workup involving labs tests, x-rays, or other tests will take time, the dysreflexia must now be treated to lower the blood pressure. Oral agents such as nifedipine, prazosin, clonidine, and phenoxybenzamine can be used to treat dysreflexia (Table 2.5). Nifedipine should be used with caution in individuals with coronary artery disease as administration of nifedipine can cause shunting of blood away from the heart and an uncontrollable drop in blood pressure. Another problem with oral agents is that there is no way to reverse the hypotensive effect. If the source of the autonomic dysreflexia is found and treated, the blood pressure may drop precipitously. Transdermal nitropaste can also be used to treat autonomic dysreflexia. One to 2 inches of nitropaste can be applied transdermally to an area about 1 inch above the level of injury. The advantage of nitropaste to oral agents is that when the source of the dysreflexia is found and the blood pressure drops, the nitropaste can be wiped off. Before autonomic dysreflexia treatment is started, the patient should be questioned about his use of sildenafil for erectile dysfunction within the previous 24 hours. Medications containing nitrites are contraindicated when sildenafil has been used within 24 hours as severe hypotension and cardiovascular collapse can occur. If sildenafil has been used, prazosin or captopril can be used effectively for treatment.

After the blood pressure is lowered to safe levels, the additional workup can be started as mentioned above. If the urinalysis indicates that a urinary

Table 2.5

Medications Used to Treat Autonomic Dysreflexia

Medication	Dose	Side effects
Nifedipine	10 mg po tid (max 30 mg tid)	Hypotension, arrhythmia
Phenoxybenzamine	10 mg po bid (max 40 mg tid)	Hypotension, tachycardia
Clonidine	0.1 mg po daily (max 0.8 mg tid)	Hypotension, sedation, withdrawal
	0.1 mg/24 hr patch (max 0.3 mg)	Withdrawal hypertension, dry mouth
Prazosin	1 mg po bid (max 5 mg tid)	Hypotension, sedation, headache
Nitropaste	1 inch topically (max 2 inch)	Hypotension, tachycardia

tract infection is present, antibiotics should be started. The use of pyridium for 3–4 days is useful in controlling dysreflexia that is caused by a urinary tract infection by blocking the pain signals in the bladder. Treatment for other conditions such as pneumonia, gastrointestinal bleeding, bladder/kidney stones, fractures, or heterotopic ossification should be treated if identified.

Patient Safety

1. The prompt and appropriate treatment of autonomic dysreflexia is essential to prevent potential effects of markedly elevated blood pressure such as brain hemorrhages and arrhythmias.
2. Nifedipine should be used with caution in individuals with coronary artery disease as administration of nifedipine can cause shunting of blood away from the heart and an uncontrollable drop in blood pressure.
3. Patients should be asked about the recent use of sidenafil prior to consideration of nitrites.
4. An advantage of using nitropaste for the treatment of autonomic dysreflexia is that it can be easily wiped off the skin if no longer indicated or side effects develop.

Patient Education

1. Patient education about the etiologies, signs and symptoms, and treatments of autonomic dysreflexia is essential.
2. The patient should be educated about the importance of maintaining a regular catheterization schedule to avoid bladder distension.
3. The importance of maintaining skin integrity and good nail grooming should be emphasized.
4. The patient needs to know about the importance of regular bowel programs to prevent impactions that can cause dysreflexia.
5. The patient should be educated about the signs and symptoms of autonomic dysreflexia such as pounding headaches, flushing of skin, and diaphoresis that can be a sign of an impending autonomic dysreflexic event.
6. The patient should be taught techniques to lower blood pressure such as loosening tight clothes, sitting up, and lowering the legs.
7. Catherization and the use of lidocaine jelly on pressure sores also can be useful techniques to lower blood pressure.
8. The patient should be educated about the potential serious side effects of autonomic dysreflexia such as brain hemorrhages and arrhythmias.

REFERENCES

1. Consortium for Spinal Cord Medicine. Acute management of autonomic dysreflexia: individuals with spinal cord injury presenting to health-care facilities. Clinical Practice Guidelines. Spinal Cord Medicine, 2nd ed., 2001. Web site www.pva.org
2. Clinical practice guidelines: acute management of autonomic dysreflexia. J Spinal Cord Med 1997; 20:284–318.
3. Braddom RL, Rocco JF. Autonomic dysreflexia: a survey of current treatment. Am J Phys Med Rehab 1991; 70:234–241.
4. Erickson RP. Autonomic hyperreflexia: pathophysiology and medical management. Arch Phys Med Rehab 1980; 610:431–440.

3 Cardiovascular System

Marinella DeFre Galea

Cardiovascular disease (CVD) is the leading cause of death in the United States and is a major cause of disability. According to the Centers for Disease Control (CDC), almost 700,000 people die of heart disease in the United States each year. That is approximately 29% of all U.S. deaths. It is estimated that in 2006 the cost of CVD and stroke was $403.1 billion.

CVD includes several more specific heart conditions, such as arteriosclerosis, coronary artery disease (CAD), heart valve disease, arrhythmia, heart failure (HF), hypertension (HTN), orthostatic hypotension, shock, endocarditis, disease of the aorta and its branches, disease of the peripheral vascular system and congenital heart disease.CVD is associated with almost all neurologic conditions, complicating diagnosis, treatment, and outcome.

Cardiovascular disease has become the leading cause of death in chronic spinal cord injury (SCI) (1). The exact prevalence of CVD in this population is unknown secondary to the high occurrence of latent heart disease and concomitance of other conditions. However, studies have consistently shown a higher prevalence of CVD in SCI versus able-bodied persons (2), with data ranging from 25 to 50% for asymptomatic disease and from 30 to 50% for symptomatic disease (3). The level and completeness of injury is also associated with CVD, with lower and complete lesions conferring a greater risk of coronary artery disease.

Each year in the Unites States 700,000 persons have a stroke; in 200,000 of these patients the strokes are recurrent. Of the 500,000 patient with a new stroke, 14% will have another stroke within one year. Few stroke patients survive for 5 years without a hospital readmission. The leading cause for readmission is another stroke, followed by acute myocardial infarction and respiratory illness (4). Stroke leads to more long-term disability than any other disease process and costs the United States $ 57.9 billion a year.

Observational studies have documented a relationship between initial stroke, vascular risk factors (hypertension, diabetes, and hyperlipidemia), and lifestyle risk factors (smoking, alcohol use, obesity, lack of physical activity). Factors associated with recurrent stroke include diabetes mellitus, previous multiple strokes, disability after initial stroke, and large artery atherosclerosis. CVD has also been shown to complicate poststroke rehabilitation. Large studies support the treatment of hypertension for the prevention of recurrent ischemic stroke (5,6). In this chapter we will include evidence-based recommendations for the control of risk factors, interventional approaches for atherosclerotic disease, antithrombotic treatments for cardioembolism, and the use of antiplatelet agents for noncardioembolic stroke.

Symptoms related to alteration of the autonomic nervous system are frequent in patients with multiple sclerosis (MS). The prevalence of cardiovascular autonomic dysfunction has been reported to be between 10 and 50%. Clinical signs such as orthostatic intolerance and fatigue have been described. The pattern of pathologic findings is highly heterogeneous, suggesting a predominantly sympathetic involvement in some patients and a predominantly parasympathetic pathology in others. Dysautonomia, or deregulation of the autonomic system, seems to occur in MS patients with more severe disability. Progression of autonomic dysfunction is correlated with progression of clinical disability.

A significant proportion of traumatic brain injury (TBI) patients have hypotension in the prehospital setting as well as in-hospital (7) (Traumatic Coma Data Bank). Hypotension increases morbidity and mortality for severe TBI. Hypotension, defined as a single observation of systemic blood pressure (SBP) of less than 90 mmHg, must be avoided if possible or rapidly corrected in severe TBI patients. At present there are no sufficient clinical data to support improved outcome with correction of hypotension.

The literature regarding TBI and CVD is scarce; this is in part due to the high heterogeneity of this population. The goal of this chapter is to provide the reader with an understanding of the assessment and treatment of CVD in adults with neurologic disabilities.

ANATOMY AND PHYSIOLOGY

SCI is associated with an increased prevalence of conventional CAD factors such as high serum concentrations of low-density lipoprotein (LDL), low serum concentration of high-density lipoprotein (HDL), diabetes mellitus, positive smoking history, elevation of inflammatory markers, obesity, and inactivity. High blood pressure or hypertension has also been reported to be more prevalent in spinal cord injuries and disorders (8), although data vary.

Changes in cardiovascular function secondary to the impairment of the autonomic pathways include orthostatic hypotension (OH), cardiac arrhythmias, autonomic dysreflexia, reduced heart rate variability (HRV), and attenuated response to activity. Addressing the risk factors, recognizing and distinguishing between CVD and autonomic dysfunction may improve morbidity and mortality in SCI.

Orthostatic Hypotension

Orthostatic hypotension (OH) is defined as a decrease in systolic blood pressure of 20 mmHg or more, in diastolic blood pressure of 10 mmHg or more, upon the assumption of an upright posture from a supine position, regardless of whether symptoms occur. Orthostatic maneuvers performed during physiotherapy and mobilization is reported to induce orthostatic hypotension in 74% of SCI patients, and symptoms of orthostatic hypotension in 59% of SCI individuals. In the able-bodied individual, with the assumption of the upright position there is an immediate redistribution of blood to the dependent circulation; venous return and central venous filling pressure are reduced, resulting in diminution of cardiac output and blood pressure. These hemodynamic alterations stimulate the baroreceptor reflex, which is mediated via the central nervous system to increase peripheral sympathetic vasomotor tone, restoring blood pressure and cardiac output within seconds to minutes. Following SCI, individuals often experience an inability to adjust to postural changes due to disruption of central command of the baroreceptor reflex, reduction in efferent sympathetic neural pathways with inadequate release of norepinephrine, lack of skeletal muscle pumps, cardiovascular deconditioning, and altered salt and water balance. Consequently, OH and symptoms of cerebral hypoperfusion may ensue.

Cardiac Arrhythmias

Bradyarrhythmias and atrioventricular (AV) blocks are common in the acute SCI phase relative to the predominance of the sympathetic tone. In chronic SCI a higher prevalence of ST elevation has been described, which is believed to be attributable to increased activity of the parasympathetic system and the vagal tone.

Autonomic Dysreflexia (AD)

AD is characterized by sympathetic hyperactivity, causing severe vasoconstriction and hypertension below the level of the lesion. This condition has been described in SCI at the thoracic level T6 or above. Its mechanism is felt to be multifactorial (disinhibition of the sympathetic system, disinhibition of sensory pathways, altered reflex responses, reinnervation by spinal interneurons, denervation hypersensitivity). AD is extremely frequent (50–90%) and can lead to severe bradycardia/tachycardia, hypertensive emergencies, ischemia and stroke. AD is discussed in greater detail in a separate chapter.

Heart Rate Variability

HRV describes the quantification of beat-to-beat variation of the R-R interval on the electrocardiogram, measured over a period of time. HRV is used to study the balance between the parasympathetic and sympathetic systems and is highly correlated to the risk of CVD. It has been shown to be decreased in SCI persons.

Attenuated Response to Activity

Peak VO_2, heart rate, and stroke volume are decreased during regular physical activity in SCI. Contributing factors include attenuated sympathetic drive, blood pooling in the lower extremities, and decreased ventilation. Sympathetic decentralization impairs the rapid acceleration of the heart rate (HR) at the onset of exercise and the rapid deceleration following exercise. Inefficient myocardial preload and contractility result in reduced stroke volume and decreased cardiac output. This mechanism impairs the ability of the heart to compensate for decreased venous return due to the lack of intermittent contraction and absence of vasoconstriction.

Restrictive pulmonary disease and blunted chemoreceptor stimulation impair ventilation and oxygen delivery causing early fatigue, decreased exercise tolerance, and increased inactivity.

Hypertension

The metabolic abnormalities commonly associated with body composition changes in SCI, including increased insulin resistance and dyslipidemia, play a significant role in the early development of hypertension. Awareness of this premature condition can prevent the development of target organ disease. The presence of concomitant autonomic dysfunctions such as orthostatic hypotension or autonomic dysreflexia can complicate the diagnosis.

Silent Ischemia

Silent ischemia has been reported in 65% of individuals with SCI based on nuclear imaging studies. There are several contributing factors to this problem, including:
- Low HDL/high LDL cholesterol
- Impaired glucose tolerance and increased insulin resistance
- Increased circulating inflammatory markers such as C-reactive protein (CRP)
- Cigarette smoking
- Decreased utilization of health preventive services
- Autonomic dysfunction such as abnormal blood pressure, HRV, arrhythmias, and blunted cardiovascular response

Abdominal Aortic Aneurysm

Reports of increased incidence of abdominal aortic aneurism (AAA) after SCI injury are sporadic. More studies are needed to determine the prevalence of this condition in the SCI population as often the lack of typical symptoms can underestimate the problem.

Deep Venous Thrombosis

Asymptomatic deep venous thrombosis (DVT) has been reported in 60–100% of persons with SCI. Predisposing factors to develop DVT in SCI include:

- Venous stasis: resulting from loss of pumping function normally provided by contracting limb muscles
- Hypercoagulable state: occurs as a result of stimulation of thrombogenic factors following injury, with resultant increase in platelet aggregation and adhesion
- Endothelial injury: may result directly from the release of vasoactive amines with trauma or surgery, or indirectly from external pressure on the paralyzed leg

Studies have shown no statistical difference in incidence of DVT between motor complete versus motor incomplete injuries, tetraplegic versus paraplegic, or traumatic versus nontraumatic causes, therefore all SCI patients are at risk of developing a DVT.

STROKE

Most strokes share pathogenetic mechanisms, although prognosis may vary, depending on their severity and cause. Definitions are dependent on the timing and degree of the diagnostic evaluation. By conventional clinical definitions, if the neurologic symptoms continue for more than 24 hours, a person has been diagnosed with a stroke; otherwise, a focal neurologic deficit lasting less than 24 hours has been defined as a transient ischemic attack (TIA). TIAs are an important determinant of stroke, with 90-day risks of stroke reported as high as 10.5%. The greatest stroke risk is apparent in the first week. Ischemic stroke is classified into different categories according to the presumed mechanism of the focal brain injury and the type and localization of the vascular lesion: 1) large-artery atherosclerotic infarction, may be extracranial or intracranial; 2) embolism from a cardiac source; small-vessel disease; 3) other determined cause such as dissection, hypercoagulable states, or sickle cell disease; and infarcts of undetermined cause.

Hypertension

Although a large amount of data from a variety of sources support the importance of treatment of hypertension for primary cardiovascular disease prevention in stroke, only limited data directly address the role of BP treatment in secondary prevention among persons with stroke or TIA. There is a general lack of definitive data to help guide the immediate management of elevated BP in the setting of acute ischemic stroke; a cautious approach has been recommended, and the optimal time to initiate therapy remains uncertain.

In the setting of acute stroke, blood pressure management must be tailored to the specific clinical situation. There are a number of reasons to avoid BP reduction.

- The cerebral blood flow autoregulation system ensures a constant influx of blood to the brain. In patients with chronic hypertension, the mean blood pressure to blood brain flow curve shifts to adapt to higher blood pressure values. At normal BP ranges their risk for hypoperfusion increases with further BP reduction.
- The "ischemic penumbra" is a region of the brain tissue surrounding an acute infarct. The blood flow in that area is just sufficient for neurons to survive, but insufficient to function. Reduction of BP may lead to hypoperfusion of the penumbra and extension of infarction.

Cardiac Arrhythmias

In stroke patients, new-onset electrocardiogram abnormalities are documented in 75% of cases, and cardiac arrhythmias account for 29%. The mechanisms of genesis of cardiac arrhythmias occurring after stroke are still not well understood. Some evidence supports the hypothesis of a "cardiac cortical rhythm control site," probably lying within the middle cerebral artery territory. Vascular damage to this area could be followed by cardiac arrhythmias related to a disinhibition of the right insular cortex with resulting increased sympathetic tone. Ischemic involvement of the right hemisphere induces a higher risk for cardiac arrhythmia occurrence than that of the left hemisphere. The most common cardiac arrhythmias are atrial fibrillation (AF) and supraventricular arrhythmias.

AF is an independent risk factor for ischemic stroke. It is classified as paroxysmal, persistent, or permanent. In-hospital and 6-month mortality rates as well as the number of patients with disabling stroke are significantly lower in paroxysmal AF than in persistent or permanent AF. More than 75,000 cases of stroke per year are attributed to AF. It has been estimated that AF affects more than 2 million Americans and becomes more frequent with age, ranking as the leading cardiac arrhythmia in the elderly. Data from the AF clinical trials show that age, recent congestive heart failure, hypertension, diabetes, and prior thrombo-embolism have been found to identify high-risk groups for arterial thrombo-embolism among patients with AF.

Extracranial Carotid Disease

Embolization is considered the most common mechanism causing ischemic strokes from atherosclerotic lesions in the carotid bulb. Thrombosis and low flow are other possible mechanisms. Ninety percent of all extracranial carotid lesions are due to atherosclerosis.

Cardiogenic Cerebral Embolism

Cardiogenic cerebral embolism derived from a diversity of cardiac disorders is responsible for 20% of ischemic strokes. There is a history of non valvular AF in about one-half the cases, of valvular heart disease in one fourth, and of left

21

ventricular (LV) mural thrombus in almost one third. Sixty percent of emboli of LV origin have been associated with acute myocardial infarction (MI). Intracavitary thrombus occurs in about one third of patients in the first 2 weeks after anterior MI and in an even greater proportion of those with large infarcts involving the LV apex. Ventricular thrombi also occur in patients with chronic ventricular dysfunction resulting from coronary disease, hypertension, or other forms of dilated cardiomyopathy. Congestive heart failure affects more than 4 million Americans and increases stroke risk by a factor of 2–3, accounting for 10% of ischemic stroke events.

LV dysfunction, left atrial size, mitral annular calcification, and left atrial thrombus by echocardiography have also been shown to predict increased thrombo-embolic risk. Overall, patients with prior stroke or TIA carry the highest stroke risk.

Acute Myocardial Infarction and Left Ventricular Thrombus

Stroke or systemic embolism is less common among uncomplicated MI patients but can occur in up to 12% of patients with acute MI complicated by a left ventricular thrombus. The rate is higher in those with anterior than those with inferior infarcts and may reach 20% of those with large antero-apical infarcts. The incidence of embolism is highest during the period of active thrombus formation in the first 1–3 months, yet the embolic risk remains substantial even beyond the acute phase in patients with persistent myocardial dysfunction, congestive heart failure, or AF.

Cardiomyopathy

When LV systolic function is impaired, the reduced stroke volume creates a condition of relative stasis within the left ventricle that may activate coagulation processes and increase the risk of thrombo-embolic events. The cause of cardiomyopathy may be ischemia or infarction based on coronary artery disease or nonischemic as a result of genetic or acquired defects of myocardial cell structure or metabolism. Stroke rate has not been found to be related to the severity of heart failure; the incidence of stroke appears to be inversely proportional to ejection fraction (EF). In patients with nonischemic dilated cardiomyopathy, the rate of stroke appears similar to that associated with cardiomyopathy resulting from ischemic heart disease. An estimated 72,000 initial stroke events per year have been associated with LV systolic dysfunction, and the 5-year recurrent stroke rate in patients with cardiac failure has been reported to be as high as 45%.

Valvular Heart Disease

Rheumatic mitral valve disease: recurrent embolism occurs in 30–65% of patients with rheumatic mitral valve disease who have a history of a previous embolic event.

Mitral valve prolapse is the most common form of valve disease in adults; it is generally innocuous. Thrombo-embolic phenomena have been reported in patients with mitral valve prolapse in whom no other source could be found. Clinically detectable systemic embolism in isolated aortic valve disease is increasingly recognized because of microthrombi or calcific emboli, which can only be visualized in the retinal artery. Prosthetic heart valves are known to cause recurrent embolism and require anticoagulation.

MULTIPLE SCLEROSIS AND TRAUMATIC BRAIN INJURY

The literature regarding CVD in MS and TBI is scarce.

Cardiovascular Autonomic Dysfunction

Cardiovascular autonomic dysfunction in patients with MS has been reported to have a prevalence between 10 and 50%, but cardiovascular symptoms are uncommon. Several studies have reported dysfunction of the left and right ventricular function in multiple sclerosis, although the pathophysiologic mechanism responsible for these abnormalities is not clear. In persons with MS the risk of developing CAD appears related to the level of inactivity.

Deep Venous Thrombosis

DVT risk is multifactorial in traumatic brain injury patients, with relative risk factor influenced by type of acquired brain injury. The risk of developing DVT in absence of prophylaxis is estimated to be 20%.after severe TBI. A few studies have identified a relative low incidence of DVT in MS; however, the literature does not support a protective effect of this condition relative to venous stasis.

PATIENT ASSESSMENT

The history and physical examination in persons with neurologic disabilities present several challenges. Motor and sensory impairment in SCI complicate the ability to properly examine the patient, obtain detailed symptom description, and interpret conventional signs such as body temperature, pulse, blood pressure, and pain. Depending on the degree of impairment, TBI and stroke patients may not be able to communicate their symptoms and/or present with the same physical barrier to being properly examined. Since the prevalence of diabetes mellitus is high in this population, the clinician must take into consideration that symptoms may be blunted secondary to peripheral nerve damage. It is important to involve the caregivers in the interview process to obtain a thorough history and also to educate them about the most common presentation of CVD, how to monitor the disease, and when to report abnormalities.

Orthostatic Hypotension

Orthostatic hypotension frequently results in cerebral hypoperfusion and symptoms of orthostatic intolerance such as lightheadedness, dizziness, blurry vision, and fatigue, nausea, ringing in the ears, cognitive impairment, and heart palpitations. It is commonly elicited by changing position from the examining bed to the wheelchair.

- It is recommended that all SCI patients be examined on a regular hospital bed which allows for Trendelenburg positioning.
- When transferring the patient from the chair to the examining table or bed, proceed in steps, gradually changing position.
- Encourage the use of elastic stockings and abdominal binders in patient with tetraplegia and/or known history of OH.

Cardiac Arrhythmias

Cardiac arrhythmias should always be suspected in stroke patients. They may be asymptomatic or have an abnormal presentation in diabetic patients.

- Identify the presence of palpitations, chest pain, lightheadedness, shortness of breath, and syncope. Triggering events, duration of symptoms, and associated symptoms should also be included in the history.
- The physical exam should
  o include pulse palpation to assess for heart rate and regularity
  o identify any underlying cause of tachyarrhythmia such as congestive heart failure, (elevated jugular venous pressure, peripheral edema, and third heart sound)

Bradycardia

In spinal cord injury persons with tetraplegia, the prevalence of vagal tone causes bradycardia, which is usually asymptomatic. Possible symptoms include palpitation, syncope, and loss of consciousness. In chronic injuries this phenomenon is less pronounced.

- Stimulation of the parasympathetic system such as tracheal stimulation, defecation, and belching can cause sinus pauses and reflex unopposed vagal activity, which precipitates bradycardia. These maneuvers should be avoided when possible or the patient should be premedicated (see below).

Cardiac Valve Dysfunction

- Mitral valve prolapse
  o Symptoms are nonspecific: fatigue, anxiety, palpitations, lightheadedness, chest pain, presyncopal and syncopal episodes.
  o A mid-systolic click followed by a mitral regurgitation murmur is pathognomonic.

- Aortic valve insufficiency
  ○ Look for a wide pulse pressure, bounding pulses, and aortic diastolic murmur.

Autonomic Dysreflexia

The typical cluster of symptoms associated with AD include hypertension, profuse sweating, headache, bradycardia, and piloerection above the level of the injury.

Hypertension

Examination should include: baseline blood pressure measurement, investigation for target organ damage or secondary cause of hypertension (carotid bruits, an S3 or S4, cardiac murmurs, additional neurologic deficit, elevated jugular venous pressure, rales, retinopathy, unequal pulses, enlarged or small kidneys, cushingoid features, and abdominal bruits).
- Blood pressure must be measured in three different occasions to make the diagnosis of HTN
- HTN is defined as:
  ○ SBP > 140 and DBP > 90 in general population
  ○ SBP > 130 and DBP > 80 in patient with diabetes mellitus
- A generally accepted normal blood pressure (<120/80 or less) can be true hypertension in a person with tetraplegia, therefore it is important to always record baseline BP.
- Autonomic dysreflexia must be excluded (see above).

Silent Ischemia

In spinal cord injury, patients with severe TBI who cannot communicate well, and persons with diabetes mellitus and neurologic disability, symptoms of ischemia are atypical. They vary from vague gastrointestinal upset to lack of any significant symptoms.
- Always suspect cervical lesion if there is no other explanation for vague symptoms. When in doubt, obtain 12 lead electrocardiogram (ECG).

Electrocardiogram Changes

Persons with longer SCI duration and at least two risk factors for CVD have a significant higher incidence of abnormal ECG.
- ST elevation abnormalities
- Left atrial abnormalities
- Left ventricular hypertrophy
- Signs of old myocardial infarction

Aortic Abdominal Aneurysm

In SCI and diabetes mellitus the typical symptoms of abdominal pain and claudication are missing. Obesity, abnormal gas pattern, incomplete bowel emptying, and abdominal spasms render the findings of a pulsating abdominal mass in the epigastrium extremely difficult.

- Follow the AAA screening guidelines (see below) and when in doubt order duplex of the abdominal aorta.

Deep Venous Thrombosis and Pulmonary Embolism

Clinical signs and symptoms for the diagnosis of DVT and pulmonary embolism (PE) may be different in SCI or TBI patients than in neurologically intact patients, therefore they are more difficult to identify. Unilateral leg swelling with pain is the hallmark of DVT, but swelling of lower extremities may be bilateral.

- Edema may be the only presenting symptom.
- In SCI leg pain is nonspecific and includes a vast differential diagnosis such as infection and pressure ulcer.
- Clinical signs and symptoms of PE may be the primary manifestation in patients with DVT. Symptoms may include pleuritic chest pain, dyspnea, hemoptysis, and feelings of impending doom.

Left Ventricular Dysfunction

The clinical manifestation of heart failure depends on the rapidity of the cardiac decompensation and may be blunted or nonspecific in the neurologically impaired patient. Consider this diagnosis in patients who present with a history of:

- Fatigue
- Exercise intolerance
- Dyspnea with or without exertion
- Orthpnea, paroxysmal nocturnal dyspnea
- Presyncope, palpitation, and possibly angina
- Peripheral edema and unexplained weight gain

The physical exam should include evaluation of heart and lung sounds, the presence of elevated jugular venous pressure, pleural and/or pericardial rub, ascites, and increasing peripheral edema. When possible the patient should be weighed.

DIAGNOSTIC TESTS

As a general principle the following measures should be undertaken when evaluating the cardiovascular status of the neurologically impaired patient. There are no specific recommendations regarding the frequency of routine tests in this population.

- BP measurement should be taken at every office visit. If not at goal it is recommended that the patient be reevaluated after each medication adjustment (usually every 4–12 weeks) until BP goal is met.
- 12 lead ECG should be recorded at least yearly or any time there is suspicion of heart rhythm irregularity. Continuous ambulatory ECG monitoring or monthly event recorder in patients with rhythm abnormalities.
- Routine laboratory tests including hematocrit, blood glucose, serum potassium, sodium, calcium, uric acid, creatinine, should be assessed yearly.
- HbA1C must be repeated every 3–6 months in patients with diabetes.
- Fasting lipid profile (including total cholesterol, triglycerides, HDL, and LDL) must be assessed yearly. If not at goal for risk factors, it has to be repeated after each therapeutic intervention. Please refer to the specific chapter for further recommendations.
- Hepatic profile has to be checked yearly or more frequently in patients who are on a lipid-lowering medication (statins, fibrate) to titrate/adjust therapy. In SCI, given the high prevalence of fatty liver disease, it is good practice to obtain a baseline hepatic profile to estimate hepatic clearance of medications.

Doppler Ultrasound for Deep Venous Thrombosis

- Commonly the initial diagnostic test
- Noninvasive and sensitive (98–100%) method for the diagnosis of proximal DVT
- Useful in patients with suspected PE with non diagnostic ventilation/perfusion (V/Q) scan

D-Dimer Assays

To be obtained for further confirmation or when Doppler ultrasound is not readily available.
- Useful adjunct to noninvasive testing for suggested DVT
- Highly sensitive
- High negative predictive value (rules out DVT if negative)

Radiocontrast Venography

It is the gold-standard for the diagnosis of DVT, but it is rarely used. Potential complications include:
- Invasive procedure that may have adverse effects, including pain
- Contraindication to venography include renal dysfunction and dye allergy

CT Venography

- Used in conjunction with spiral CT to diagnose PE
- Less sensitivity and specificity than Doppler ultrasound
- Less sensitive to incomplete obstruction of vein by DVT
- Extrinsic compression may give positive result.

Ventilation/Perfusion Lung Scan for Pulmonary Embolism

- This scan is indicated as part of diagnostic evaluation of PE.
  - ○ Definitive diagnosis occurs if results are normal or there is high probability, especially if clinical suspicion is confirmed.
- Low or intermediate probability scan results require further evaluation, such as lower extremity Doppler ultrasound or pulmonary angiography.

TREATMENT

Preventive and Screening Measures

General preventive measures to be applied to the neurologically impaired population include the following.

Annual Evaluation
- Blood pressure monitoring, evaluation of end target organ complication
- Annual eye exam for all patients with diabetes and/or hypertension
- Foot exam in patient with diabetes or insensate
- Laboratory exam including hematocrit, lipid profile, blood glucose, renal function, urine analysis
- Body mass index (BMI) (goal 18.9–24.9) must be calculated yearly. In the SCI population, however, BMI is an insensitive marker of obesity. This may be due to potential measurement error and to the inability of BMI to distinguish between fat and fat-free mass and to measure body fat distribution. It is recommended that 10% of BMI be added to calculated value to adjust for SCI.
- Thyroid-stimulating hormone, to be checked yearly, will help to differentiate vague symptoms of fatigue and or poor appetite, unexplained weight loss or gain.
- Glomerular filtration rate should be calculated yearly and trend recorded to ensure safe administration of medications. Consider that in SCI persons this value may overestimate renal function secondary to the decrease of muscle mass.
- 24-hour urine collection for total volume, microalbumin and/or protein, and creatinine is recommended yearly in SCI persons to better estimate renal function for safe medication administration, to estimate grade of proteinuria, if present, and progression of heart failure, if present.
- An oral glucose tolerance test (OGTT) or alternatively an HbA1C can be obtained on a yearly basis to identify patient at increased risk of diabetes mellitus.

Diet
The appropriate diet should address the different co morbidities, such as:
- 2 g Na diet in patients with hypertension
- ADA diet in patients with diabetes mellitus
- Low-cholesterol diet in patients with hyperlipidemia

The patient should always receive a consult with a nutritionist to reinforce compliance and education.

Exercise

When possible, all patients should be encouraged to follow an exercise program:

- A cardiac stress test is commonly prescribed in patients who intend to participate in an exercise program and have one or more risk factors. Patients who are unable to exercise should undergo a pharmacological stress test.
- In SCI individuals, radionuclide myocardial perfusion imaging after upper body ergometry exercise has been shown to reveal latent coronary artery disease. This test is not available in most centers and requires coordination of care. Can only be performed by individuals who can exercise.
- Tilt table test has to be performed in individuals with suspected orthostatic hypotension prior to initiation of a therapy program.

Smoking Cessation

Particular effort should be made to promote smoking cessation:

- Ask every patient about tobacco use
- Assess the level of tobacco dependence by using the heavy smoking index
- Advise the patient to quit and provide education (tobaccoinfo@cdc.gov)
- Assess readiness to quit smoking
- Consider nicotine replacement product and oral medication such as Bupropion and Varenicline:
  - Nicotine replacement therapy (NRT): reduces cravings. In recommended doses, NRT is safe for most patients, including those with stable heart disease. To be used in combination with Bupropion. NRT is available in several forms, including patches, gum, lozenges, an oral inhaler, and nasal spray. Patches, gum, and lozenges are available over the counter (OTC). The nasal spray and nicotine inhaler are dispensed by prescription only. The once-a-day OTC nicotine patch is the most effective and convenient form of NRT for most smokers.
    - 14 mg/24 hr patch for those who smoke 10–15 cigarettes/day; 21 mg/24 hr patch for those who smoke 16–20 cigarettes/day
  - Bupropion SR: increases quit rates. Marketed as Zyban® for smoking cessation treatment. Due to its antidepressant effects, it is the best choice for patients with history of depression. Contraindications include history of seizure, bipolar, or eating disorder.
    - Start 1–2 weeks before quit date, 150 mg PO daily, 12 weeks to 6 months depending of success of therapy.
    - Side effects include insomnia, dry mouth, and anxiety
  - Varenicline (Chantix®): eliminates the pleasurable effects of smoking a cigarette. 0.1 mg starting dose, 1 mg continuation. To be used alone.
    - Days 1–3: 0.5 mg tablet every morning
    - Days 4–7: 0.5 mg tablet twice daily
    - Days 8 to end of week 4: 1 mg tablet twice daily
    - "Continuing Month Pak:"
    - Week 5 to end of treatment, 1 mg tablet twice daily.
    - Side effects include nausea, insomnia, abnormal dreams, and headache

Carotiod Artery Stenosis Screening

- The U.S. Preventive Service Task Force (USPSTF) recommends against screening for asymptomatic carotid artery stenosis (9).

Aortic Abdominal Aneurysm (AAA) Screening

- Men ages 65–75 who have ever smoked should be screened one time for AAA by abdominal ultrasonography. The USPSTF found that there is little benefit to repeat screening in men who have a negative ultrasound and that men over age 75 are unlikely to benefit from screening.
- Because the prevalence of AAA is very low in men ages 65–75 who have never smoked, and thus any harms of screening are likely similar to the benefits, the USPSTF does not recommend for or against screening in such men.
- The USPSTF recommends against screening for AAA in women.

Treatments for Specific Conditions

Orthostatic Hypotension

There are currently two classes of drugs used to treat and/or prevent orthostatic hypotension in SCI: mineralcorticoid and -adrenergic medications.

- Mineralocorticoid drugs expand plasma volume, but slow titration and careful monitoring is required since they can cause electrolytes abnormalities including hypokalemia. Fludrocortisone is a commonly used mineralcorticoid drug which causes sodium retention over few days and increases BP.
  - Starting dose is 0.1 mg daily. It is important to check baseline potassium level, then 48 hours after initiation of therapy, then after one week; if normal can check every month. Usually requires potassium supplementation (20 mEq daily or more according to blood levels). If BP is not at goal or the patient is still symptomatic, gradual increase up to 0.4 mg daily is recommended.
- α-Adrenergic medications increase blood pressure by means of vasoconstriction. Ephedrine sulfate and midodrine hydrochloride, both α_1-receptor agonists, are recommended for the treatment of postural hypotension in SCI.
  - Phenylephrine is a selective α-agonist drug which is marketed in a convenient intranasal formulation. The usual dose is 1–2 sprays 5 minutes prior to sitting. Side effects include bitter taste and palpitation.
  - Midodrine comes in oral formulation. Starting dose should be 2.5 mg given 30 minutes prior to sitting up. Gradual increments of 2.5 mg up to 10 mg Q4-6H PRN change in position can be made to titrate to desired BP value or to the patient's symptoms. Patients can have hyperresponsiveness to sympathomimetics drugs.

Individuals should be educated about the mechanisms underlying orthostatic hypotension and common factors likely to provoke an episode. Further advice should include:

- Ensure adequate salt and fluid intake (needs to be individualized for each patient).

- Avoid diuretics such as alcohol and caffeine.
- Slow change in position from supine to sitting, possibly allowing first the lower extremities to dangle off the bed. There is no recommendation on how long to wait before completing each passage toward reaching the sitting position. The patient should be monitored and the inclination augmented according to his or her comfort. Consider placing the patient in Trendelenburg if he or she develops symptomatic hypotension while supine.
- Use abdominal binders or supportive stockings to restrict venous pooling in the splanchnic region and dependent limbs when out of bed to chair. These medical devices should be removed when the patient returns to bed and the skin monitored for integrity. It is recommended that the patient be appropriately measured by a prosthetic specialist to ensure correct fit. Consider supportive stockings with zipper and adaptive devices such as hooks and pullers to facilitate placement and promote independence.
- Avoid vasodilatatory stresses such as heat stress. Always suggest the use of sunscreen, light clothing, and hats when outside, educate the patient to drink approximately 2 liters of fluid per day.
- Take regular small meals to minimize post-prandial hypotension.
- Plan any exercise program in the afternoon.
- Assume a recumbent or semi-recumbent position should symptoms of orthostatic hypotension occur.

Bradycardia

- Anticholinergic drugs can be used prior to specific maneuvers to avoid the reflex vagal activity. Pretreatment with atropine 0.1–1 mg given intravenously or endotracheally 1–5 minutes before suctioning if needed. Heart rate monitoring is required.
- The use of methylxanthines in the treatment of SCI- associated bradycardia has been studied. Although there is limited evidence, aminophylline intravenously and then orally has been used. More data are needed to validate these preliminary findings.
- Severe symptomatic bradycardia (HR < 50 associated with dizziness, syncope, loss of consciousness, palpitation, chest pain, etc.) and heart block require placement of a temporary pacemaker. An increased risk has been associated with this procedure in SCI, but the literature is scarce.

Hypertension

Table 3.1 summarizes the recommendations from the Seventh Report of the Joint National Committee on Prevention, Detection, Evaluation, and Treatment of High Blood Pressure (JNC7) (10).

Studies have shown that, depending on the patient's ethnicity, comorbidities, and severity of hypertension, some antihypertensive medications are more effective than others.

Table 3.1

Recommendations of the Joint National Committee on the Treatment of High Blood Pressure

Blood pressure values	Associated risks	Intervention
Normal BP: 120/80 mmHg		No pharmacological intervention
Prehypertension: 120–39/80–89 mmHg	0–1 risk factor except diabetes or end-organ damage[a]	Lifestyle modifications
Prehypertension: 120–139/80–89 mmHg	Diabetes or end-organ damage	Lifestyle modifications + Pharmacological therapy
Stage I hypertension: 140–159/90–99 mmHg		Lifestyle modification + pharmacological therapy
Stage II hypertension: >160/>100 mmHg		Lifestyle modification + pharmacological therapy
Hypertensive emergencies: diastolic 120–130 mmHg	Optic disk edema Progressive end-organ complications Severe perioperative hypertension	Pharmacological therapy with BP reduction within several hours
Accelerated hypertension: Systolic BP > 210 mmHg Diastolic BP >130 mmHg	Headaches Blurred vision Focal neurologic symptoms	Pharmacological therapy to reduce BP by 20–25%
Malignant hypertension: systolic BP >210 mmHg diastolic BP >130 mmHg	Papilledema present	Pharmacological therapy to reduce BP by 20–25%
Isolate systolic hypertension: systolic BP >140 mmHg		Careful pharmacological therapy and frequent follow-up

[a]Target organ damage includes: left ventricular hypertrophy, angina or prior myocardial infarction, prior coronary revascularization, heart failure, stroke or TIA, chronic kidney disease, peripheral artery disease, and retinopathy.

This is a brief summary of the therapeutic intervention recommended by the JNC7 as well as a compendium of the most common observation in our practice. It is recommended that:

- The patient be started on the lowest possible dose of an antihypertensive medication.
- Another class of medication be added, if BP control is not achieved, to enhance the effectiveness of the first drug and reach an additive effect.
- The frequency of follow-up after initiation of therapy should range from 4 to 12 weeks according to the initial stage of HTN as well as response to the medication regimen.

Thiazide-type diuretics should be the first line of therapy, as shown by the Antihypertensive and Lipid-Lowering Treatment to Prevent Heart Attack Trial (ALLHAT) (11). Thiazide-type diuretics block sodium reabsorption mainly in the distal convolute tubule by inhibition of the thiazide-sensitive Na/Cl transporter.

- Hydrochlorothiazide 12.5 mg PO daily usual dose 50 mg daily
- Chlorthalidone 12.5 mg PO daily usual dose 50 mg daily
  (Side effects include weakness, muscle cramps, and impotence.)

Inhibitors of the Renin-Angiotensin System

Angiotensin-converting enzyme inhibitors (ACE-I) are indicated in patients with diabetes and/or proteinuria and/or congestive heart failure (CHF).

- Captopril 25 mg PO bid-tid increment by 25 mg up to 450 mg daily
- Fosinopril 5 mg PO daily increment by 5 mg up to 40 mg daily
- Lisinopril 5 mg PO daily increment by 5 mg up to 40 mg daily
- Quinapril 5 mg PO daily increment by 5 mg up to 80 mg daily
- Ramipril 1.25 mg PO daily increment by 2.5 mg up to 20 mg daily
  (Side effects include dry cough, angioneurotic edema and hypotension.)

Note: This class of medication requires caution when used in persons with cervical SCI who depend on the angiotensin-converting system to maintain adequate blood pressure when upright. ACE-I cause vasodilatation of the efferent arteriole in the kidney; therefore, worsening renal function may occur in patients who have decreased renal perfusion or who have preexisting severe renal insufficiency. Furthermore, in SCI persons serum creatinine does not adequately reflect renal function. These individuals have an increased risk of developing renal disease and hyperkalemia if their renal function is overestimated. It is important to obtain 24-hour creatinine clearance and monitor the renal function while on this class of medications. These drugs are effective in reducing microalbuminuria regardless of diabetic status—an important consideration in persons who are at risk to develop skin wounds and need to maintain an adequate plasma protein level. Experimental evidence has linked the renin-angiotensin system (RAS) to the development and progression of cerebrovascular disease. Inhibition of the RAS has beneficial cerebrovascular effects and may reduce the risk of stroke independently from the alterations of BP. Some clinical trials suggest that ACE-I and angiotensin II type 1 receptor antagonists may have cerebro-protective effects beyond BP lowering, but the evidence is controversial. The JNC7 report suggested that recurrent stroke rates are lowered by the combination of an ACE-I and thiazide-type diuretic.

Angiotensin receptor inhibitors are an alternative in patients with mild to moderate hypertension intolerant to ACE-I and/or have CHF.

- Valsartan 40mg PO daily, increment by 40 mg up to 320 mg daily
- Losartan 25 mg PO daily, increment by 25 mg up to 100 mg daily
  (Can cause angioedema, allergic reaction, and rash.)

β-Blockers (BB) have been shown to decrease the incidence of stroke, myocardial infarction, and heart failure. Individuals with prior history of CAD or with risk factors for heart disease (cigarette smoking, hyperlipidemia, HTN, obesity) should be placed on this class of drugs. The mechanism of action is competitive inhibition of the effects of the catecholamines at α-adrenergic receptors, which decrease heart rate and cardiac output. They are divided into different categories: cardio-selective, with primarily β_1-blocking effects (recommended in patient with mild chronic obstructive pulmonary disease, diabetes or peripheral vascular disease), nonselective, with β_1- and β_2-blocking effects, and α- and β-antagonists.

For cardio-selective BB:

- Atenolol 25 mg PO daily, increment by 25 mg up to 100 mg daily
- Metoprolol 25 mg PO bid, increment by 25 mg up to 200 mg bid
- Metoprolol XL 25 mg PO daily, increment by 25 mg up to 400 mg daily

For nonselective BB:

- Propranolol 20 mg PO BID, increment by 20 mg up to 120 mg bid
  (Side effects include ventricular block, congestive heart failure, Raynaud phenomenon, and impotence.) In high SCI lesion the sympathetic output is blunted below the level of the injury, causing bradycardia, therefore HR should not be used as the sole parameter to titrate the medication.

Selective α-agonist drugs are not recommended as first-line therapy as they have been shown to be less efficacious than other classes of drugs in reducing mortality and morbidity. However, Terazosin is recommended when the patient has both a diagnosis of HTN and benign prostatic hyperplasia (BPH) as it relaxes the external urethral sphincter allowing dual effect with one drug.

- Terazosin 1 mg PO bedtime increase by 1–2 mg to 20 mg bid
  (Side effects include syncope, OH, dizziness, headache, and drowsiness.)

These drugs should be used with caution in SCI individuals who are prone to lower extremities blood pooling. Change in position may cause severe blood pressure fluctuation resulting in cerebral hypoperfusion.

α- and β-Antagonists: Carvedilol has been mostly used in patients with CHF to block the cardiac effect of chronic adrenergic stimulation This medication should be instituted at low dose and titrated with careful attention to BP and heart rate.

- Labetalol 50 mg PO BID, increment by 50 mg up to 600 mg bid
- Carvedilol 3.25 mg PO bid, increment by 3.25 mg up to 25 mg bid
  (Side effects of Labetalol include hepatocellular damage, postural hypotension, positive anti-nuclear antibody test, lupus-like syndrome, and tremors. Carvedilol has the same side effects as BB; it can cause volume retention and worsening CHF symptoms, reflex tachycardia can occur.)

Calcium channel antagonists are effective agents in the treatment of HTN. Although the old-generation, short-acting dihydrophyridine calcium channel antagonists have been shown to possibly increase the number of ischemic cardiac events, long-acting agents appear to be safe. Second-generation drugs such as Amlopidine and Felodipine are more vasoselective and present less negative cardiac inotropic effects. These medications should not be initiated in patients immediately after a myocardial infarction.

- Amlodipine 5 mg PO daily, increase by 2.5 mg to 10 mg daily
- Diltiazem 30 mg PO qid, increase by 15 mg to 90 mg qid
- Diltiazem SR 60 mg PO bid, increase by 30 mg to 180 mg bid
- Verapamil 40 mg PO tid, increase by 20 mg to 160 mg tid
- Verapamil SR 60 mg PO daily, increase by 30 mg to 480 mg daily
  (Side effects include constipation, nausea, headache, and orthostatic hypotension.)

Centrally acting adrenergic agents are potent antihypertensive agents with significant side effects, particularly in neurologically impaired patients, that can cause extreme blood pressure variation. The patch formulation allows for better drug distribution and avoids the complications of acute withdrawal syndrome (HTN, tachycardia, and diaphoresis), which were frequently observed in the past. They are not first-line agents, and their use should be reserved for when other classes of drugs or combination have failed to normalize BP.

- Clonidine 0.1 mg PO bid, increase by 0.1 mg to 0.6 mg bid
- Clonidine patch transdermal therapeutic system 1/week, can be increased up to 0.3 mg week
  (Side effects include bradycardia, drowsiness, dry mouth, OH, galactorrhea, sexual dysfunction, and rash.)

Note: In SCI persons clonidine has been historically used to treat spasticity where other medications have failed. With the advent of new-generation antispasticity medications, clinicians have distanced themselves from this medication.

Stroke Prevention

Antithrombotic Therapy

Antithrombotic agents include antiplatelet agents (aspirin, ticlopidine, clopidogrel, and dipyridamole) and the anticoagulant warfarin (Coumadin).

- Aspirin: a wide range of aspirin dosages (30–1300 mg per day) have been studied. High dosage (325 mg per day) and low dosage (50–166 mg per day) have similar effectiveness in preventing vascular events, but higher dosages are associated with more gastrointestinal side effects and bleeding episodes. Aspirin is not recommended for patients with uncontrolled hypertension. It is widely used in primary prevention and post–myocardial infarction.
- Clopidogrel (75 mg) is approved by the U.S. Food and Drug Administration for the prevention of recurrent vascular events when aspirin has failed. Side effects include rash and bleeding.
- Clopidogrel and aspirin combination therapy does not appear to be more effective than Clopidrogel alone in preventing ischemic stroke, MI, vascular death, or rehospitalization for ischemic events. Patients who underwent drug-eluting

stent placement after MI require at least one year of dual therapy, and evidence shows that the abrupt interruption of Clopidogrel significantly increases mortality in the following 90 days. Side effects include risk of life-threatening bleeding and major bleeding.

- Dipyridamole and aspirin extended-release combination therapy is approved (Aggrenox) for the prevention of recurrent stroke. The combination decreases the risk of death from all vascular causes and nonfatal stroke. At the same time it does not increase the risk of major or minor bleeding.
- Warfarin it is commonly recommended for the prevention of stroke in patients with atrial fibrillation, but it has a lesser role in the prevention of noncardioembolic ischemic stroke. Given the risk/benefit ratio, cost of monitoring therapy, and difficulty in maintaining a therapeutic INR in a community setting, antiplatelet agents are preferred over warfarin for prevention of recurrent ischemic stroke.

The choice of antithrombotic therapy for the prevention of recurrent ischemic stroke should be made based on the safety, tolerability, effectiveness, and price of each agent.

- Aspirin has low cost and good effectiveness.
- Aspirin plus dipyridamole increases effectiveness over aspirin alone with excellent side effect profile.
- In patients intolerant to aspirin and/or with aspirin allergy or who experience headaches with dipyridamole, clopidrogel is an appropriate alternative.
- Warfarin should be reserved for patients who cannot tolerate antiplatelet agents.
- Expert opinion recommends switching to dipyridamole and aspirin or clopidogrel in patients who experience an ischemic stroke while taking aspirin.

Role of Endarterectomy for Treatment of Carotid Artery Disease

Among patients with TIA or stroke and documented carotid stenosis, a number of randomized trials have compared endarterectomy plus medical therapy with medical therapy alone. For patients with symptomatic atherosclerotic carotid stenosis >70%, as defined using the North American Symptomatic Carotid Endarterectomy Trial (NASCET) criteria, the value of carotid endarterectomy (CEA) has been clearly established. For patients with carotid stenosis <50%, there is no significant benefit of surgery. For those with symptomatic carotid stenosis in the moderate category (50–69% stenosis), there is some uncertainty. Various comorbid features altered the benefit-to-risk ratio for CEA for moderate carotid stenosis. Benefits were greatest among those with more severe stenosis, those 75 years of age, men, patients with recent stroke (rather than TIA), and patients with hemispheric symptoms rather than transient monocular blindness. Gender and age differences, as well as comorbidity, must be considered when treatment options are evaluated in patients with stenosis between 50 and 69%, because the absolute benefit of surgery is less than that for more severe degrees of stenosis.

DVT Prophylaxis

Pharmacological
Patients who are hospitalized because of an acute illness and have significant risk factors such as advanced age, previous venous thrombo-embolism, trauma, obesity, malignancy, pregnancy, inflammatory bowel disease, coagulation factor deficiency, severe respiratory disease, and congestive heart failure should be given prophylactic dosing of low-dose unfractionated heparin (UFH) or low molecular weight heparin (LMWH).

In SCI patients treatment with enoxaparin 30 mg SC twice daily for VTE prophylaxis is recommended. Subcutaneous enoxaparin administered once or twice daily is equally effective for the prevention of venous TE disease. Both dosing strategies are associated with a low incidence of bleeding in patients with SCI who are undergoing rehabilitation.

In patients with TBI, either UFH or LMWH should be used in combination with mechanical prophylaxis. There is insufficient evidence to support recommendations regarding the preferred agent, timing, or dose of pharmacologic prophylaxis in DVT. In the TBI population there is an increased risk of expansion of intracranial hemorrhage.

Nonpharmacological
Note: Prior to applying mechanical compression, tests to exclude the presence of lower extremity DVT should be undertaken.
Compression hose (elastic stockings):
- Apply a uniform distribution of pressure over the extremity
- Improve lower extremity venous return
- Help to control edema
- Underlying skin should be examined daily for integrity
- No study is known to evaluate the difference in the incidence of thigh-length versus calf-length elastic stockings

External pneumatic devices are graded for sequential, multicompartment uniform pressure or single-chamber uniform pressure:
- Improve lower extremity venous return
- May be knee or thigh length
- Contraindicated in patients with severe arterial insufficiency

Range-of-motion exercises (ROM):
- Active and passive ROM daily reduces lower extremity stasis.
- Some indirect evidence exists that ROM could be beneficial in the prevention of DVT.

Note: In SCI mechanical compression modalities used in combination with pharmacological prophylaxis in the first 2 weeks after injury have been shown to be effective for reducing the incidence of DVT in acute SCI patients. Venous foot pumps have not been studied in larger trials or in SCI patients, so efficacy in prevention of DVT in this population has not been established.

DVT treatment

The goal of VTE therapy is to prevent recurrent VTE, consequences of VTE, such as postphlebitis syndrome, and pulmonary arterial hypertension, as well as complication of therapy (bleeding). After obtaining baseline CBC and PT/aPTT, the treatment consists of the following:

1. Parenteral anticoagulation with IV unfractionated (UFH), or SC LMWH or SC pentasaccharide (fondaparinux). LMWH has been shown to be superior to unfractionated heparin for the initial treatment of DVT (12), particularly for reducing mortality and reducing the risk for major bleeding during initial therapy.
   - UFH is usually administered IV with a bolus followed by continuous infusion. Normogram-driven weight-based dosing provides reliable prolongation of the aPTT into therapeutic ranges (60–94). aPTT has to be repeated every 6 hours after any bolus or change in infusion rate.
   - Fondaparinux 5 mg SC daily for weight <50 kg, 7.5 mg SC daily for weight 50–10 kg, and 10 mg SC daily for weight >100 kg.
   - Enoxaparin
     - outpatient: 1 mg/kg SC q12
     - inpatient: 1 mg/kg SC q12H or 1.5 mg /kg q24H
2. If oral therapy with warfarin is recommended, then the typical starting dose is 5 mg PO daily on day 1 of parenteral anticoagulation, which is gradually increased every 72 hours with a target INR of 2.5 (therapeutic range is 2–3). Patients with mechanical heart valves require INR 2.5–3.5. There are no recommended dose adjustments for elderly patients.
3. If oral therapy with warfarin is recommended and the patient is currently receiving UH or LMWH, then these medications should be continued for at least 4–5 days or until INR reaches 2.0 on 2 consecutive days with warfarin therapy.
4. INR should be frequently monitored during the first month, but once stable can be monitored every 4 weeks.

Outpatient treatment of DVT, and possibly pulmonary embolism, with LMWH is safe and cost-effective for carefully selected patients, and should be considered if the required support services are in place.

1. Compression stockings should be used routinely to prevent postthrombotic syndrome, beginning within 1 month of diagnosis of proximal DVT and continuing for a minimum of 1 year after diagnosis.
2. There is insufficient evidence to make specific recommendations for types of anticoagulation management of VTE in pregnant women.
3. Anticoagulation should be maintained for 3–6 months for VTE secondary to transient risk factors and for more than 12 months for recurrent VTE.
4. In SCI persons anticoagulation should be continued for at least 3 months; 6 months is recommended.

Patient Safety

The following are important patient safety principles:
1. Given the high prevalence of cardiac disease (i.e., CAD, arrhythmias, silent ischemia.) in adults with SCI, clinicians should actively evaluate for it.
2. Silent ischemia can be particularly challenging to diagnose in SCI and in TBI/noncommunicative patients. Symptoms are often vague. When in doubt, obtain a 12 lead ECG.
3. Given the high prevalence of DVT in bedridden adults with neurologic disabilities, DVT prophylaxis with medications and/or mechanical compression is highly recommended if not contraindicated.
4. Medications commonly used by adults with neurologic disabilities can have a detrimental effect on underlying cardiovascular conditions. For example, tizanidine, opioids, and tricyclic antidepressants can all cause hypotension.
5. Phosphodiesterase inhibitors used for erectile dysfunction should be used with caution in patients receiving α-blocking agents since the combination of both might lead to excessive vasodilatation and hypotension.
6. Nondepolarizing neuromuscular blocking agents such as succinylcholine induces rapid development of hyperkalemia, which can lead to cardiac arrest.
7. A combination of nonsteroidal anti-inflammatory drugs and ACE inhibitors can lead to a worsening of renal function.
8. During rehabilitation sessions with therapists, vital signs should be monitored before, during, and after therapy. Evidence of hypotension or hypertension—especially if associated with symptoms—should be reported to the treating physician and appropriate interventions initiated. Use of Borg/Rate of Perceived Exertion scales during therapy sessions can be very beneficial as well.

Patient Education

The following are important patient education principles:
1. Patients and their caregivers should be educated about the impact of their neurologic disability on cardiovascular function.
2. Given the high prevalence of coronary artery disease in adults with neurologic disabilities, it is important that patients and their caregivers be educated on strategies to reduce risk factors (i.e., weight reduction, exercise, nutrition, smoking cessation).
3. Patients and their caregivers should be educated about early recognition of symptoms of autonomic dysreflexia and implementation of preventive measures.

4. Patients and their caregivers should be educated on their medications. This includes name, indications, administration schedules, common side effects, significant side effects, significant drug–drug interactions.

5. Education should be provided about symptoms of hypotension as well as interventions to prevent or minimize the risk of its occurrence. These include:

- Adequate salt and fluid intake
- Avoidance of diuretics such as alcohol and caffeine
- Slow change in position from supine to sitting, possibly allowing first the lower extremities to dangle off the bed
- Use of abdominal binders or supportive stockings to restrict venous pooling in dependent limbs when out of bed to chair
- In warm weather, use sunscreen, wear light clothing and a hat, and drink approximately 2 liters of fluid per day
- Take regular small meals to minimize postprandial hypotension
- Plan any exercise program in the afternoon
- Assumption of the recumbent or semi-recumbent position should symptoms of orthostatic hypotension occur

REFERENCES

1. Garshick E, Kelly A, Cohen SA, et al. A prospective assessment of mortality in chronic spinal cord injury. Spinal Cord 2005; 43:408–416.

2. Phillips WT, Kirati BJ, Sarkati M, et al. Effect of spinal cord injury on the heart and cardiovascular fitness. Curr Probl Cardiol 1988; 23:641–720.

3. Washburn RA, Figoni SF. Physical activity and chronic cardiovascular disease prevention in spinal cord injury: a comprehensive literature review. Top Spinal Cord Inj Rehabil 1998; 3:16–32.

4. Bravata DM, Ho S-Y, Meehan TP, Brass LM, Concato J. Readmission and death after hospitalization for acute ischemic stroke: 5-year follow-up in the medicare population. Stroke 2007; 38(6):1899–1904.

5. Yusuj S, Sleight P, Pogue J, et al. Effects of angiotensin-converting enzyme inhibitor, ramipril, on ardiovascular events in high-risk patients: the Heart Outcomes Prevention Evaluation Study Investigators. N Engl J Med 2000; 42:145–153.

6. Progress Collaborative Group. Randomized trial of a perinopril based blood pressure lowering regimen among 6105 individuals with previous stroke or transient ischemic attack. Lancet. 2001; 358:1033–1041.

7. Guidelines for the treatment of severe traumatic brain injury. J Neurotrauma 2007; 24 S1.

8. Weaver FM, La Vela SL. Preventive care in spinal cord injuries and disorders: examples of research and implementation. Phys Med Rehabil Clin N Am 2007; 18:297–316.

9. Wolff T, Guirguis-Blake J, Miller T, Gillespie M, Harris R. Screening for carotid artery stenosis: an update of the evidence for the U.S. Preventive Service Task Force. Ann Intern Med 2007 Dec 18; 147(12):860–870.

10. Chobanian AV, Bakris GL, Black HR, et al., for the National Heart, Lung, and Blood Institute Joint National Committee on Prevention, Detection, Evaluation, and Treatment of High Blood Pressure; National High Blood Pressure Education Program Coordinating

Committee. The Seventh Report of the Joint National Committee on Prevention, Detection, Evaluation, and Treatment of High Blood Pressure: the JNC 7 Report. *JAMA* 2003; 289: 2560–2571.

11. Davis BR, Cutler JA, Gordon DJ, et al. Rationale and design for the Antihypertensive and Lipid Lowering Treatment to Prevent Heart Attack Trial (ALLHAT). Am J Hypertens 1996; 9:342–360.

12. Snow V, Qaseem A, Barry P, et al. Management of venous thromboembolism: a clinical practice guideline from the American College of Physicians and the American Academy of Family Physicians. Ann Fam Med 2007; 5(1):74–80.

4 | Cerebral Palsy

Danielle M. Kerkovich
Mindy Aisen

Cerebral palsy (CP) is the result of a one-time neurologic insult to the brain during development. The etiology of the injury can vary from infection, trauma, hemorrhage, ischemia, and other factors but always occurs prenatally during infancy or early childhood before age 3 and causes an impairment of muscle tone (1).

The exact number of children and adults living with CP in the United States is unknown. However, this number is widely believed to be increasing due to improvements in the survival of low and very low birthweight infants (2). Estimates of CP prevalence in the Western world range from 2 to 4.4 cases per 1000 live births (3). Incidence increased 20% from the mid-1960s to the mid-1980s. Decades ago there were far fewer middle-aged (and older) people with CP, but in 2008 the number of adults with CP is roughly equal to the number of children with CP.

Longitudinal studies indicate that 87–93% of children born with CP are surviving into adulthood across a range of disability (4). Today, the survival rate for 10-year-old children with quadriplegia—the most severe form of CP—is 80% of their able-bodied counterparts (5). For those who reach the age of 20, the prognosis for reaching the age of 60 is well above 90% (6). It is estimated that there are 700,000 persons with CP between 1 and 50 years old living in the United States.

ANATOMY AND PHYSIOLOGY

A recently published report defines CP as "a group of permanent disorders of the development of movement and posture." CP is thought to be a non-progressive neurologic injury in that the patho-physiological mechanisms that lead to it are from a single or discrete series of events that are not active at the time of diagnosis. This injury results in a disruption of normal brain structure and function, which, over time, may be associated with changing or additional clinical manifestations. CP is defined by motor dysfunction and is described by muscle tone, coordination, and body part involvement.

41

The three major types of CP are spastic, athetoid, and ataxic. Seventy to 80 percent of patients with CP have spastic clinical features. Affected limbs may demonstrate increased deep tendon reflexes, tremors, hypertonicity, weakness and a characteristic scissors gait with toe-walking.

Although CP is defined by abnormal tone resulting in motor dysfunction, poor coordination, and balance problems, there are several co-occurring conditions associated with or found at higher rates in individuals with CP. These conditions, believed to occur due to increased susceptibility to trauma of the central nervous system, include epilepsy, mental retardation, learning disabilities, autism, and sensory impairments (1). Risk factors including exposure to toxins, prematurity, and anoxia are similar in both sensory impaired individuals and individuals with CP.

ASSESSMENT

Individuals with CP surviving into adulthood face unique physical and medical problems related to their underlying condition. Young adults (18–25 years) report worsening of their physical condition (weakness, spasticity, fatigue) after leaving high school. Differences in tone, flexibility, and posture lead to inefficient and overuse injuries, falls, and a lack of healthy muscle tone. Indeed, aging adults with CP experience an early, multifactorial decline in function.

Adults with CP experience medical and physical problems that nondisabled adults do not experience until much later in life. Physical difficulties associated with CP become increasingly more pronounced. In addition, there are many secondary musculoskeletal problems associated with CP, including subluxations, hip dislocations, scoliosis, osteoarthritis, and osteoporosis, which often lead to pain, dysfunction, and disuse over time (7). Bowel and bladder dysfunction are common in persons with CP. Incontinence and urinary urgency have been reported in up to 50% of persons with moderate to severe CP (8). Adults who have trouble voiding are susceptible to urinary tract infections and impacted bowels. A lack of mobility may exacerbate these problems over time, further exacerbated by increased difficulty in physically accessing the facilities.

Excruciating pain has been reported by many individuals with CP, and chronic pain has been reported in 67–84% of adults with CP (9). The extent to which pain affects function in CP adults has not been widely studied. However, one study of pain and mobility indicated that of 75% of 101 individuals with CP who were ambulatory stopped walking by age 25 due to fatigue and walking inefficiency, and the majority of the remaining subjects stopped walking by age 45 due to joint pain (10). Long-term immobilization increases one's risk for cardiovascular disease, obesity, hypertension, diabetes, osteoporosis, and other potentially life-threatening conditions.

When dealing with an adult with CP, it is critically important to obtain a current medical history and to perform a thorough physical examination. In addition to discussing factors associated with current symptoms, it is necessary for the physician to inquire about issues such as musculoskeletal pain, functionality, depression, hearing loss, visual problems, communication, dental problems, falls, weight gain, cardiac risk factors, diet, acid reflux, etc. Otherwise one is apt to miss CP-related issues that could be addressed early before exacerbation leads to decreased functionality. Tables 4.1 and 4.2 list some key points of the medical history and physical examination as they apply to the patient with CP.

Table 4.1

Pertinent Physical Examination

1. Cognitive Evaluation (if applicable)
   a. Orientation
   b. Memory—immediate and delayed
   c. Concentration
   d. Ability to follow instructions
2. Body Habitus
3. Musculoskeletal System
   a. Range of motion of major joints in the upper and lower extremities
   b. Presence of pain or tenderness with movement or palpation of extremities
   c. Motor strength of key muscle groups in the upper and lower extremities
   d. Presence of contractures in upper and lower extremities
   e. Functional abilities (e.g., use of hands to grasp objects, transfer, ambulate with/without assistive device)
4. Communication
   a. Ability to express needs effectively with or without communicative device
5. Oral Cavity
   a. Evidence of food pocketing in the cheeks
   b. Evidence of drooling
   c. Gingival hyperplasia
   d. Evidence of poor oral hygiene, tooth decay, abscess, tender teeth, poorly coordinated tongue movements
6. Swallowing—Ability to Swallow Solid Food and/or Liquids
7. Vision
   a. Snellen chart
   b. Peripheral vision
   c. Accommodation
   d. Presence of nystagmus
8. Hearing—Evidence of Hearing Loss
9. Skin—Evidence of Pressure Ulcers (buttocks, sacral area, heels, occiput)
10. Braces and Wheelchairs
    a. Good or poor fit of braces
    b. Evidence of skin breakdown under braces
    c. How well do the braces support and/or assist the weakened limb?
    d. If patient uses a wheelchair, how well does the patient fit in the wheelchair? Is it too big? Is it too small?
11. Spasticity
    a. Ashworth spasticity scale score
    b. Location of spasticity
12. Bladder/Bowel Function—Evidence of Incontinence

Table 4.2

Pertinent Medical History

1. Review of Systems
   a. Fatigue—mental and physical
   b. Weakness
   c. Vision problems
      i. Double vision, blurry vision
      ii. Difficulty reading
      iii. Photosensitivity
   d. Dental problems
      i. Last dental checkup
      ii. Dry mouth
      iii. Frequency of oral hygiene and who performs the oral hygiene (patient or caregiver)
   e. Swallowing problems
   f. Communication problems
   g. Spasticity
      i. Current management (e.g., medications, intrathecal Baclofen pump, botulinum toxin injections)
      ii. Frequency of spasms
      iii. Impact of spasticity on work, social interactions
      iv. Does the spasticity negatively impact on hygiene?
   h. Depression, anxiety
   i. Weight gain or weight loss
   j. Nutrition
   k. Bladder function:
      i. Current bladder routine (e.g., intermittent catherization, indwelling catheter, timed voiding, suprapubic catheter)
      ii. Urinary incontinence
   l. Bowel function
      i. Current bowel routine
      ii. Constipation
      iii. Fecal accidents
   m. Pain—musculoskeletal:
      i. Location, intensity, quality, radiation, aggravating factors, alleviating factors
      ii. Diagnostic tests performed
      iii. Treatments tried for the alleviation of pain
2. Past Medical History
   a. Seizure disorder
   b. Coronary artery disease, diabetes, hypertension, hyperlipidemia
   c. Immunization and vaccination history
   d. Depression, mental illness
3. Past Surgical History
   a. Tendon lengthening
   b. Selective dorsal rhizotomy
4. Allergies
5. Medications
   a. Medications with cognitive impairment
   b. Antiseizure medications

Table 4.2 (*Continued*)

6. Functional History
   a. Mobility
      i. Distance ambulated during a typical day.
      ii. Assistive devices used for ambulation and their effectiveness
      iii. Wheelchair use and problems with wheelchair
      iv. Falls or near-falls
   b. Adaptive equipment to prevent falls in the home
7. Social History
   a. Living arrangements (alone, lives with family member or friend)
      i. Any recent changes to living arrangements or support system.
   b. Work history (if applicable)
   c. Substance abuse (e.g., cocaine, marijuana)
   d. Alcoholism

TREATMENT

Interventional strategies in individuals with CP are largely empirical. The effects of growth and development, limited validated outcome measures, and the absence of techniques assessing central nervous system organization and function have confounded analysis of treatment modalities in CP. In order to accurately assess the efficacy of these interventions, new techniques in brain imaging such as functional magnetic resonance imaging (fMRI), transcranial magnetic stimulation (TMS), and diffusion tensor imaging (DTI) are needed to understand underlying cortical motor function abnormalities in CP.

There also appears to be a lack of high-quality studies guiding the care of the various medical problems facing adults with CP. Many of the principles of good care are based on expert opinion or extrapolated from the care rendered to children with CP, adults with other neurologic disabilities, or the general population. This section will briefly discuss some of the treatment principles of key medical issues facing adults with CP. These include: 1) dental problems, 2) communication and swallowing problems, 3) seizure disorders, 4) hearing loss, 5) musculoskeletal pain, 7) mobility-related problems, 8) osteoporosis, 9) spasticity, 10) communication and swallowing, 11) nutrition and the gastro-intestinal system, and 12) preventative care.

Dental Care

A combination of poor oral hygiene, often limited dental care, and dry mouth can all lead to dental problems such as caries and periodontal disease. In addition, seizures can be associated with lacerations (tongue, cheeks and lips), broken teeth (increased risk of aspiration), and gingival hyperplasia (side effects of phenytoin). Appropriate and timely dental care and oral hygiene are important to the preservation of teeth. This, in turn, is important to ensure adequate nutritional intake and an aesthetic facial appearance. The reader is referred to the dental care chapter in this book for more information.

Seizure Disorders

The incidence of seizure disorder is greater in individuals with CP (30–50%) than in those without neurologic damage (5%). In patients with CP, seizure activity is more likely to occur in certain areas of the brain, including the motor and temporal cortices and the hippocampus (11). Those with spastic hemiparesis are usually highly functional, while those with spastic quadriplegia have more severe impairment accompanied by these associated conditions (12).

Hearing Loss

Fifteen percent of children and adults with CP also have either a conductive or sensori-neural hearing disorder. It is recommended that adults with CP have their hearing checked periodically to ensure that hearing loss is appropriately addressed with hearing aids and/or adaptive equipment for the home

Musculoskeletal Pain

Osteoarthritis is a secondary condition that is very underreported (7) and often cited as a major cause of pain in individuals with CP. Atypical and sometimes excessive joint compression from the imbalance of muscle activation across the joint, the abnormal timing of muscle activation, and cessation and the abnormal relationship of joint surfaces in CP can lead to the early degeneration of the articular cartilage and bony deformities of joint surfaces. Researchers examining the health status of 149 adolescents and young adults with CP between the ages of 15 and 25 years found clinical evidence of arthritis in 27% of subjects versus 4% in normal population (13). Repeated stress on surgically altered joint mechanisms can also result in the development of arthritis, the formation of bony deformities, and pain.

It is important for clinicians to inquire about musculoskeletal pain at regularly scheduled outpatient visits as well as during hospital admissions. Inquiries about its location, duration, quality, inciting factors, aggravating factors, alleviating factors, and impact on functionality and treatments tried should all be documented. Interventions typically range from noninvasive (e.g., physical therapy, physical modalities such as ice, heat, electrical stimulation), adaptive (e.g., gait aids, wheelchairs), pharmacological (nonsteroidal anti-inflammatory drugs, antidepressants, antiseizure medications, opioids), and invasive (e.g., peripheral joint injections, botulinum toxin injections, epidural steroids) depending on etiology. Treatment plans should emphasize the maintenance and/or restoration of function and reduction of pain. Given the communicative and/or cognitive impairments of many adults with CP, all attempts should be made to minimize potential harm to the patient, and vigilance is key. Some examples of potential harm are the application of heat modalities over an insensate area in a noncommunicative patient or the administration of medications with cognitive- or balance-impairing side effects.

Mobility Training

With advancing age, ambulatory adults with CP face new challenges to walking. The combination of a sedentary lifestyle, possible obesity, and arthritic changes in lower extremity joints can all affect the quality, speed, and distance of ambulation.

Clinicians need to be aware of these challenges and proactively try to address them. Lower extremity orthotic devices, which may have been effective in the past, need to be reevaluated for proper fit and function. Ambulatory aids such as canes and crutches may cease to be effective, with subsequent falls or near falls being reported. Walkers, wheelchairs, and motorized wheelchairs may be more appropriate in some adults with CP and impaired mobility.

If a patient is already in a wheelchair, it is important to assess the wheelchair for proper function and fit. It is not uncommon for sedentary adults to gain weight, necessitating a larger wheelchair, a different seat cushion, or support system for contracted limbs and poor trunk control. The implications of a poorly fitting wheelchair can include pressure ulcers and pain. Clinicians should consider referral to a local wheelchair clinic.

Weakness in lower extremities may also become more apparent due to a more sedentary lifestyle and would subsequently benefit from a course of physical therapy to strengthen paretic limbs. Minimizing the risk of falls in the home is also paramount, and a home safety evaluation could prove very beneficial. Items such as tub benches, grab bars, and handheld showers accompanied by a "refresher" course in activities of daily living (ADLs) could be very effective.

New Technologies

Recent developments in neuro-rehabilitation have been stimulated by information on neuronal recovery processes and their modulation by various physical and pharmacologic interventions. There is a growing body of evidence demonstrating that the adult human brain is capable of significant recovery (plasticity) after injury providing that the amount and frequency of treatments are applied appropriately. In addition to quantity, the quality of the intervention is equally important, with task-specific interventions enhancing neural reorganization and behavioral recovery.

Innovations in clinical robotics technology, together with new understanding of the neurologic recovery process in chronic stroke, have led to new task-specific, robot-assisted neuro-rehabilitation therapies for the upper limbs, lower limbs, and hands. Task-oriented rehabilitative modalities include robot-assisted body weight–supported treadmill training (BWSTT) for the lower limbs and robots such as the MIT-Manus for upper limb training. These devices enable severely affected individuals to follow principles of motor learning and acquire new skills. Several studies have shown the potential of

BWSTT to improve walking ability in patients after stroke, spinal cord injuries, and in children with CP (14–16). A recent meta-analysis of the effectiveness of robot-assisted BWSTT in stroke patients indicated that this treatment modality combined with usual care significantly increased the odds of walking independently and significantly increased walking capacity as compared to usual care alone. It is reasonable to assume that the adult with CP would have the same ability to learn new motor skills as the stroke patient. Clinical studies using task-specific rehabilitation modalities in the adult with CP are therefore warranted.

These task-specific techniques, while promising, require many hours of progressive practice that engage and challenge the patient. Virtual reality (VR) technology can alleviate this problem by providing an environment where the presentation of stimuli (e.g., a video game) can be controlled systematically for adapting task difficulty as performance improves as well as by providing positive feedback. VR has shown promise in improving upper and lower limb function in stroke and CP patients when used in conjunction with neuro-rehabilitation modalities as discussed above.

In addition, haptic technology has been recently employed in many VR rehabilitation techniques. Haptic refers to the science of touch and force feedback in human–computer interactions. Similar to existing robotic therapy devices, these devices can simulate the sense of touch and movement and apply therapeutic patterns of forces to the hand and arm as the user attempts to move. Finally, a new virtual reality-based motor neuro-rehabilitation system uses the concept of "mirror neurons" to facilitate motor relearning and improve functional recovery after loss from brain injury. It is based on the hypotheses that 1) observed actions correlated with intended actions engage mirror neurons and 2) activation in damaged parts of motor cortex can be enhanced by viewing mirrored movements of nonparetic limbs (17).

Because CP may lead to profound muscle weakness in the affected extremities due to large deficits in voluntary contractions (16), there may not be sufficient force to induce muscle growth during training exercises. It has been demonstrated that neuromuscular electrical stimulation (NMES) used in conjunction with a 12-week isometric strength training program produces a significantly greater normalized force production for the quadriceps (muscle strength) and greater walking speed posttraining than strength training without NMES (18). To date, NMES used in conjunction with BWSTT has not been reported in CP patients. However, it has been shown to be more effective in restoring gait in stroke patients than BWSTT alone (19). NMES may enhance the benefits of BWSTT already demonstrated in CP children by recruiting and strengthening muscles that are needed to complete normal gait cycles.

Osteoporosis, Sarcopenia, and Fractures

Immobilization of the musculoskeletal system, as experienced by persons with CP, often results in sarcopenia and the loss of muscle mass, which is soon followed by osteopenia, leading to further immobilization. The combination of an altered gait in ambulatory adults with CP, risk of falling, and the presence of osteoporosis can all increase the risk of a fracture.

It has been reported that reduced mobility and subsequent reduced muscle load is the major etiologic factor for bone fragility in children with CP (20). Chronic immobility results in low bone mass and abnormal bone architecture that is unable to withstand occasional mechanical challenges. Fracture rates in adults with CP have not been well documented, and few studies have been performed on bone density of adults with CP. However, King et al. (18) reported the effects on bone mass in children and adults with spastic quadriplegia, with a median age of 15, the oldest patient being 48 years old. Both the children and adults had significantly lower bone mineral densities than the normal population, and the deficiency continued to worsen with age. Studies of ambulatory and nonambulatory adolescents and children with CP have demonstrated increases in bone mineral accrual and bone size when they participate in weight-bearing activities as well as biomechanics-based therapies (20). It is reasonable to assume that these therapies would benefit the adult with CP, although clinical studies to assess efficacy in the adult have not been done.

Recent studies have shown that vibration therapy may prevent these immobilizing conditions. Whole body vibration therapy (WBV) has been shown to prevent bone loss in immobilized adults by improving muscular coordination through the induction of frequent muscle contractions of agonists and antagonist of the musculoskeletal system (21). Several recent studies have shown that vibration therapy improves bone health and mobility and decreases spasticity in the disabled, showing success in persons with osteogenesis imperfecta, spina bifida, and CP (21) through these noninvasive low-level mechanical signals. These vibrations create vertical oscillations that generate strain or deformations in bone, effectively promoting bone formation (22), enhancing bone morphology (23), and decreasing bone catabolism (24).

One study found that WBV training in adults decreased spasticity in knee extensors and increased the Gross Motor Function Measure and isokinetic muscle strength after only 8 weeks of therapy (25). Another study found that WBV decreased spasticity, increased functionality of limbs, and allowed the postponement of surgical interventions. A study that observed disabled children standing on a vibrating platform for an average of only 4.4 minutes a day, 5 days a week, for 6 months showed an average of more than 6% increase in BMD of the tibia, while the controls who stood on a nonvibrating platform showed an almost 12% loss in BMD (24).

In addition to improving bone health and mobility, extremely low-magnitude mechanical signals have been shown to inhibit adipogenesis (23) and influence bone resorption in mice, which could potentially be very beneficial for overweight adults with CP. These findings could have huge implications for the CP population, from simultaneously preventing obesity and osteoporosis (23) to decreasing susceptibility to metabolic syndrome.

Spasticity

To improve gait and mobility, spasticity is the most often treated condition in children with CP and is managed through the administration of physical therapy, chemo-denervation using compounds such as botulinum toxin A or phenol, continuous intrathecal baclofen, neurosurgical procedures, and orthopedic surgeries such as tendon transfer. A recent meta-analysis of studies in which an intervention was used to improve gait found that overall there was significant improvement in gait after an intervention, but when broken down by type of intervention (e.g., tendon transfer, rhizotomy, physical therapy) there was not enough data to make a clinical recommendation regarding one intervention over another (26).

Several studies support the use of botulinum toxin A in the treatment of equine spasticity during walking, but a systematic review of trials (27) did not find strong evidence to support or refute its use for treatment of leg spasticity in patients with CP.

Selective dorsal rhizotomy (SDR) is a neurosurgical procedure used to reduce spasticity by selectively cutting dorsal rootlets from spinal cord segments L1 to S2. Its use in children has been well described (28), but its role in adults has not yet been defined.

Intrathecal Baclofen has been used successfully for the treatment of spasticity in SCI and TBI, and there is some literature describing its benefits and limitations in CP-related spasticity (29), but its role in the treatment of adults with CP-related spasticity remains undefined.

For a further description of the assessment and treatment of spasticity in adults with neurologic diseases, the reader is referred to the spasticity chapter in this book.

Nutrition and Gastrointestinal Problems

Poor coordination and spasticity of facial muscles along with mandibular joint contractures can make it difficult for some with CP to self-feed. Even with assistance, feeding, chewing, and even swallowing can lead to fatigue, reducing the amount of nutritional intake. Over time, poor nutrition can lead to weight loss and its deleterious effects on the body.

As we age, it is important that we eat more fiber, calcium, iron, protein, and vitamins A and C and folic acid. For example, dietary fiber, not increased use of laxatives, helps maintain normal bowel function and decreases one's risk for intestinal inflammation. Calcium and vitamin D protect against osteoporosis. Medications used to control diseases such as hypertension or heart disease can alter the need for electrolytes such as sodium or potassium and interfere with many vitamins. Vitamin C, zinc, iron, and copper are all enzyme cofactors in collagen synthesis important for the prevention of ulcers. Water, often overlooked as a component of nutrition, is also important for skin integrity and the prevention of ulcers as well as promoting healthy bladder and bowel function. Nutritional deficiencies in an adult with CP may not be obvious.

Nutritional assessment of an adult with CP is recommended to quantify caloric intake as well intake of protein, fats, carbohydrates, and water and key vitamins. This is especially important if the person has either gained or lost a significant amount of weight. Key interventions should follow depending on the problem identified.

Some estimates that claim over 90% of individuals with CP present with gastrointestinal symptoms, including difficulty swallowing, regurgitation, and constipation or bowel obstruction. Constipation or abnormal bowel movements may be caused by delayed gastric emptying, abnormal autonomic control of gastrointestinal mobility, or prolonged colonic transit. Some medications used in the treatment of adults with CP (i.e., opioids) can have constipation as a significant side effect. Clinicians should review the medication list and limit medications with this side effect or proactively try to prevent it from occurring.

Adults with CP have a higher incidence of acid reflux disease leading to increased risk for ulcers of the esophagus or Barrett's esophagus in which the cells lining the esophagus either change or are replaced with abnormal cells. It is critically important to incorporate necessary screening techniques into CP plans of care as individuals with Barrett's esophagus have a 30- to 125-fold increased risk for developing esophageal adenocarcinoma.

Preventive Care

As children with CP enter adulthood, they are at increased risk of developing similar diseases to their non-CP counterparts. These include increased risk of coronary artery disease (as a result of, e.g., sedentary lifestyle, poor diet, hypertension, obesity, and hyperlipidemia) and diabetes mellitus, among others. Adults with CP should receive the same preventive care measures as their non-CP counterparts. The reader is referred to the preventive care chapter in this book as well as to other pertinent chapters.

Patient Safety

Difficulties with communication and cognitive impairments place adults with CP at risk for iatrogenic events in inpatient and outpatient medical settings. Clinicians must ensure adequate understanding of medical care issues by the patient and/or caregivers prior to them being carried out. All attempts must be made to simplify treatment plans and minimize medications with cognitive side effects.

Patient Education

Patients with CP and their caregivers should be educated on general preventative measures and screenings that are recommended for the general population: 1) maintaining stable body weight, 2) age and gender appropriate cancer screenings, 3) the importance of a nutritionally sound diet and exercise program (if applicable), and 4) regular checkups with physicians and dentists, with screenings for coronary artery disease risk factors and diabetes. In addition, they should be counseled on ways to maintain their functional levels in spite of age and comorbid disease-related impairments.

REFERENCES

1. Bax M, Goldstein M, Rosenbaum P, et al. Executive Committee for the Definition of Cerebral Palsy, Proposed definition and classification of cerebral palsy. Dev Med Child Neurol 2005.
2. Colver AF, Gibson M, Hey EN, Jarvis SN, Mackie PC, Richmond S. Increasing rates of cerebral palsy across the severity spectrum in north-east England 1964–1993. 2000 The North of England Collaborative Cerebral Palsy Survey. Arch Dis Child Fetal Neonatal Ed 2000; 83(1):F7–F12.
3. Surveillance of Cerebral Palsy in Europe (SCPE). Prevalence and characteristics of children with cerebral palsy in Europe. Dev Med Child Neurol 2002; 44:663–640.
4. Hutton JL, Pharoah POD. Life expectancy in severe cerebral palsy. Arch Dis Childhood 2006; 91:254–258.
5. Crichton JU, Mackinnon M, White CP. The life expectancy of persons with cerebral palsy. Dev Med Child Neurol 1995; 37(7):567–576.
6. Strauss DJ, Shavelle RM, Reynolds RJ, Rosenbloom L, Day SM. Survival in cerebral palsy in the last 20 years: Signs of improvement? Dev Med Child Neurol 2007; 49:86–92.
7. Gajdosik CG, Cicirello N. Secondary conditions of the musculoskeletal system in adolescents and adults with cerebral palsy. Phys Occup Ther Pediatr 2001; 21:49–68.
8. Karaman MI, Kaya C, Caskurlu T, et al. Urodynamic findings in children with cerebral palsy. Int J Urol 2005; 12:717–720.
9. Liptak GS. Health and well being of adults with cerebral palsy. Curr Opin Neurol 2008; 21(2):136–142.
10. Murphy KP, Molnar GE, Lankasky K. Medical and functional status of adults with cerebral palsy. Dev Med Child Neurol 1995; 37(12):1075–1084.
11. Zgorzalewicz B, Mieszczanek T, Zgorzalewicz M. Descriptive epidemiology of cerebral palsy. Ortop Traumatol Rahabil 2001; 3(4):467–471.
12. Krigger KW. Cerebral palsy: an overview. Am Fam Phys 2006; 73(1):91–100.
13. Cathels BA, Reddihough DS. The health care of young adults with cerebral palsy. Med J Aust 1993; 159(7):444–446.
14. Maltais DB, Pierrynowski MR, Galea VA, de Bruin H, Al-Mutawaly N, Bar-Or O. Minute-by-minute differences in co-activation during treadmill walking in cerebral palsy. Electromyogr Clin Neurophysiol 2004; 44(8):477–487.
15. Provost B, Dieruf K, Burtner PA, et al. Endurance and gait in children with cerebral palsy after intensive body weight-supported treadmill training. Pediatr Phys Ther 2007; 19(1): 2–10.

16. Begnoche DM, Pitetti KH. Effects of traditional treatment and partial body weight treadmill training on the motor skills of children with spastic cerebral palsy. A pilot study. Pediatr Phys Ther 2007; 19(1):11–19.
17. Eng K, Siekierka E, Pyk P, et al. Interactive visuo-motor therapy system for stroke rehabilitation. Med Biol Eng Comput 2007; 45(9):901–907.
18. King W, Levin R, Schmidt R, Oestreich A, Heubi JE. Prevalence of reduced bone mass in children and adults with spastic quadriplegia. Dev Med Child Neurol 2003; 45(1):12–16.
19. Daly JJ, Ruff RL. Construction of efficacious gait and upper limb functional interventions based on brain plasticity evidence and model-based measures for stroke patients. Sci World J 2007; 7:2031–2045.
20. Munns CF, Cowell CT. Prevention and treatment of osteoporosis in chronically ill children. J Musculoskelet Neuronal Interact 2005; 5(3):262–272.
21. Semler O, Fricke O, Vezyroglou K, Stark C, Schoenau E. Preliminary results on the mobility after whole body vibration in immobilized children and adolescents. J Musculoskelet Neuronal Interact 2007; 7(1):77–81.
22. Judex S, Donahue LR, Rubin C. Genetic predisposition to low bone mass is paralleled by an enhanced sensitivity to signals anabolic to the skeleton. FASEB J 2002; 16(10):1280–1282. Epub 2002 Jun 21.
23. Rubin MA, Jasiuk I, Taylor J, Rubin J, Ganey T, Apkarian RP. TEM analysis of the nanostructure of normal and osteoporotic human trabecular bone. Bone 2003; 33(3):270–282.
24. Ward K, Alsop C, Caulton J, Rubin C, Adams J, Mughal Z. Low magnitude mechanical loading is osteogenic in children with disabling conditions. J Bone Miner Res 2004; 19(3):360–369.
25. Ahlborg L, Andersson C, Julin P. Whole body vibration training compared with resistance training: effect on spasticity. J Rehabil Med 2006; 38(5):302–308.
26. Paul SM, Siegel KL, Malley J, Jaeger RJ. Evaluating interventions to improve gait in cerebral palsy: a meta-analysis of spatiotemporal measures. Dev Med Child Neurol 2007; 49(7):542–549.
27. Ade-Hall RA, Moore AP. Botulinum toxin type A in the treatment of lower limb spasticity in cerebral palsy. Cochrane Database Syst Rev 2000; (2):CD001408.
28. Golan JD, Hall JA, O'Gorman G, et al. Spinal deformities following selective dorsal rhizotomy. J Neurosurg 2007; 106(6 Suppl):441–449.
29. Butler C, Campbell S. Evidence of the effects of intrathecal baclofen for spastic and dystonic cerebral palsy. AACPDM Treatment Outcomes Committee Review Panel. Dev Med Child Neurol 2000; 42(9):634–645.

5 | Dental Care

Daniela Spector
Yuval Spector

Dental problems are very common in adults living with neurologic disabilities such as spinal cord injury (SCI), traumatic brain injury (TBI), stroke (CVA), and multiple sclerosis (MS) They are commonly attributed to 1) impaired cognition, 2) impaired hand strength and control, 3) poor oral hygiene, 4) lack of access to appropriate dental care, and 5) side effects of medications. They can have a considerable impact on the nutritional, communicative, emotional, as well as dental well-being of the person afflicted (1–5).

Dental problems are common in stroke survivors. The lack of adequate tongue control and strength combined with difficulties in swallowing can predispose to the accumulation of food on one side of the mouth, under the tongue, and around the teeth, thereby promoting tooth decay. A flaccid tongue and cheek can also be traumatized during chewing. Problems with speech and cognition can make it difficult for the patient to communicate dental pain to family and caregivers. Problems with dentition can lead to avoidance of food that is difficult to chew, which can subsequently adversely affect adequate nutritional intake.

Patients with traumatic brain injuries pose several dental problems. The impaired cognition and communication and swallowing dysfunction commonly seen in severe brain injuries can also adversely affect dental care for the reasons mentioned above. Seizure disorders are also common in severe brain injuries and can pose additional challenges to teeth and gums. Teeth, tongue, lips, and cheeks can be traumatized during seizures. Teeth can break, with potential aspiration of tooth and crown particles. Gingival overgrowth commonly seen with some antiseizure medications can make oral hygiene difficult.

Oral manifestations occur in 2–3% of patients with MS. These include periorbital paresthesias, orofacial numbness, trigeminal neuralgia, and dysarthria.

Adults with the above-mentioned diagnoses are frequently treated with multiple medications, many of which have xerostomia (dry mouth) as a side effect. Adequate hydration of the oral cavity is essential to dental well-being, and xerostomia can increase the incidence of dental decay (Table 5.1).

Table 5.1

Medications That Can Adversely Affect Dental Care and Dental Health

---

Aspirin
Warfarin
Steroids
Antiseizure medications (e.g., phenytoin)
Oxybutinin
Tricyclic antidepressants (amitriptyline, nortriptyline)
Clozapine

The goal of this chapter is to provide an overview of the assessment and treatment of dental conditions typically seen in adults with neurologic disabilities as well as to provide the reader with pertinent information about patient safety issues and patient education. Clinicians should refer patients to dentists for individualized patient care.

ANATOMY AND PHYSIOLOGY

The tooth is made up of a crown, enamel, dentin, pulp, and root. The crown is the hardest part of the tooth. Dentin is below the enamel, and the pulp is at the center of the tooth. The root makes up most of the tooth and anchors the tooth to the jaw (6).

The oral cavity is divided into four quadrants: upper left, upper right, lower left, and lower right. Adults generally start with 32 teeth. The shape of the teeth varies, as different teeth serve different functions. The largest teeth are the molars. There are three molars in each of the four quadrants. The molars are wide enough to tackle strong mastication forces and assure adequate grinding and crushing of food. They are located in the posterior section of the mouth.

In front of the molars are smaller versions of the molars, called the premolars. There are two in each quadrant and eight in total. They start the grinding of the food before passing it on to the molars. The canines are in front of the premolars, and there are four in number. They are very strong and long, with the longest roots in the mouth. They have the very important function of grabbing and tearing the food. They also keep the food steady as it is chewed inside the oral cavity and help guide the jaw in lateral movements and keep the generated forces symmetric. Dentists rely on these strong teeth for support in many prosthetic situations such as anchoring dentures.

The most anterior teeth in the mouth are called the incisors. They are eight in number, two in each quadrant. These teeth are also used to tear and maintain the food in the mouth. They also keep saliva and food particles in the oral cavity and are very important for phonetics. The tongue rests on these teeth, and speech is dictated by their position and shape. Due to their prominence, they play a very important role in the self-esteem of the patient.

Posterior teeth help maintain the vertical dimension of the face, which also can make a person look younger or older. Losing one's vertical dimension from posterior tooth loss also will cause pooling of saliva in the commisures of the mouth, causing painful sores and infections for the patient.

With normal progression of age, wear patterns on teeth are noted. This may come from grinding of teeth (often due to stress) or poor symmetry of balance throughout the mouth. This phenomenon is slightly more exaggerated in people who have lost their back teeth and are overusing their front teeth and traumatizing them. An equilibrated mouth, where the masticatory (chewing) forces are evenly distributed among the quadrants, is a healthy mouth.

PATIENT ASSESSMENT

Aside from the general medical examination, there are many collateral questions that apply to the dental management of the patient.

History of Present Illness

- *Tooth pain*: What are the location, frequency, and quality of the pain? Is the pain brought on by a direct stimulation or present without any stimulation? When did pain start? Is it getting worse? Is it fleeting pain or long lasting? What makes the pain go away? Does food get caught between the teeth?
- *Limitations of oral function*: Is there an impaired ability to chew and/or swallow? Is there a sensation of choking? Difficulty with speech/communication?
- *Oral hygiene routine*: What is the frequency of brushing and flossing? Does the patient use an antimicrobial rinse? If yes, how often? For denture wearers: Does the patient sleep with the denture? How often do they wash the denture and with what material? Do they wear adhesives? Do they clean the adhesive? How often is adhesive changed?

Past Medical History

- *Hospitalization and surgical history*: It is important to note the presence of any metal prosthetics in the body as this would determine the need of prophylactic antibiotics.

Review of Systems

- *Cognitive limitations*: how is patient handling them as it pertains to oral care
- *Oral side effects*: Burning or dry mouth? Sticky tongue? Painful, bleeding gums? How often do gums bleed—provoked bleeding or passive bleeding? Do they wake up with blood on their pillow? Any notable pus or draining of the gums? Bad breath noted? Any mouth lesions? What makes the lesions go away? Biting of cheeks?

Allergies

- *History of allergies*: Latex, dental anesthesia, antibiotics.

Medications

- It is important to obtain a list of all current medications being taken by the patient, including aspirin products and warfarin, as this increases the risk of bleeding with dental work. The dose of the medications (including recent changes), indications, frequency of use, and dosing route should be recorded. Use of over-the-counter medications, nutritional supplements, vitamins, and herbal preparations should also be noted. For example, vitamin E and omega-3 can have blood-thinning properties.
- Intravenous bisphosphonate use: Patients who have received this medication are at risk for complications after routine dental surgeries. They are prone to necrosis of the jaw.

Table 5.2 provides a list of some commonly asked questions.

Table 5.2

Dental History Questionnaire

Do you have a history of smoking or chewing tobacco?
Do you have a history of drinking alcohol excessively?
Do you have any allergies?
When was your last dental visit?
When was your last dental cleaning?
When were your last full-mouth x-rays?
How often do you brush your teeth?
If you don't brush your teeth, who assists you and how much assistance do you require?
What other dental aides do you use (e.g., floss or waterpik electric brush)?
Are your teeth sensitive to hot/cold/sweets/chewing?
Have you noticed any mouth odors or bad tastes?
Do your gums bleed or hurt?
Do you have any loose teeth?
Have you lost any teeth before?
Does food get caught between the teeth?
Do you bite your lips or cheeks often?
Do you have any broken teeth that cut your tongue or cheeks?
Do you tend to breathe through your mouth?
Do you smoke or use any tobacco products?
Do you have a history of cancer? If yes, any history of cancer of the mouth or throat?
Do you have a history of cancer in the family?
Do you have difficulty opening and closing your mouth?
Do you have pain in the facial muscles when you wake up?

Table 5.2 (*Continued*)

Do you wear a denture? If yes, do you sleep with it? How often do you clean it?

Do you feel nervous about dental treatments?

Have you had any upsetting dental experiences?

Do you use any of the following medications: aspirin, warfarin, steroids, intravenous biphosphonates?

Have you had any metal prostheses implanted in your body?

The physical examination should focus on the oral cavity as well as pertinent neurologic and musculoskeletal examinations that could adversely impact
on dental care.

Generally speaking, the oral cavity examination should assess for any loose
or missing teeth, tooth pain, abscesses, gingival hypertrophy, dry mouth,
lesions, lacerations of the cheeks and lips, evidence of food pocketing, and
drooling. Percussion tests, tongue evaluation, temperomandibular joint (TMJ)
evaluation, and use of illuminating lights can also be very helpful.

Percussion tests: These are used to determine if the pain is coming from a particular tooth. An instrument such as a dental mirror is used to tap on the tooth.
A report of pain may indicate need for a root canal procedure.

Tongue evaluation: The tip of the tongue is wrapped in 2" × 2" gauze and is pulled
gently to the right and to the left to evaluate the lateral borders of the tongue. This
is the most prevalent area for oral cancer. It also allows for a better visualization
under the lateral borders of the tongue where the floor of the mouth is sometimes
hard to see. Using a tongue depressor, the patient is then asked to sing a note
to visualize the back of the throat. The palate is checked, as well as the cheeks.
Lesions are typically red or white in color, and they may be indurated or ulcerated. They may or may not be painful to touch. If lesions are identified it is best
to send the patient to an oral surgeon for evaluation. The tongue should also be
evaluated for lacerations, strength, and symmetry of movements in all directions.

Temporal mandibular joint (TMJ) evaluation: The physician's two middle fingers are placed in front of the ears and the patient is asked to open the mouth
as wide as possible, and then to close slowly. A click or a deviation is typically
felt with opening or closing the mouth. TMJ dysfunction can be associated with
headaches and, in severe cases, even lockjaw. Lockjaw is a condition in which
the person opens his or her mouth and is unable to close it afterwards.

Illuminating lights: These are sometimes used to identify cavities between teeth
that are not apparent on the clinical exam. This is accomplished by shining a
light beam near the teeth where they connect with one another.

Pertinent neurologic and musculoskeletal evaluations include range of
motion in the upper extremities, presence of contractures, strength testing
including hand grip, finger dexterity, and coordination of movements—all of
which are necessary for the use of toothbrushes and adaptive aids. Cognition,
ability to follow instructions, and vision should also be evaluated.

Key elements of the pertinent physical evaluation are listed in Table 5.3.

Table 5.3

Physical Examination

Oral Cavity
   Teeth: any missing, loose, black, broken teeth?
   If patient is wearing dentures: Are the dentures loose? Are they ill-fitting?
   Gingival hyperplasia
   Dry mouth
   Lacerations of the cheeks, lips
   Tongue evaluation:
      Lesions on the sides and the base of the tongue
      Lacerations
      Strength
      Symmetry of movements in all directions
   Any evidence of pocketing of foods, drooling, or coughing?
   Any lesions in the oral cavity?
   Halitosis
   TMJ evaluation
Upper Extremities
   Range of motion of shoulders, elbows, wrists, and fingers
   Any contractures?
   Strength of the muscles of the upper extremities
   Hand grip strength and coordination of finger movements
Cognition
   Is patient able to follow 1-2-3 step instructions?
   Is patient oriented to name, place, and time?
   Check for memory (immediate and delayed) and concentration deficits

X-Rays

X-rays are primarily used by dentists to determine tooth decay after the clinical exam is completed. However, they often reveal additional important information, such as: 1) the size and proximity of the cavity to the nerve, 2) bone height, which is used to evaluate the severity of periodontal disease, 3) bone lesions, such as cancer, cysts, or impacted teeth, and 4) potential sinus problems. Interestingly, large panoramic x-rays have also shown carotid artery calcifications.

TREATMENTS OF COMMON DENTAL PROBLEMS

Prevention

Many of the dental problems commonly seen in adults with neurologic disabilities stem from lack of adequate oral hygiene and preventative dental care. It is very important that adults with neurologic disabilities have an adequate daily oral hygiene routine that includes brushing of teeth, flossing, and use of mouth rinses, as well as regular dental checkups and professional cleanings every 3 months. Fluoride has been shown to strengthen teeth and can be taken as an oral supplement or as a mouth rinse or administered in the dentist's office.

For patients with seizure disorders who are at risk for broken teeth with subsequent potential risk of aspiration, simple treatment plans, without many crowns or small removable appliances, can be very beneficial.

Periodontal disease is commonly known as gum disease. It is an infection of the gum and bone and, if left untreated, can lead to bone loss. When bone is lost, the basic foundation and support of the tooth is gone, which in turn can lead to tooth loss. Periodontal disease in the early stages is a painless disease, and one is not aware that one has it until it is severe. Once it is very severe, it is usually impossible to save a lot of teeth, rendering the patient edentulous.

Patients who have a hard time maintaining their oral hygiene are very prone to periodontal disease. Dental check-ups and dental cleanings should be every 3 months for this population. Signs of periodontal disease are 1) bleeding upon brushing or flossing or eating, 2) halitosis, and 3) detached gingivae and swollen gums that easily bleed.

The treatment for periodontal disease varies with the degree of severity. The first step in the treatment is to evaluate the extent of the inflammation. The next step is to do a deep cleaning (e.g., scaling and root planning) using local anesthesia. In this procedure calculus (mineralized bacteria) is scraped off the teeth. This step typically takes two visits.

If the scaling and root planning does not work , and the inflammation of the tissue does not get better, then a periodontist or a gum surgeon will be asked to step in and remove some excess tissue and further clean the region. Sometimes subgingival antibiotic therapy is used to prevent further bacterial infection of the area.

If the patient presents with excessive swelling of the gum and an abscess, an incision and possibly a drain is placed if the abscess is large enough. The patient is placed on systemic antibiotics and reevaluated three days later.

Reversible Pulpitis (Tooth Pain from Simple Cavities)

These are toothaches patients get when simple fillings fall out or break. Patients may also have teeth that were never filled and have dental decay. These teeth hurt when eating sweets and sometimes when they drink a cold drink. Usually, the pain is short lived and goes away when the stimulus is taken away.

These "cavities" are actually called carious lesions, and the hole in the tooth is infiltrated with food and bacteria. This problem is usually remedied by cleansing the area, removing and filling the opening, and applying a sedative packing and possibly a silver filling, depending on the severity of the pain. The temporary inflammation of the pulp (nerve inside the tooth) is usually reversible. The treatment for cavities can vary depending on the size of the cavity. Some small cavities that cause pain are drilled and filled with amalgam or acrylic. For cavities that are very large, a sedative filling is first placed and the tooth is placed under observation. The patient goes home with that sedative filling and returns in 2–4 weeks. If the tooth is not hurting the patient, a permanent filling is then placed, while leaving a base of the medication under it.

If a filling will not hold because of lack of tooth structure, a crown is placed. The tooth is shaved down to a dome shape and a mold is taken and sent to a lab. A crown is made at the lab utilizing metal and porcelain or just porcelain. This procedure typically takes two visits.

Nonreversible Pulpitis

These are very bad toothaches in which there is a severe attack on the nerve structure inside of the tooth. Bacteria have eaten to the substructure of the tooth where the nerve is housed with subsequent inflammation of the nerve itself.

During such an attack a root canal procedure is performed if the tooth has a chance at being restored. A root canal is performed by achieving local anesthesia and cleansing the tooth from the inside out. The nerve is removed using a small barbed instrument. The canal is then irrigated with antimicrobial agents, and a filling material is packed tightly in the space where the nerve used to be. Once the tooth has healed (generally about 2 weeks' time), it is restored mostly with a crown to replace all the missing tooth structure, thereby rendering it useful again for mastication. Sometimes the decay is so extensive that performing a root canal successfully will be impossible and an extraction may be recommended.

When the nerve to a tooth has been compromised by tooth decay, the nerve must be removed to be able to save the tooth. Local anesthesia is administered and the nerve is removed with a barbed instrument. The nerve space is cleaned well and disinfected and instrumented into a special shape. The canal is then filled with a special cement and clay. This will take two or three visits. The patient is sent home to heal for 2 weeks after which a crown is placed on the tooth to give strength to this nonviable tooth. Nonviable teeth are very prone to fracture because they are dry and brittle and too weak to withstand the strong masticator pressures placed on them.

Restorative dentistry is perofrmed to restore the function of a tooth or a group of teeth in one area. Teeth can be rebuilt in a few ways. Large silver fillings used to be the treatment of choice. Today teeth can also be restored with crowns, which are shells of metal and porcelain, and the cover pieces of tooth that remain after large carious lesions are cleaned out.

Some patients request acrylic white fillings to be placed, since they are more aesthetic. These fillings are generally not as strong as amalgam fillings or crowns. Sometimes they tend to get secondary decay and cause more sensitivity.

Crowns are usually performed after a root canal treatment is completed and healed. Crowns are also done on live teeth that have not been treated with root canal if the decay or breakage was extensive. Sometimes a person is missing a few teeth and does not want to wear a denture. If it is possible, and the teeth allow it, a few crowns are connected together to close up a gap and a bridge is created. If patients do not have enough teeth to allow that to happen, the denture is either made or an implant is paced in that gap, and a crown is attached to that. An implant is a titanium screw that is placed in the bone, which, when it heals, is topped off with a crown.

When the tooth is severely decayed, broken down, or abscessed, it needs to be removed. This is usually a simple procedure, but the complications can vary from minor to major. The patient is administered a local anesthetic injection with or without intravenous sedation or nitrous oxide and the tooth is removed. Antibiotics may be administered (e.g., in an immunocompromised patient or if the patient had an abscess there previously).

Halitosis, also known as "bad breath," is generally caused by an accumulation of bacteria in the oral cavity. There are many reasons for halitosis. Bacterial proliferation under the gums (periodontal disease), around the teeth, or on the tongue and caries are common causes. The use of medications that dry the mouth render it more susceptible to bacterial overgrowth. Other causes include medications or diseases of the digestive tract. Proper treatment of halitosis depends on its underlying cause. Proper care of dentures, brushing of the tongue, treatment of caries and periodontal disease, and adequate oral hydration will all decrease the bacteria and reduce halitosis.

Dry mouth is commonly due to 1) side effects of medications that decrease salivary flow, 2) mouth breathing due to a deviated septum or severe allergies, and 3) an open bite (due to skeletal and dental malformations at a young age), with the end result being adherence of food to oral structures and subsequent bacterial overgrowth. Clinicians should minimize the use of medications with anticholinergic side effects and encourage their patients to drink sips of water throughout the day. If these are not effective, chewing sugar-free gum and using over-the-counter medications that increase salivary flow are recommended. For persons with mouth breathing or severe allergies, referral to an ear, nose, and throat specialist is recommended.

Oral lesions are commonly caused by trauma from broken teeth and crowns. These structures are sharp and tend to cut and irritate the surrounding soft tissues. Lacerations to the tongue and roof of the mouth can be caused by food, especially in the person with a dry mouth.

Dentures that are loose or ill-fitting can also be a source of irritations, which can subsequently become infected. They can also cause canker sores or apthous ulcers.

Some lesions may be precancerous or cancerous, especially in a patient with a history of smoking or chewing tobacco. Referral to an oral surgeon for evaluation and biopsy is recommended.

Treatment of oral lesions depends on the underlying cause. Often, rinsing with warm salt water helps these lesions heal quickly. Additionally, there are over-the-counter products that alleviate pain (i.e., topical anesthesia) as well as antimicrobial rinses that are very affective.

Adaptive Equipment

There are many special devices available to make dental care easier for patients who have neurologic disabilities.

1. Oral irrigators help dislodge food particles in tight to reach areas.
2. Battery-operated toothbrushes are very effective and easier to use that conventional brushes.
3. Battery-operated flossers can be used to aid with flossing.
4. Toothbrush holders shaped like a softball or a bike handle can make holding a toothbrush easier.
5. Proxy brushes are tiny toothbrushes that can be used when there is too much space between the teeth.

Patient Safety

1. Patients with a history of seizure disorders are at risk for broken teeth, lacerations of the tongue, cheeks, and lips, as well as aspiration of tooth or crown materials.
2. Adults with neurologic disabilities are at risk for poor dental health due to 1) impaired cognition, 2) impaired hand strength and control, 3) poor oral hygiene, 4) lack of access to appropriate dental care, and 5) side effects of medications. Poor dental care can have a significant impact on the nutritional, communicative, emotional, as well as dental well-being of the person afflicted.

Patient Education

- See dentist/hygienist every 3–6 months.
- Brush, floss, and use waterpik twice per day.
- Avoid caries-inducing foods like sticky candy, sugar drinks or energy drinks
- Use saliva substitute for a dry and burning mouth.
- Keep mouth hydrated—drink about 2 liters of water per day
- Prevent tooth fracture—don't chew bones or popcorn kernels
- Any small cavity is to be taken care of quickly before it becomes larger
- Avoid excessive alcohol consumption since it can cause dry mouth and infections
- Avoid smoking since it can cause dry mouth and slow down healing rate, causing gum disease to worsen and oral cancer

- Plan long visits to the dentist, so that much can be done at a slow and careful pace, explaining home care techniques until they are understood by patient and/or caregiver
- Remove dentures daily at night and cleanse well
- Do not sleep with dentures
- Cuts and fissures of the mouth should be taken care of promptly before an infection can occur

REFERENCES

1. Lancashire P, Janzen J, Zach GA, Addy M. The oral hygiene and gingival health of paraplegic inpatients—a cross-sectional survey. J Clin Periodontol 1997; 24(3):198–200.
2. Fiske J, Griffiths J, Thompson S. Multiple sclerosis and oral care. Dent Update 2002; 29(6):273–283.
3. Talbot A, Brady M, Furlanetto DL, Frenkel H, Williams BO. Oral care and stroke units. Gerontology 2005; 22(2):77–83.
4. Stiefel DJ, Truelove EL, Persson RS, Chin MM, Mandel LS. A comparison of oral health in spinal cord injury and other disability groups. Spec 1993; 13(6):229–235.
5. Zasler ND, Devany CW, Jarman AL, Friedman R, Dinius A. Oral hygiene following traumatic brain injury: a programme to promote dental health. Brain 1993; 7(4):339–345.
6. www.colgate.com
7. www.ada.org

6 Diabetes Mellitus and Lipid Disorders

Marinella Defre Galea

Diabetes is becoming more common in the United States. According to the Centers for Disease Control and Prevention (CDC), from 1980 through 2005 the number of Americans with diabetes increased from 5.6 to 15.8 million. Regardless of race/ethnicity and sex, prevalence tended to be highest among persons aged 65 years or older. Hyperlipidemia is a major risk factor for heart disease, the leading cause of death in the United States. About 17% of adult Americans have high blood cholesterol, defined as 240 mg/dL or more total cholesterol.

The prevalence of diabetes in spinal cord injury (SCI) has been reported as high as 19% compared to 7% in the general population (1). Other studies have reported rates between 13 and 22%. Veterans with SCI between the ages of 45 and 59 years have a higher prevalence of diabetes compared to able-bodied veterans of similar age. One fourth of the persons with an SCI and diabetes reported that diabetes affected their eyes or that they had retinopathy (25%), and 41% had foot sores that took more than 4 weeks to heal.

Individuals with SCI have been shown to have elevated low-density lipoprotein (LDL) cholesterol and depressed high-density lipoprotein (HDL) cholesterol. Studies have shown that approximately 24–40% of SCI persons have HDL <35 mg/dL compared to 10% of the general U.S. population, while approximately 25% of SCI persons have elevated LDL.

Diabetes and hyperlipidemia can also occur in adults with other neurologic disabilities, such as stroke, multiple sclerosis, and severe traumatic brain injury, possibly due to a more sedentary lifestyle that can lead to obesity and glucose intolerance. Insulin resistance and glucose intolerance are highly prevalent after stroke (27%), contributing to worsening cardiovascular disease risk and a predisposition to recurrent stroke. The metabolic syndrome has also been associated with an increased risk of prevalent stroke. In selected population with genetic inheritance of multiple sclerosis, an increased prevalence of type I diabetes mellitus has been reported, but these findings cannot be extended to the general multiple sclerosis population. These patients remain at increased risk to develop obesity, insulin resistance, glucose intolerance, and hyperlipidemia as consequence of a sedentary lifestyle.

Obesity, glucose intolerance, hypertension, and dyslipidemia have been shown to increase the risk of developing heart disease. The clustering of these cardiovascular disease risk factors has been known alternatively as the metabolic syndrome, or insulin resistance syndrome or syndrome X, and the term metabolic syndrome has been adopted by various organizations, such as the World Health Organization (WHO) (2) and the Third Report of the National Cholesterol Education Program's Adult Treatment Panel (ATP III) (3).

Of the various risk factors mentioned above, five essential components, according to ATP III, comprise the metabolic syndrome and are defined by the following parameters:

- Central obesity: waist circumference >40 inches in males and >35 inches in females and/or body mass index (BMI) >25 kg/m²
- Glucose intolerance: fasting glucose level of >100 mg/dl or a 120-minute post–glucose challenge value of 140–200 mg/dl.
- Blood pressure >130/85 mmHg
- Atherogenic dyslipidemia: HDL cholesterol <40 mg/dl for men and <50 mg/dl for women
- Triglyceride levels >150 mg/dl

WHO takes a different view toward defining the metabolic syndrome, using the following parameters:

- Diabetes, insulin fasting glucose (IFG), insulin glucose tolerance (IGT), or insulin resistance (assessed by clamp studies) and at least two of the following criteria:
  o Waist-to-hip ratio >0.90 in men or >0.85 in women
  o Serum triglycerides >1.7 mmol/l or HDL cholesterol <0.9 mmol/l in men and <1.0 mmol/l in women
  o Blood pressure >140/90 mmHg
  o Urinary albumin excretion rate >20 μg/min or albumin-to-creatinine ratio >30 mg/g

The term preferred by the American Diabetes Association for the clustering of cardiovascular disease risk factors is cardiometabolic risk (Figure 6.1) (4).

ANATOMY AND PHYSIOLOGY

Spinal Cord Injury

The mechanism of carbohydrate and lipids disorders (Figure 6.2) in SCI persons can be explained as follows:

- Denervation of skeletal muscle, which can lead to insulin resistance
- Inactivity, which leads to body compositional changes including decreased skeletal muscle with a relative increase in adiposity

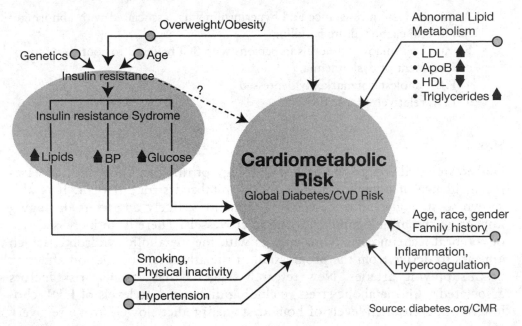

Figure 6.1. Factors contributing to cardiometabolic risk.

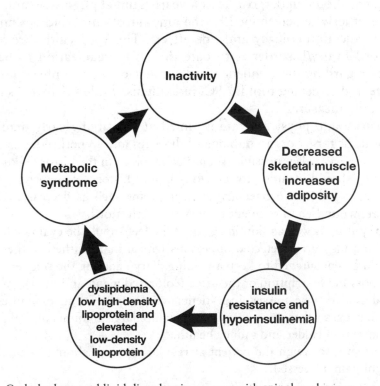

Figure 6.2. Carbohydrate and lipid disorders in persons with spinal cord injury.

- A state of insulin resistance and hyperinsulinemia, associated with abnormalities in oral carbohydrate handling
- Elevated plasma insulin levels in persons with SCI believed to contribute to the development of dyslipidemia
  - HDL cholesterol markedly depressed
  - LDL relatively elevated

Stroke

Diabetes contributes to the pathophysiology of this condition and increases the incidence of complications in the hospitalized stroke patient. It is also shown to strongly influence cognitive functions, likely due to its damaging impact on the brain's capillaries and microvessels. There is an increased risk of cerebral ischemic events in patients with the metabolic syndrome, which appears to derive from the progression of the atherosclerotic lesion affecting brain-supplying arteries. New research suggests that vascular risk factors associated with metabolic stress, including diabetes, low levels of HDL cholesterol, and elevated levels of homocysteine, predict slower stroke recovery (5).

PATIENT ASSESSMENT

Every patient should undergo at least a yearly annual physical exam; frequency should be otherwise determined by the amount of comorbidities and need to monitor medication efficacy and side effects. The VA HealthCare System for Spinal Cord Injury/Disorder is to date the only organization to have issued guidelines regarding the frequency and content of routine physical exam as a preventive and screening tool for SCI individuals. Table 6.1 reviews preventive and screening measures.

The history and physical exam is aimed at identifying early manifestation, progression, or target organ damage of diabetes and hyperlipidemia.

- The caregiver, when possible, should be involved in the history taking process.
- History should include any previous family history of diabetes or hyperlipidemia as well as uncover atypical symptoms such as decreased vision, skin rashes, wounds, and frequent urinary tract infections.
- Pedal pulses as well as skin integrity of the feet should be evaluated.
- Polyuria may go undetected in persons with urinary catheters; therefore, they should be encouraged to keep a voiding diary detailing the frequency, amount, and possibly description of the urine (color, sediment, and odor).
- Polidypsia can be missed in patients who believe in an old misconception, which suggests that persons with SCI require large amounts of oral fluid intake to maintain bladder and kidney health.
- An attempt to weigh the patient at regular intervals should be made and any weight gain addressed.

Table 6.1

Preventive and Screening Measures

The following tests should be repeated at least yearly or more often when noted:
1. Fasting lipid profile
2. Hepatic (alanine aminotransferase [ALT/SGPT], aspartate aminotransferase [AST/SGOT], serum albumin, alkaline phosphatase, total protein, total bilirubin) and renal (serum albumin, calcium, carbon dioxide, chloride, creatinine, glucose, phosphorus, potassium, sodium) function panels
3. Assessment of renal function: acceptable methods include renal ultrasound or computed tomography and 24-hour urine collection for volume, creatinine, microalbumin, and/or protein
4. Weight and calculated BMI at every office visit and yearly, to be adjusted for SCI (minus 10% of ideal body weight)
5. Nutrition consults for patients and caregivers to provide education, reinforcement, and weight management

Patients with a diagnosis of DM also require:
1. Annual retinal exam to detect early diabetic retinopathy
2. HbA1C every 6 months in stable patients, more often if noncompliance or complications ensue
3. Foot exam with monofilament testing in patients with sensation in lower extremities
4. Podiatric evaluation and evaluation for appropriate footwear
5. Rehab evaluation to assess for possible functional decline and need for assistive devices

Note: Persons with SCI and multiple sclerosis may not manifest the typical symptoms of diabetes including diaphoresis and tachycardia. Physical and financial barriers affect preventive health care and often the patients seek medical attention only when complication of diabetes ensue (diabetic retinopathy, renal insufficiency, coronary artery disease). Stroke and traumatic brain injury patients may not be able to complain of symptoms of hyper- or hypoglycemia depending on the level of neurologic impairment.

Diagnostic Tests

Diabetes

- Plasma glucose is 126 mg/dl or greater after an overnight fast.
- Symptoms of diabetes exist with a plasma glucose of 200 mg/dl or greater.
- The oral glucose tolerance test (OGTT) shows a plasma glucose of ≥200 mg/dl at 2 hours after a 75 g glucose load. This test should be performed in all SCI persons who do not have a diagnosis of diabetes mellitus at least once and later as the time of the injury/disability increases.

The diagnosis of IFG is established by:
- Fasting plasma glucose between 100 and 125 mg/dl
- OGGT values between 140 and 199 mg/dl

HbA1C:
- Provides an integrated measure of blood glucose profile over the preceding 2–3 months; should be obtained every 3 months or at least twice a year in a well-controlled patient
- Normal HbA1C levels in population studies 4–6% using the Diabetes Control Complication Trial assay

Hyperlipidemia

According to the National Cholesterol Education Program Adult Treatment Panel III Guidelines (6), in all adults aged 20 years or older, a fasting lipo-protein profile (total cholesterol, LDL cholesterol, HDL cholesterol, and trig-lycerides) should be obtained once every 5 years. If the testing opportunity is nonfasting, only the values for total cholesterol and HDL cholesterol will be usable. In such a case, if total cholesterol is 200 mg/dL or HDL is <40 mg/dL, a follow-up lipoprotein profile is needed for appropriate management based on LDL.

Major risk factors that modify low density lipoprotein cholesterol goals are:
- Cigarette smoking
- Hypertension (blood pressure ≥140/90 mmHg or on antihypertensive medications)
- Family history of premature cardiac heart disease (CHD). CHD in male first-degree relative <55 years; CHD in female first degree relative <65 years
- Low HDL cholesterol (<40 mg/dL)
- Age: men ≥45 years, women ≥55 years
- CAD
- Coronary heart disease equivalent
  - Carotid artery disease
  - Peripheral vascular disease
  - Abdominal aortic aneurysm
  - Estimated 10-year risk of CAD is performed in patients with two or more risk factors using Framingham score tables (7)
  - Very high risk (LDL < 60) is defined as established vascular disease and additional conditions, including
    - multiple risk factors (especially diabetes)
    - severe and poorly controlled risk factors
    - metabolic syndrome
    - acute coronary syndrome

TREATMENT

Diabetes

Lifestyle Interventions

The major environmental factors that increase the risk of type 2 diabetes are overnutrition and a sedentary lifestyle, with consequent overweight and obesity.

While there is still active debate regarding the most beneficial types of diet and exercise, weight loss almost always improves glycemic levels. In addition to the beneficial effects of weight loss on glycemia, weight loss and exercise improve coincident CVD risk factors, such as blood pressure and atherogenic lipid profiles. Evidence shows that the long-term success of lifestyle programs to maintain glycemic goals in patients with type 2 diabetes is limited. The vast majority of patients will require the addition of medications over the course of their diabetes.

Pharmacological

In this section the major classes of antihyperglycemic medications, their mode of action, safety profile, side effects, and complications will be described. This description does not intend to be exhaustive; moreover, the recent controversy on the use of some of these medications (see Rosiglitazone and ACCORD trial with increased number of deaths) calls for more clinical trials to study the effects of these drugs in large populations, especially the elderly and patients with multiple comorbidities and target organ damage.

The choice of specific antihyperglycemic agent depends on their effectiveness in lowering glucose and on the adjunctive effects that may reduce long-term complications, safety profiles, tolerability, and expense (8).

Metformin

- Is the only biguanide available in most of the world.
- Decreases hepatic glucose output and lowers fasting glycemia.
- As a monotherapy can lower HgA1C by ~1.5 percentage points.
- Prior to initiation of therapy a renal function panel (creatinine, blood urea nitrogen [BUN], potassium, phosphorus, carbon dioxide) must be checked. A serum creatinine ≥ 1.5 mg/dl in men and ≥ 1.4 mg/dl in women or a glomerular filtration rate <70 mL/min are contraindication to use.
- Metformin should be avoided or discontinued in cardiogenic or septic shock, congestive heart failure, liver disease, pulmonary insufficiency, and hypoxia.
- Metformin should be discontinued at the time of the radiographic contrast procedure and not restarted for 48 hours.
- Starting dose: 500 mg po daily, increased every 4 weeks by 500 mg up to 1000 mg tid.
- It is generally well tolerated, with the most common adverse effects being gastrointestinal. Lactic acidosis has an incidence of 3 per 100,000 patient-years. Risk factors include renal dysfunction, hypovolemia, tissue hypoxia, infection, alcoholism, and cardiopulmonary disease.
- It is contraindicated when serum creatinine level >1.5.
- As monotherapy usually not accompanied by hypoglycemia and has been safely used.
- Major nonglycemic effect of metformin is either weight stability or modest weight loss.

Sulfonylureas

- Sulfonylureas lower glycemia by enhancing insulin secretion.
- They can lower HgA1C by ~1.5 percentage points.
- These agents should always be taken 30–60 minutes before food and should never be administered to fasting patients.
- The initial dose of glyburide is 2.5 mg po daily. It can be increased in increments of 2.5–5mg every 4–6 weeks to a maximum dose of 20 mg bid.
- Major adverse side effects—severe hypoglycemia, characterized by need for assistance, coma, or seizure—are infrequent. These episodes are more frequent in the elderly and in patients with impaired renal function.
- Weight gain of ~2 kg is common with the initiation of sulfonylurea therapy.

Glinides

- Similar to the sulfonylureas, the glinides stimulate insulin secretion, although they bind to a different site within the sulfonylurea receptor.
- They have shorter circulating half-life than the sulfonylureas and must be administered more frequently.
- Of the two glinides currently available in the United States, repaglinide is almost as effective, decreasing A1C by 1.5 percentage points. Nateglinide is somewhat less effective in lowering A1C than repaglinide when used as monotherapy or in combination therapy.
- Repaglinide initial dose is 1 mg daily, can be incremented by 1–2 mg every 4–6 weeks to a maximum of 4 mg qid or 8 mg bid.
- The glinides have a similar risk for weight gain as the sulfonylureas, but hypoglycemia may be less frequent.

Glucosidase Inhibitors

- Glucosidase inhibitors reduce the rate of digestion of polysaccharides in the proximal small intestine, primarily lowering postprandial glucose levels without causing hypoglycemia.
- They are less effective in lowering glycemia than metformin or the sulfonylureas, reducing HgA1C by 0.5–0.8 percentage points.
- The initial dose of acarbose is 25 mg tid, which can be gradually titrated in increments of 25–50 mg to a maximum dose of 30 mg.
- Since carbohydrate is absorbed more distally, malabsorption and weight loss do not occur; however, increased delivery of carbohydrate to the colon commonly results in increased gas production and gastrointestinal symptoms.

Thiazolidinediones

- Thiazolidinediones increase the sensitivity of muscle, fat, and liver to endogenous and exogenous insulin ("insulin sensitizers").
- When used as monotherapy, there is a 0.5–1.4% decrease in HgA1C.
- The use of these drugs should be monitored frequently, at least during the first 12 months of therapy (4-week intervals) and their effect revaluated at each visit; significant side effects include congestive heart failure and hepatotoxicity.

- The initial dose of Rosiglitazone is 4 mg po daily, which can be advanced to 8 mg po daily after 12 weeks if glycemic control is inadequate.
- There is a potential drug interaction with Phenobarbital, Rifampin, Amiodarone, and Fluconazole.

Insulin
- Insulin is the most effective diabetes medication for lowering glycemia.
- It is recommended for patients a) in whom oral agents have failed to sustain glycemic control, b) in diabetic ketoacidosis, c) in nonketotic hyperosmolar crisis, and d) newly diagnosed with severe hyperglycemia.
- Insulin is also used in pregnancy when oral agents are contraindicated.
- When used in adequate doses, it can decrease any level of elevated HgA1C to, or close to, the therapeutic goal.
- The success of insulin therapy depends on the use of sufficient doses (0.6 to >1.0 Units/kg of body weight per day) to achieve normoglycemia.
- Although initial therapy is aimed at increasing basal insulin supply (usually with intermediate- or long-acting insulin), patients may also require prandial therapy with short- or rapid-acting insulins as well.
- Insulin therapy has beneficial effects on triglyceride and HDL cholesterol levels, but it can be associated with weight gain of ~2–4 kg.
- Severe hypoglycemic episodes (defined as requiring help from another person to treat) occur at a rate of 1–3 per 100 patient-years.
- Insulin analogs with longer, nonpeaking profiles may decrease the risk of hypoglycemia compared with NPH, and analogs with very short durations of action may reduce the risk of hypoglycemia compared with regular insulin. Inhaled insulin was approved in the United States in 2006 for the treatment of type 2 diabetes. More clinical studies are needed to evaluate its role as monotherapy.

Glucagonlike Peptide 1 Agonists
- Exenatide is a naturally occurring glucagonlike peptide produced by the L-cells of the small intestine, which stimulates insulin secretion.
- It is administered twice per day by subcutaneous injection.
- It appears to lower Hg A1C by 0.5–1 percentage points, mainly by lowering postprandial blood glucose levels.
- Exenatide also suppresses glucagon secretion and slows gastric motility.
- Exenatide is not associated with hypoglycemia but has a relatively high frequency of gastrointestinal side effects, with 30–45% of treated patients experiencing one or more episodes of nausea, vomiting, or diarrhea.

Amylin Agonists
- Pramlintide is a synthetic analog of the β-cell hormone amylin and inhibits glucagon production, decreasing postprandial glucose excursions.
- It is approved for use in the United States only as adjunctive therapy with insulin and is injected before meals.
- It is administered subcutaneously before meals and slows gastric emptying.

- HgA1C has been decreased by 0.5–0.7 percentage points.
- Major clinical side effects of this drug are gastrointestinal in nature, mostly nausea. Weight loss associated with this medication is ~1–1.5 kg over 6 months.

Suggested Algorithm to Initiate Therapy

In the treatment of diabetes it is important to define the targets of effective glucose management. Typically the values are:

1. Fasting and preprandial plasma or capillary glucose levels between 70 and 130 mg/dl (3.89 and 7.22 mmol/l)
2. Postprandial levels (usually measured 90–120 minutes after a meal) less than 180 mg/dl (10 mmol/l)
3. HbA1C values less than 7.3

Patients should be taught how to self-monitor blood glucose since this is an important element in adjusting or adding new interventions and, in particular, in titrating insulin doses. Figure 6.3 outlines a suggested algorithm for the treatment of diabetes.

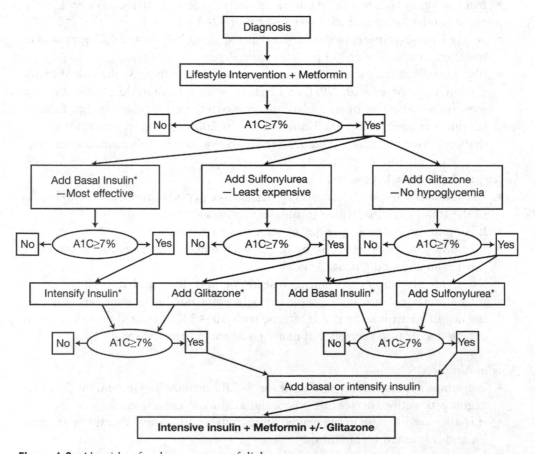

Figure 6.3. Algorithm for the treatment of diabetes.

1. Lifestyle interventions should be initiated as the first step in treating new-onset type 2 diabetes. In most individuals lifestyle interventions fail to achieve or maintain metabolic goals, either because of failure to lose weight, weight regain, progressive disease, or a combination of factors.

2. Metformin therapy should then be initiated, in the absence of specific contra-indications (active congestive heart failure). Treatment should be titrated to its maximally effective dose over 1–2 months, as tolerated.

3. A second medication should be added within 2–3 months of the initiation of therapy or at any time when A1C goal is not achieved. There is no strong consensus regarding the second medication added after metformin other than to choose among insulin, a sulfonylurea, or a TZD. A1C level will determine in part which agent is selected next, with consideration given to the more effective glycemia-lowering agent, insulin, for patients with A1C >8.5% or with symptoms secondary to hyperglycemia. Insulin can be initiated with a basal (intermediate- or long-acting) insulin. The relative increased cost of the newer agents that are only available as brand medications must be balanced against their relative benefits.

4. If lifestyle modification, metformin, and a second medication do not result in goal glycemia, the next step should be to start, or intensify, insulin therapy. When A1C is close to goal, addition of a third oral agent could be considered; however, this approach is relatively more costly and potentially not as effective in lowering glycemia compared with adding or intensifying insulin. Intensification of insulin therapy usually consists of additional injections that might include a short- or rapid-acting insulin given before selected meals to reduce postprandial glucose excursions. Insulin secretagogues (sulfonylurea or glinides) should be discontinued, or tapered and then discontinued, since they are not considered synergistic with administered insulin.

Hyperlipidemia

Nonpharmacological

It is important to educate patients on sound principles of nutrition to reduce their risk for hyperlipidemia, and a referral to a nutritionist is recommended. Basic principles of nutrition in adults with neurologic disabilities are also covered elsewhere in the text.

Pharmacological

Although no prospective clinical trials are available to justify the early consideration of lipid-lowering therapy in SCI persons, they remain at higher risk to develop the metabolic syndrome, early atherosclerosis, and asymptomatic heart disease. The threshold for initiation of therapy should be low, and a specific effort should be made to identify early risk factors such as prediabetes, obesity, and smoking.

It is also helpful to identify the goal for the treatment of hyperlipidemia prior to the initiation of medications and to also monitor lipid profiles with periodic blood tests. Table 6.2 provides an outline of the various risk categories, appropriate LDL goals, and guidance on the initiation of therapy. In very high-risk patients an LDL goal of <70 mg/dl should be considered.

The benefits of the various drug classes used to treat hyperlipidemia, major side effects, contraindications, and clinical trial results are outlined in Table 6.3.

1. HMG-CoA reductase inhibitors (statins) increase hepatic LDL receptor activity and accelerated clearance of circulating LDL, resulting in a dose-dependent reduction in plasma LDL-C. Statins also exert a number of vasculo-protective actions that include improvement of endothelial function, increased nitric oxide (NO) bioavailability, antioxidant properties, stabilization of atherosclerotic plaques, regulation of progenitor cells, inhibition of inflammatory responses and immunomodulatory actions. They appear to confer neuroprotection, prevent strokes, reduce dementia and may have a clinical impact in a number of non-vascular conditions including multiple sclerosis.

   • Simvastatin 5–10 mg initial dose can be incremented 5–10 mg every 4–12 weeks to achieve desired LDL goal

Side effects include dyspepsia, headaches, fatigue, hepatitis, and muscle or joint pains. Severe myopathy and rhabdomyolysis can occur rarely. The risk of myopathy is increased by the presence of renal insufficiency and by coadministration of drugs that interfere with the metabolism of HMG-CoA reductase.

   • Muscle symptoms: The plasma creatine phosphokinase (CPK) level should be obtained to document the myopathy, but serum CPK levels do not need to be monitored on a routine basis as an elevated CPK in the absence of symptoms does not predict the development of myopathy and does not necessarily suggest the need for discontinuing the drug.

   • Hepatitis: Liver transaminases (ALT and AST) should be checked before starting therapy, at 8 weeks, and then every 6 months. Substantial (>3 × upper limit of normal) elevation in transaminases is relatively rare, and mild to moderate (1 to 3 × normal). In the absence of symptoms, elevation in transaminases does not mandate discontinuation of therapy.

Table 6.2

LDL Goals and Initiation of Therapy

Risk category	LDL goal	LDL level at which to initiate therapeutic lifestyle changes	LDL level at which to consider drug therapy
CHD and CHD risk equivalent, DM	<100 mg/dl	≥ 100 mg/dl	≥130 mg/dl (100–129 mg/dl: drug optional)
2+ risk factors (10-yr risk ≤ 20%)	<130 mg/dl	≥ 130 mg /dl	<160
0–1 risk factor	<160 mg/dl	≥ 160 mg/dl	≥ 190 mg/dl (160–189 mg/dl: LDL-lowering drug optional)

Table 6.3

Lipid-Lowering Medications

Drug class	Lipid effect	Side effects	Contraindications	Clinical trial results
HMG-CoA 5 reductase inhibitor Statins	LDL ↓ 18–55% HDL ↑ 5–15% TG ↓ 7–30%	Myopathy Increased liver enzymes	Absolute: • Active or chronic liver disease Relative: • Concomitant use of certain drugs	Reduced major coronary events, CHD deaths, need for coronary procedures, stroke, and total mortality
Bile acid sequestrants	LDL ↓ 15–30% HDL ↑ 3–5% TG no change or increase	Gastrointestinal distress Constipation Decreased absorption of other drugs	Absolute: • Dysbetalipoproteinemia • TG > 400 mg/dl Relative: • TG >200 mg/dl	Reduced major coronary events and CHD deaths
Nicotinic acid	LDL ↓ 5–25% HDL ↑ 15–35% TG ↓ 20–50%	Flushing Hyperglycemia Hyperuricemia (or gout) Upper GI distress Hepatotoxicity	Absolute: • Chronic liver disease • Severe gout Relative: • Diabetes • Hyperuricemia • Peptic ulcer disease	Reduced major coronary events, and possibly total mortality
Fibric acids	LDL ↓ 5–20% (may be increased in patients with high TG) HDL ↑ 0–20% TG ↓ 20–50%	Dyspepsia Gallstones Miopathy	Absolute: • Severe renal disease • Severe hepatic disease	Reduced major coronary events

2. Bile acid sequestrants bind bile acids in the intestine and promote their excretion in the stool. In order to maintain an adequate bile acid pool, the liver diverts cholesterol to bile acid synthesis. The decreased hepatic intracellular cholesterol content upregulates the LDL receptor and enhances LDL clearance from the plasma. Cholestyramine, colestipol, and colesevelam can increase plasma triglycerides. Therefore, patients with hypertriglyceridemia should not be treated with bile acid–binding resins.
   - Cholestyramine and colestipol are insoluble resins that must be mixed with liquids.
   - Colestipol is also available in large tablets, but multiple tablets must be taken to achieve significant lowering of plasma LDL cholesterol levels.
   - Colesevelam is a new bile acid sequestrant that comes in smaller tablets, and fewer tablets per day are required.

Side effects of resins are gastrointestinal with bloating and constipation. Bile acid sequestrants can also interfere with the absorption of other drugs such as digoxin and warfarin.

3. Nicotinic acid, or niacin, is a B-complex vitamin that reduces plasma triglyceride and LDL cholesterol levels and raises the plasma HDL cholesterol.
   - Niacin starting dose is 100 mg po tid, must be taken with meals to delay absorption. The dose of niacin should be increased every 4–7 days by 100 mg until a dose of 500 mg tid is obtained. After 1 month on this dose, lipids and pertinent chemistries (glucose, uric acid, hepatic transaminases) should be measured. The dose can be further increased as needed up to a total dose of 6 g/day.
   - Niacin is the drug of choice to selectively elevate HDL in patients with low levels (<60 mg/dl).

Side effects: The most frequent side effect is cutaneous flushing, but this improves with continued administration. In many patients, taking an aspirin 30 min prior to the niacin prevents flushing.

4. Fibric acid derivatives, or fibrates, are agonists of PPAR, a nuclear receptor involved in the regulation of carbohydrate and lipid metabolism. They are the most effective drugs available for reducing triglyceride levels, and they also raise HDL cholesterol levels.
   - Gemfibrozil 600 mg po bid starting dose is also the therapeutic dose. Lipids and hepatic transaminases should be checked in 4 weeks, then every 12 weeks or if any sign or symptoms of muscle pain, cramps, or jaundice.
   - Fibrates are the drug class of choice in patients with severe hypertriglyceridemia and are a reasonable consideration in patients with moderate hypertriglyceridemia.
   - Fibrates can potentiate the effect of warfarin and some oral hypoglycemic agents; the anticoagulation status and plasma glucose levels should be monitored every 4–12 weeks in patients on these agents.

Side effects: The most common side effect is dyspepsia. Myopathy and hepatitis occur rarely in the absence of other lipid-lowering agents (statin). Fibrates promote cholesterol secretion into bile and are associated with an increased risk of gallstones.

5. Fish oil supplements can be used in combination with fibrates, niacin, or statins to treat hypertriglyceridemia.
   - Fish oils starting dose is 500–1000 mg bid, which can be titrated according to desired level of triglyceride up to 3 g total per day.

Side effects: The large numbers of capsules required for a therapeutic effect, the associated dyspepsia, and fishy aftertaste have limited the clinical use of these agents. Although fish oil administration is associated with a prolongation in the bleeding time, no increase in bleeding has been seen in clinical trials.

Patient Safety

Much of the patient safety concerns in the treatment of diabetes have to do with minimizing the risks for side effects of commonly used medications, including the risk of hypoglycemia. Some specific examples include:

1. Increased risk of severe hypoglycemia with sulfonylureas (i.e., glyburide), especially in elderly patients and patients with impaired renal function.
2. Fluid retention and congestive heart failure in patients receiving thiazolidinediones (specifically rosiglitazone), which can be especially problematic in patients with dependent edema and restrictive lung disease.
3. Metformin requires monitoring of renal function; always consider decreasing dose or hold if patient develops urinary tract infection, or stop the day prior to any test that require requires intravenous contrast.
4. Insulin therapy presents problems related to self-administration: consider prefilled syringes.
5. Rehabilitation therapists need to be aware of the possible atypical manifestation of glucose abnormality, especially in SCI and stroke patients. Hypoglycemia during exercise is frequent and can manifest as generalized malaise and fatigue. The rapid evaluation and assessment of the patient may avoid dramatic consequences. Patients should be encouraged to bring glucose tablets with them to rapidly address hypoglycemia and avoid catastrophic consequences.

Patient safety concerns in hyperlipidemia are also mostly related to the side effects of commonly used medications. Some examples include:

1. Hepatitis, myopathy, and rhabdomyolysis have been associated with the use of HMG-CoA reductase inhibitors (statins). Caution should be used in prescribing them to patients with renal insufficiency. Liver function tests should also be performed prior to start of therapy, at 8 weeks, and then every 6 months.
2. Bile acid sequestrants can interfere with the absorption of drugs such as digoxin and warfarin.
3. Fibrates can potentiate the effect of warfarin and some oral hypoglycemic agents; therefore, close monitoring of INR and glucose levels in patients taking fibrates is recommended.

Patient Education

- Patients with diabetes should be educated about this disease and its potential adverse effect on other parts of the body (i.e., heart, eyes, nerves, peripheral circulation, etc.). They should be educated on the medications commonly used for the treatment of diabetes, including insulin administration (if indicated), dosages, common side effects, significant side effects, and strategies to minimize the risk of hypoglycemia.
- Diabetics should also be educated on the importance of periodic checkups (i.e., eye exams, foot exams) as well as strategies to minimize the risk of limb loss. Some of these strategies include:
  - Wear proper footwear (wide and high toe box) and socks.
  - Don't walk barefoot.
  - Check the foot daily for evidence of skin breakdown, ingrown toenails, or irritation (especially bottom of feet and in between toes).
- Patients with diabetes and/or hyperlipidemia should be educated on an appropriate diet for their condition. Referral to a nutritionist to customize this diet according to the patient's preferences and food availability is strongly recommended.

REFERENCES

1. Weaver FM, La Vela SL. Preventive care in spinal cord injuries and disoders: examples of research and implementation. Phys Med Rehabil Clin N Am 2007; 18:297–316.
2. Definition, Diagnosis, and Classification of Diabetes Mellitus and its Complications: Report of a WHO Consultation. Geneva: World Health Organization, 1999.
3. Grundy SM, Brewer HB, Jr., Cleeman JI, Smith SC, Jr., Lenfant C. Definition of metabolic syndrome: report of the National Heart, Lung, and Blood Institute/American Heart Association conference on scientific issues related to definition. Circulation 2004; 109: 433–438.
4. Kahn R, Buse J, Ferrannini E, Stern M. The metabolic syndrome: time for a critical appraisal: joint statement from the American Diabetes Association and the European Association for the Study of Diabetes. Diabetes Care 2005; 28:2289–2304.
5. Newman GC, Bang H, Hussain SI, Toole JF. Association of diabetes, homocysteine, and HDL with cognition and disability after stroke. Neurology 2007; 69:2054–2062.
6. Executive Summary of The Third Report of The National Cholesterol Education Program (NCEP) Expert Panel on Detection, Evaluation, and Treatment of High Blood Cholesterol In Adults (Adult Treatment Panel III). JAMA 2001; 285(19):2486–2489.
7. www.nhlbi.nih.gov/guidelines/cholesterol/risk
8. Nathan DM, Buse JB, Davidson MB, Heine RJ, Holman RR, Sherwin R, Zinman B. Management of hyperglycemia in type 2 diabetes: a consensus algorithm for the initiation and adjustment of therapy: a consensus statement from the American Diabetes Association and the European Association for the Study of Diabetes. Diabetes Care 2006; 29:1963–1972.

7 | Dysphagia

Uri S. Adler
Susan A. Laskoski
Maria D. McNish

The goal of all feeding is adequate and safe nutrition and hydration. This normally occurs by ingestion of food and liquid into the mouth, passing through the pharynx and esophagus and then into the stomach.

The simplest definition of dysphagia is difficulty moving food and liquid from the mouth to the stomach. A more expansive definition includes "all behavioral, sensory and preliminary motor acts in preparation for the swallow, including cognitive awareness of the upcoming eating situation, visual recognition of food, and of other physiologic responses to the smell and presence of food such as increase salivation" (1). This provides a picture of all considerations that should be taken into account when evaluating and treating patients with this disorder (8).

Dysphagia requires attention because of the risks associated with it. These include aspiration of material into the trachea and lungs, aspiration-induced pneumonia and/or pnuemonitis, airway obstruction, malnutrition, and dehydration. We also should be sensitive to the impact dysphagia may have on social interactions.

Ingestion of food and liquid is usually divided into three stages or phases: oral, pharyngeal, and esophageal. Keeping in mind that dysfunction in any of these phases is characterized as dysphagia, it is understandable that the diagnosis of dysphagia is a heterogeneous one and requires elucidation as to the exact nature of the specific problem(s). In this chapter we will discuss common neurologic and nonneurologic causes of dysphagia. It is important to understand a few key definitions regarding this diagnosis, anatomy and physiology, and normal and abnormal swallowing.

For the purposes of management and follow-up of dysphagia, it is important to separate the disorders in which dysphagia appears into two categories. In disorders that occur as result of a sudden injury, such as stroke, traumatic brain injury, and cervical spinal cord injury, one can expect gradual improvement over time with the proper therapies and intervention. In diseases that are progressive in nature, such as multiple sclerosis, dementia, and Parkinson's disease, partial recovery may occur, but the long-term prognosis and course of the disease should be anticipated (8).

When the word dysphagia is mentioned, stroke is probably the disorder that first comes to mind. Partly because of the broad definition of dysphagia (and the different ways to diagnose it) and partly because of the heterogeneity of strokes, the incidence ranges from 19 to 81%, but most likely it occurs in 60–70% of strokes. The incidence of pneumonia in those with dysphagia after stroke ranges from 7 to 28%. Recurrent strokes increase the incidence of dysphagia and often confound the treatment. Brainstem strokes typically have the highest incidence of dysphagia and often are the most challenging to treat (2).

In those serious enough to be admitted to inpatient rehabilitation with a traumatic brain injury, dysphagia occurs in 25–60%. Because of the nature of the disorder—behavioral as well as physical manifestations—the incidence can be as high as 90% in those with severe traumatic brain injury.

The incidence of dysphagia in adults with spinal cord injury ranges from 8 to 48%, with an overall incidence or approximately 16% in those suffering from traumatic cervical spinal injury. Higher risk for dysphagia occurs in those with tracheostomy tubes or with a history of anterior cervical surgical approach. The highest incidence occurs in those with both. Contributing to the dysphagia is the injury to the neck itself, postoperative cervical edema, and immobilization of the cervical structures by bracing or surgery and the mechanical interference of the tracheostomy tube (3).

The incidence of dysphagia in those with MS ranges from 34 to 43%. As in many with dysphagia, it is often not recognized by the patient or clinician until instrumental evaluations are performed.

Dysphagia occurs in about 50% of those with Parkinson's disease. It usually becomes clinically significant later in the disease course. Reevaluation is warranted as the disease progresses.

Studies show that some type of dysphagia occurs in 7–10% of those over 50 years of age. Difficulties in mealtime management are noticed in close to 90% of the elderly who are residents of homes for the elderly. It is not practical to screen this entire population, but healthcare providers should have a low threshold for formal evaluation if signs or symptoms of dysphagia are present.

Aspiration is a necessary but not sufficient condition to develop aspiration pneumonia. In the above-mentioned diseases, aspiration pneumonia is more prevalent in those dependent on others for feeding, with poor oral hygiene, and/or with reduced activity levels. The complexity of medical comorbidities also contributes greatly to the risk of aspiration pneumonia (4).

ANATOMY AND PHYSIOLOGY

The anatomic structures involved in deglutition (swallowing) include the oral cavity (mouth), larynx, pharynx, and esophagus.

The Oral Cavity (Mouth)

The oral cavity includes the lips, teeth, hard palate, soft palate, uvula, and mandible, floor of the mouth, tongue, and faucial arches. The musculature that forms the floor of the mouth includes the myelohyoid, geniohyoid, and anterior belly of the digastric muscles. The roof of the mouth is formed by the maxilla (hard palate), velum (soft palate), and uvula. The two lateral walls of the mouth are formed by the teeth and cheeks. The anterior wall of the mouth is formed by the lips and anterior teeth. The posterior border of the mouth is demarcated by the faucial arches. The tongue is comprised of an oral portion (tip, blade, front, center, and back) and a pharyngeal portion (begins at the circumvallate papillae and extends to the hyoid bone). Three large salivary glands are located in the oral cavity: the sublingual, parotid, and submandibular glands. Saliva has an important function in assisting deglutition by maintaining oral moisture and acting as a natural neutralizer of stomach acid (that may reflux into the esophagus).

The Larynx

The epiglottis is the uppermost area of the larynx. It deflects during the swallow to protect the airway. Between the epiglottis and the base of tongue is a space referred to as the vallecula. This is a potential site of pooling or residue. The opening of the larynx is referred to as the laryngeal vestibule. The false vocal folds are superior to the true vocal folds. They close off the larynx to protect against tracheal aspiration. The hyoid bone acts as an anchor for the tongue and suspends the larynx.

The Pharynx

There are three posterior constrictors that form the pharyngeal walls. The pyriform sinuses are potential sites for pooling and residue. They are side pockets in the pharynx, superolateral to the cricopharyngeus muscle. The cricopharyngeus muscle helps to form the upper esophageal sphincter (UES). It forms a valve that regulates entrance of food and liquids into the esophagus.

The Esophagus

The esophagus is approximately 25 cm long and is made up of striated and smooth muscles with the upper esophageal sphincter superiorly and the lower esophageal sphincter (LES) inferiorly.

Physiology of the Normal Swallow

The physiology of swallowing is complex but is generally divided into three stages (Table 7.1). While this is a basic classification, it is important to note

Table 7.1

Stages of Swallowing

Oral stage	The bolus is accepted into the mouth, manipulated into a bolus, and propelled (principally by the tongue) from the anterior to posterior part of the oral cavity.
Pharyngeal stage	The pharyngeal swallow is triggered, propelling the bolus through the pharynx.
Esophageal stage	The bolus passes through the UES. Esophageal peristalsis carries the bolus through the cervical and the thoracic esophagus and into the stomach via the LES.

that the stages are interconnected and that impairment in one stage may negatively impact the others.

Oral Stage

The oral preparatory stage begins when food enters the mouth. This stage is volitional and requires anticipation of the bolus. Sensory recognition of food and liquid approaching the mouth is the initial step of the swallow. Once the oral cavity is "aware" of the bolus, oral preparatory movements are initiated. During bolus preparation closure of the lips contains the bolus and builds up intraoral pressure. At this time, the nasal passageways open for respiration so the lips can remain closed during mastication (chewing).

Movement patterns in the oral cavity and oral transit time vary depending on the consistency of the bolus. The bolus is chewed, manipulated, and mixed with saliva before being propelled posteriorly by the tongue. Mastication occurs via a rotary lateral movement of the tongue and mandible. Peripheral feedback is important for coordinated mastication, positioning of the bolus on the teeth, and prevention of injury to the tongue during chewing. The act of swallowing transitions from volitional to reflexive once the bolus reaches the anterior faucial arches. The pharyngeal swallow is triggered when the bolus reaches the base of tongue and the angle of the ramus of the mandible.

Pharyngeal Stage

The pharyngeal stage of the swallow begins with the triggering of the pharyngeal swallow. This stage is involuntary and acts as the most critical stage in airway closure and protection of the trachea when eating. Sensory input from the posterior portion of the oral cavity is sent to the swallowing center in the brain. The velum is raised to close off the nasopharynx. This prevents nasal regurgitation during the swallow. The base of tongue retracts to prevent food from reentering the mouth. The larynx and hyoid are then pulled upward and forward to enlarge the pharynx and initiate opening of the cricopharyngeal muscle.

Closure of the airway occurs at three levels, which are, in chronological order: the true vocal folds (cords), the false vocal folds, and the epiglottis. Once the hyoid elevates, the epiglottis deflects to further protect the airway and divert the bolus past the larynx and pyriform sinuses.

Rhythmic, top to bottom, contraction of the pharyngeal constrictors facilitates clearance of any pharyngeal residue. The pharyngeal stage ends once the opening of the cricopharyngeal sphincter allows material to pass from the pharynx to the esophagus.

Esophageal Stage

The esophageal stage normally lasts between 3 and 20 seconds. After food and/or liquid pass the UES, it is propelled trough the esophagus via gravity and a series of peristaltic waves. It eventually reaches the LES, where it empties into the stomach.

Physiology of the Abnormal Swallow

A few essential terms need to be defined before describing the abnormal swallow: aspiration, penetration, and residue. Aspiration is the passage and entry of food or liquid below the level of the true vocal folds into the trachea. Penetration is the passage of food or liquid into the larynx but not through the true vocal folds. Residue is food or liquid that is inadequately cleared from the mouth or pharynx.

Table 7.2 lists some of the common abnormal findings in each of the stages of swallowing.

PATIENT ASSESSMENT

The evaluation of swallowing function is divided into two broad areas: 1) noninstrumental and 2) instrumental.

A noninstrumental clinical evaluation (NICE), also known as a bedside dysphagia evaluation, should be performed on any patient: 1) with suspicion or evidence of dysphagia, 2) who is not taking oral feeding (NPO), and 3) with a history of dysphagia. The evaluation is usually performed by a speech–language pathologist, but may also be performed by a physician or nurse experienced in dysphagia evaluation (8).

The NICE is used to: 1) gather pertinent medical information, 2) identify signs and symptoms of dysphagia, 3) provide recommendations for diet modifications, 4) assist with treatment planning, and 5) evaluate compensatory strategy use or potential.

Medical History

The clinical evaluation begins with a detailed medical history inclusive of current diagnoses, past medical history, and/or comorbidities. This can be obtained by reviewing the patient's medical chart and speaking to the patient and family members. Onset, duration, progression, and severity of the dysphagia should

Table 7.2

Stages of Dysphagia

Oral Stage Dysphagia
- Poor recognition of food/liquids
- Delayed onset of oral prep due to reduced coordination or sensation
- Inability to hold food/liquids in the mouth
- Spillage of foods/liquids into pockets of cheeks
- Inability to form a cohesive bolus
- Prolonged oral transit time
- Premature spillage to the pharynx
- Inability to transport bolus front to back of mouth
- Residue in the mouth after swallowing

Pharyngeal Stage Dysphagia
- Nasal leakage
- Penetration
- Aspiration
- Osteophytes (bony outgrowth from cervical vertebrae impacting swallow)
- Delayed trigger of the pharyngeal swallow
- Diffuse residue in the pharynx
- Residue in the vallecula
- Residue in the pyriform sinus
- Reduced laryngeal closure

Esophageal Stage Dysphagia
- GERD (gastroesophageal reflux disease)
- Reduced peristalsis
- Tracheoesophageal fistula
- Zenker's diverticulum
- UES/LES dysfunction
- Esophageal cancer

be identified. Important consideration should be given to the patient's general health, present diet, nutritional status, appetite, unexplained weight loss, and any changes in eating habits. History of a recent pneumonia may be indicative of aspiration. A list of the patient's current medications should be reviewed as certain drugs may interfere with swallowing (Table 7.3). The patient's subjective description and complaints of the swallowing problem should be obtained if possible. Areas of inquiry may include asking the patient the following questions:

Do you experience the feeling of food sticking in your throat?
What specifically happens when you try to swallow?
Do you cough?
Does this occur with any particular food or liquid consistency?

Complaints of reflux, heartburn, belching, or globus sensation (the feeling that something is stuck in your throat or chest) may be indicative of an esophageal problem. The patient interview can add valuable information in determining

Table 7.3

Common Medications and Their Effect on Swallowing

Effect	Medications
Xerostomia (reduced saliva production)	Anticholinergics
	Antihistamines
	Antipsychotics
	Opioids
	Diuretics
Sedation	Anticonvulsants
Weakness	Benzodiazepines
	Neuroleptics
	Opioids
Impaired esophageal motility	Anticholinergics
	Calcium channel blockers
	Theophylline

what specific components and stages of swallowing are involved. It is also important to keep in mind that patients may have little or no insight into their swallowing difficulties.

Esophageal cancer is a relatively rare form of cancer that can present with difficulty and/or painful swallowing, pain radiating to the chest and back, vomiting, and weight loss.

Physical Examination

An assessment of the patient's level of alertness and cognitive status is an integral part of the physical examination. Attention, comprehension, memory, awareness of deficits, and observed behavior provide important information regarding safety and ability to utilize compensatory swallowing strategies (9).

Common signs of dysphagia are described below and listed in Table 7.4.

Table 7.4

Signs of Dysphagia

- Drooling, decreased ability to manage secretions
- Oral leakage of food/liquids from the mouth
- Decreased ability to propel food/liquid from the mouth to the pharynx
- Pocketing of food in the cheek
- Coughing, choking or throat clearing before, during or after the swallow
- Sensation of food sticking in the throat
- "Wet" or "gurgled" vocal quality with saliva or after swallowing food/liquids
- Nasal regurgitation of food/liquids
- Dysphonia

Guidelines for the Assessment of Oral Anatomy and Function

1. Direct observation and assessment of the strength, mobility, coordination and sensation of the face, cheeks, lips, jaw, tongue, hard palate, soft palate as well as status of dentition should be performed.
2. Labial function: Lip closure is important for maintaining the bolus in the mouth and initiating the swallow. Note if there is a facial droop, drooling of saliva, or evidence of oral apraxia (difficulty with initiation of movements). Ask the patient to: 1) pucker and retract the lips into a smile and 2) close the mouth tightly, and produce bilabial sounds such as /Pa/ or /Ba/.
3. Jaw control: This can be assessed by asking the patient to open and close the jaw.
4. Lingual function: Limitation of tongue function may affect the ability to propel food or liquids from the mouth to the base of the tongue and pharynx for initiation of the swallow reflex. This can be assessed by asking the patient to extend, retract, lateralize, and elevate the tongue. Ask for sound production of /Ta/ for anterior function and /Ka/ for posterior function.
5. Soft palate (velar) symmetry and elevation: Velopharyngeal insufficiency can result in nasal regurgitation of food or liquid. This can be assessed by asking the patient to say and sustain /Ah/.
6. Sensitivity of the oral structures: Decreased sensitivity can cause lack of awareness of food or liquid in the mouth affecting the timing of oral movement and swallowing. This can be assessed by tactile stimulation.

Guidelines for the Assessment of Laryngeal Function

Changes in vocal quality during speaking can lead one to suspect dysphagia. A breathy or hoarse vocal quality may indicate decreased vocal fold closure, resulting in decreased airway protection during the swallow. A "wet" or "gurgled" vocal quality may be related to poor management of secretions and risk of aspiration due to fluid resting on the true vocal folds. Asking the patient to volitionally cough or clear his or her throat can provide information regarding the patient's ability to clear potentially aspirated material or expectorate material if needed. A weak or absent cough may indicate poor airway protection.

Respiratory Function

Observe for signs of labored breathing, shortness of breath, and lack of coordination between breathing and swallowing. Patients with a compromised respiratory status may fatigue easily, putting them at higher risk for aspiration. Use of a pulse oximeter can assist in evaluation of respiratory compromise in dysphagia.

Trials of Liquids and Solids

Based on the information gathered, the clinician decides if the patient is ready for oral trials. If so, further decisions such as consistencies to be used (e.g., thin liquids versus nectar thick), volumes to be given (e.g., teaspoon versus sips), and method of delivery (e.g., cup versus straw) should be made.

The decision to defer oral trials may be based on: 1) poor arousal, 2) decreased awareness of food in the mouth, 3) acute illness, 4) compromised respiratory status, 5) weak or absent throat clear and cough, and/or 6) poor oral function with decreased ability to manage ones own saliva. In some cases the patient may be referred directly for an instrumental examination or may receive dysphagia therapy prior to initiation of oral trials of food and liquids.

If deemed safe enough for oral trials, the clinician will provide foods and liquids of various consistencies and volumes (see next section for more detail). There are no hard and fast rules for determining which consistencies may be best tolerated by each individual patient.

The clinician should be alerted to any signs of dysphagia occurring with any particular consistency and/or volume. Patients are then placed on the least restrictive but safest diet.

Instrumental Assessments

Upon completion of the NICE, the patient with suspected or overt signs of dysphagia is referred for an instrumental assessment. Referral criteria for instrumental testing include: 1) exhibition of signs of a pharyngeal dysphagia, 2) history of silent aspiration, 3) history of pneumonia, 4) demonstration of potential for a diet upgrade, 5) NPO, 6) tracheostomy, and 7) degenerative medical conditions or medically complex history that suggests potential for pharyngeal dysphagia.

The most common instrumental assessments are the Videofluoroscopic Swallow Study (VFSS) and the Flexible Endoscopic Evaluation of Swallowing (FEES).

Videofluoroscopic Swallow Study
VFSS or modified barium swallow (MBS) is very frequently used and is considered by many to be the gold standard to view the oral, pharyngeal, and early esophageal stages of swallowing.

The VFSS is a real-time, radiographic study of swallowing performed by administering trials of liquids and foods of varying consistencies and volumes. The patient is usually seated in an upright position (90°). The oral cavity, pharynx, larynx, and esophagus can be examined in both the lateral and anterior/posterior (AP) planes. The VFSS allows identification of motility problems at all stages of swallowing and penetration and aspiration as they occur. It can also provide information concerning the "why" someone is aspirating and the underlying causes of the dysphagia. Compensatory strategies and postures can be introduced during the study to determine the safest and most efficient mode of swallowing.

The VFSS is a noninvasive procedure that most patients tolerate quite well. Patients are exposed to a minimal amount of radiation. The VFSS may not be indicated in patients who: 1) are not alert enough to participate, 2) cannot tolerate sitting for at least 10 minutes, and 3) are too critically ill to be moved to an x-ray room.

Flexible Endoscopic Examination of Swallowing

FEES is an endoscopic examination of the velopharynx, hypopharynx, pharynx, and larynx. Oral and esophageal phases of swallowing are not evaluated with this procedure. A narrow, flexible, fiberoptic tube is inserted through the nasal cavity and down to the pharynx. Here, the tip of the scope hangs just above the epiglottis so that the hypopharynx and larynx can be visualized. The endoscope is left in this position most of the time, but after each swallow it is lowered into the laryngeal vestibule so the vocal folds can be visualized and into the subglottic region to see if any material has been aspirated (foods and liquids are dyed blue or green for easier visualization). A variation of FEES has been developed called flexible endoscopic evaluation of swallowing with sensory testing (FEEST). FEEST adds further testing of pharyngeal sensation by blowing air through the endoscope onto pharyngeal structures and assessing the patient's response (for the remainder of the chapter, the term FEES will refer also to FEEST) (5,6).

This allows the structures and function of the larynx to be observed. The patient's ability to manage his own secretions can be observed. Tolerance of various food and liquid consistencies and volumes can be assessed via presentation with the scope in place. The FEES allows visualization of:
- Premature spillage of the bolus over the back of the tongue
- Residue in the vallecula or pyriform sinuses
- Delays in swallow initiation
- Timing of airway and velopharyngeal closure

The main advantage FEES has over VFSS is that it can assess sensation in the pharynx and larynx. As with the VFSS, compensatory strategies and postural changes can be observed with FEES. FEES may be more suitable for the patient who is too ill to be moved or where videofluoroscopy is not available.

A shortcoming of the FEES is the "whiteout phase." The moment the swallow is triggered the pharynx closes around the tube, obliterating the view during the swallow. We can view what happens immediately before and after the swallow but not during the swallow itself (unlike VFSS). In addition, FEES is more invasive than VFSS and may cause more discomfort, laryngospasm, vasovagal response, and/or epistaxis. Caution should be displayed in individuals with cardiac arrhythmias, recent respiratory distress, or bleeding disorders.

The two procedures yield similar but not identical information. Decisions on which test to use should be based on patient factors, availability of the test, and clinician comfort with the test.

TREATMENT

Treatment of dysphagia varies depending on the nature of the dysfunction. However, the goals are always to achieve the safest and most efficient swallowing while optimizing the nutrition and hydration of the patient (9).

Swallowing therapy may be compensatory and/or rehabilitative in nature. Compensatory techniques aim to reduce/prevent aspiration and/or pharyngeal pooling/residue (postural changes), whereas rehabilitative techniques aim to improve the swallow itself either indirectly (facilitating techniques/exercises) or directly (maneuvers).

Dysphagia treatment can be categorized into five main types. These are: 1) alterations in the consistency of the bolus, 2) limitations of the volumes of the bolus, 3) postural changes and maneuvers to help the swallow, 4) therapeutic modalities to rehabilitate the swallow, and 5) procedural and surgical intervention.

Alterations of Consistency

The most common management approach to dysphagia is to change diet consistencies. Decisions regarding the safest diet are based on the functional and structural impairments as observed at bedside or during instrumental evaluations. The dysphagia diet must meet the patient's individual needs depending on the nature of oropharyngeal impairment.

Patients with poor oral control and/or a delayed swallow may better tolerate a thicker consistency liquid (which is more cohesive) and a pureed solid (which requires less lingual and masticatory demands).

Solids

The National Dysphagia Diet (NDD), published in 2002 by the American Dietetic Association, aims to establish standardized terminology regarding diet consistencies. This terminology is briefly described in Table 7.5.

When deciding solid food diet consistencies, the decisions are generally based on the oral phase. The more impaired the oral phase, the lower level the diet. For example:

Table 7.5

Diet Consistency Terminology

NDD	Lay description	Definition	Example
I	Puree	Blended to a pudding-like consistency	Applesauce
II	Moist fine-chopped	Moist and minced to pieces no larger than ¼ inch	Egg salad
III	Bite size soft	Nearly regular textures with the exception of very hard, sticky, or crunchy	Moist breads, sliced meat
	Regular	All solid foods allowed	Lettuce, toast

A diet of pureed foods may be recommended for a patient with an oral stage dysphagia who demonstrates decreased lingual strength and control or who demonstrates excessive or incomplete chewing of harder solids.

Patients with a weakened cough or throat-clear may be better suited to swallow foods that are softer and of smaller size per bite.

Liquids

Liquid consistencies are classified as thin, nectar thick, and honey thick. Liquid consistencies can be altered by commercially available thickening agents. One can also purchase ready-to-serve thickened liquid products.

In general, the thicker the liquid, the easier it is to control during the swallow. This can help prevent premature spillage or dumping into the pharynx or larynx and may also prevent aspiration or penetration. A thicker liquid, however, can lead to increased pharyngeal residue, which is also a risk for aspiration. For example:

Patients with a delayed pharyngeal component may do better with a thickened liquid (which maintains cohesiveness) than with a thin liquid (which may prematurely spill into the pharynx).

Patients with severe pharyngeal residue may have a safer swallow with a thinner consistency.

It is important to factor into the decision-making process the fact that, along with tolerance of food and liquid consistencies, patients need to be monitored for adequate hydration and nutrition. Patients with diet alterations often drink and eat less than their requirements. Calorie and fluid intake monitoring is essential, and IV fluids and/or nutritional supplements are often needed.

To enhance oral intake and psychological well-being, the diet should retain as many "normal" characteristics as possible. It is therefore important to carefully decide which is the least restrictive but safest diet (taking into account risk for aspiration and caloric and hydration needs).

The decision to advance the diet is made based on clinical evaluation and/or repeat instrumental evaluation (VFSS or FEES).

Alteration in Volumes

Liquids can be administered by 3cc (approximately 1/2 teaspoon), 5 cc (1 teaspoon), small sips, or "normal" sips. Often, smaller volumes are safer for neurogenic dysphagia. However, there are those, such as those with oral apraxia, who perform better with larger volumes. Patient compliance and social acceptance is better with sips as opposed to spoonfuls.

For solids there are usually no volume restrictions per se.

Postural Changes, Strategies, and Maneuvers

Certain head/neck positions and alterations in the swallow do increase the safety of the swallow (Table 7.6).

Table 7.6

Head and Neck Positions and Alterations in Swallowing to Increase Patient Safety in Swallowing

A. Postural change	Used in	What it does	Tell the patient to
Chin tuck	Delayed swallow	Widens vallecula, narrows opening to airway	"Swallow with your chin flexed to your chest"
Head turn (paretic side)	1. Pyriform pooling/residue	Closes off weakened pyriform sinus, guides food down stronger side, and decreases pooling/residue	"Swallow with your head turned to the right or the left side"
	2. Unilateral vocal fold weakness	Helps vocal fold adduction	
Head Tilt (to stronger side)	Pharyngeal pooling/residue	Guides bolus away from weakened pharynx	"Touch your ear to your shoulder"

B. Strategy	Used in	What it does	Tell the patient to
Oral clear	Oral residue	Empties residue from mouth	"Clear food by using your tongue or finger"
Throat clear	Penetration and pharyngeal pooling or residue	Removes material that potentially can aspirate	"Clear your throat on purpose after you swallow"
Multiple swallows	Vallecula and pharyngeal pooling or residue	Clears residue	"Swallow more than once per bite or sip"

C. Altered swallow	Helps by		Tell the patient to
Controlled swallow	Coordinating swallow sequencing		"Gather the bolus together and swallow as one unit"
Effortful swallow	Clearing pharyngeal residue		"Swallow by squeezing the muscles in your throat as hard as you can"
Supra-glottic swallow	Increasing airway protection		"Hold your breath while you swallow and then immediately cough"
Mendelsohn's maneuver	Increasing swallow coordination and cricopharyngeal opening		"Swallow with your Adam's apple up as high as possible"

Rehabilitation of the Swallow

Swallowing Exercises

These include oral, pharyngeal, and laryngeal exercises to improve strength, range of motion, and coordination of the muscles for swallowing. Examples include:

1. Lips: Repetitions of puckering and smiling.
2. Tongue: Repetitively moving the tongue to each corner of the mouth and back.
3. Vocal folds: Pushing down on the arms of a chair while sustaining "ah."
4. Tactile and thermal stimulation: The clinician applies an iced dental mirror to the anterior faucial arches. This sensitizes the oral cavity to properly trigger and increase the speed of the swallow.

Neuromuscular Electrical Stimulation (VitalStim™)

Under the direction of a trained clinician, a small electrical current is transcutaneously delivered to the musculature involved in swallowing. This strengthens and improves coordination of the swallowing mechanism.

Deep Pharyngeal Neuromuscular Stimulation (DPNS)

This involves stimulation of three key reflex sites (tongue, soft palate, and pharynx) with frozen probes or swabs. It aims to improve base of tongue retraction and palatal elevation and improve pharyngeal peristaltic movement.

Procedural and Surgical Intervention

This is rarely indicated in patients with oropharyngeal dysphagia but may be effective for selected patients. It is usually pursued only after failure of more conservative measures has persisted for at least 6 months. The following is a description of a few procedures used for dysphagia:

1. Botulinum toxin injection for cricopharyngeal dysfunction: The cricopharyngeus muscle (major component of the UES) can be injected with botulinum toxin. This relaxes the muscle and eases the passage of food into the esophagus. This procedure should be considered when traditional and noninvasive therapies have failed, and there is definitive evidence of cricopharyngeal dysfunction by instrumental evaluation. Approximately 25 units can be used and can be injected percutaneously or endoscopically. Some reports require reinjection on an average of every 4 months, while others describe no need for reinjection at the 24-month reevaluation (7).
2. Cricopharyngeal myotomy: This can be performed in those with refractory cricopharyngeal dysfunction. This relaxes the UES and allows food and liquid to pass from the pharynx and into the esophagus.
3. Zenker's diverticulectomy: Aspiration can stem from a Zenker's diverticulum, an abnormal outpouching caused by weakening of the posterior pharyngeal or esophageal wall. Closing of the diverticulum can correct this problem.
4. Vocal fold augmentation: When paralyzed or weakened a vocal fold can be augmented with substances such as collagen or Teflon. This allows the nonparetic vocal fold's adduction to close off the airway during the swallow.

Nonoral Feeding

Even with all interventions mentioned above, there remain cases where patients are unable to maintain adequate and safe oral nutrition and hydration. In these cases alternative means of nutrition and hydration have to be considered. It should be explained to the patient and caregivers that these options:

- Are reversible when the ability to safely swallow returns
- Can be used as primary or supplemental means of nutrition
- Are often beneficial as a bridge to oral feeding (if the patient is not taking sufficient calories in, he or she may not be able to strengthen the swallowing musculature)

Due to the complications associated with them (sinusitis, aspiration, frequent dislodging, patient discomfort, etc.), nasogastric tubes should be inserted only as temporary measures. If long-term enteral feeds are needed, a gastrostomy tube should be inserted. Gastrostomy tubes are most commonly placed percutaneously and under local anesthesia (PEG).

REFERENCES

1. Leopold NA, Kagel MC. Prepharyngeal dysphagia in Parkinson's disease. Dysphagia 1996; 11(1):14–22.
2. Meng NH, Wang TG, Lien IN. Dysphagia in patients with brainstem stroke: incidence and outcome. Am J Phys Med Rehabil 2000; 79(2):170–175.
3. Kirshblum S, Johnston MV, Brown J, O'Connor KC, Jarosz P. Predictors of dysphagia after spinal cord injury. Arch Phys Med Rehabil 1999; 80(9):1101–1105.
4. Langmore SE, Terpenning MS, Schork A, et al. Predictors of aspiration pneumonia: how important is dysphagia. Dysphagia 1998; 13(2):69–81.
5. Langmore SE, Schatz K, Olsen N. Fiberoptic endoscopic examination of swallowing safety: a new procedure. Dysphagia 1988; 2(4):216–219.
6. Aviv JE, Kim T, Sacco RL, et al. FEESST: a new bedside endoscopic test of the motor and sensory components of swallowing. Ann Otol Rhinol Laryngol 1998; 107(5 Pt 1):378–387.
7. Masiero S, Briani C, Marchese-Ragona R, Giacometti P, Costantini M, Zaninotto G. Successful treatment of long-standing post-stroke dysphagia with botulinum toxin and rehabilitation. J Rehabil Med 2006; 38:201–203.
8. Logemann JA. Evaluation and Treatment of Swallowing Disorders, 2nd ed. Austin, TX: Pro-ed, 1998.
9. Palmer JB, Drennan JC, Baba M. Evaluation and treatment of swallowing impairments. Am Fam Phys Review 2000; Apr 15 61(8):2453–2462.

8 | Endocrinology

Michael A. Via
Jeffrey I. Mechanick

The endocrine system has evolved as the major control mechanism for homeostasis and metabolic regulation in multicellular organisms, including humans. Hormone signals released by endocrine glands affect end organs and tissues throughout the body in a variety of ways. This chapter aims to review the major hormone axes, their disruption in disease states common to patients with neurologic disease, and the metabolic disorders that ensue.

ANATOMY AND PHYSIOLOGY

The pituitary gland, or hypophysis, is located within the sella turcica, inferior to the optic chiasm, and is often described as "the size of a pea." It is divided functionally and anatomically into anterior and posterior sections. Although much of its function is controlled by the hypothalamus, the pituitary is considered the master gland for its role in regulating many of the other endocrine glands.

The anterior pituitary secretes six major peptide hormones: growth hormone (GH), prolactin (PRL), thryroid-stimulating hormone (TSH), adrenocorticotrophic hormone (ACTH), leutinizing hormone (LH), and follicle-stimulating hormone (FSH). The secretion of each of these hormones is pulsatile with a pattern that varies by circadian rhythm. For example, GH is secreted mostly at night, whereas ACTH peaks early in the morning. TSH also tends to be highest before noon. LH and FSH levels fluctuate at different times in the menstrual cycle and become persistently elevated during menopause. The secretion of these hormones from the anterior pituitary is governed by hormonal stimulation or neural modulation (in the case of PRL) from the hypothalamus and by negative feedback from hormonal products of the downstream endocrine organs: the thyroid, adrenal cortex, and gonads.

Prolactin synthesis is regulated by inhibitory dopaminergic neurons of the hypothalamus. The other peptide hormones of the pituitary are synthesized in response to stimulatory hormones secreted by the hypothalamus. Thus, any process that disrupts hypothalamic–pituitary signaling tends to yield high levels of PRL from loss of inhibition and low levels of the other hormones. Antidopaminergic compounds such as antipsychotic medications and metoclopramide can also raise the levels of PRL. Conversely, levodopa treatment for Parkinson's disease can lower circulating levels of PRL.

The posterior pituitary releases two peptide hormones: antidiuretic hormone and oxytocin. These hormones are synthesized in neuronal cell bodies located in the hypothalamus and transported axonally to the posterior pituitary for release into the bloodstream.

Hypopituitarism

Pituitary activity can be altered in a variety of disease states, often leading to a partial or complete loss of function. The clinical features of pituitary dysfunction, including fatigue, weakness, and hair loss, are nonspecific and insidious in onset. Premenopausal women may manifest early by menstrual cycle changes (Table 8.1).

The most common cause of hypopituitarism is a nonfunctioning pituitary tumor. Other important etiologies include head trauma, subarachnoid hemorrhage, brain irradiation, and neurosurgical procedures.

Head Trauma

Recently it has been recognized that up to of 35% of patients with traumatic brain injury develop pituitary dysfunction (1). The most common hormones affected are GH, LH, and FSH. Several small open-label studies suggest that treatment of these patients with recombinant human growth hormone improves cognition, memory, depression, anxiety, and fatigue, although such treatment is not currently standard practice (2). Approximately half of pituitary hormone deficiencies resolve spontaneously after 1 year.

Table 8.1

Signs and Symptoms of Anterior Pituitary Dysfunction

Adrenal Axis
  • Weakness, fatigue, nausea, vomiting, lightheadedness, hair loss, orthostatic hypotension, hypoglycemia

Thyroid Axis
  • Weight gain, cold intolerance, fatigue, bradycardia, dry skin

Gonadal Axis
  • Women: Oligomenorrhea or amenorrhea, hot flashes
  • Men: Decline in sperm count, erectile dysfunction
  • Both: Decrease libido, osteoporosis, weakness, fatigue

Growth Hormone Axis
  • Fatigue, depression, hypoglycemia

Prolactin Hypersecretion
  • Breast tenderness, galactorrhea, symptoms of hypogonadism

Subarachnoid Hemorrhage

Similar to head trauma, patients with subarachnoid hemorrhage have a high prevalence of pituitary dysfunction. Almost half of these patients have pituitary hormone deficiencies that have been noted to persist after 2 years of follow-up (3).

Brain Irradiation

Approximately 40% of patients receiving irradiation for nonpituitary brain tumors eventually develop hypopituitarism. This process is slow, and these patients typically do not manifest pituitary deficiency until 10 years after radiation treatment.

Neurosurgery

Patients who undergo pituitary surgery for adenoma, Rathke's cleft cyst, or craniopharyngioma are at risk for developing hypopituitarism. The rate of hypopituitarism following surgery depends on preoperative pituitary function, the surgeon's experience, and the type of pituitary mass. A case series of 721 patients that had resection of nonfunctioning pituitary adenomas at experienced neurosurgical centers showed that nearly 50% had permanent deficiency of at least one hormone axis (4). Patients who underwent resection of craniopharyngioma had total hypopituitarism about 40% of the time (5). Some studies indicate that surgical resection of a pituitary adenoma may improve pituitary function, but this remains to be confirmed (4).

Neurosurgical resection of nonpituitary brain tumors such as glioma, meningioma, or schwannoma has also been associated with hypopituitarism. Several case series show the incidence of hypopituitarism is about 40% at 3 months after surgery, which improves to 20% at 1 year (6,7). The most common hormone deficiency is that of GH.

Screening for Hypopituitarism

In patients with one of the neurologic conditions mentioned above, it is reasonable to screen for pituitary dysfunction. For head trauma, intracranial hemorrhage or postop neurosurgical patients, pituitary function should be assessed 6–8 weeks after the event (see section on diagnostic approach and treatment for appropriate blood tests). For patients with brain irradiation, pituitary function should not be tested until at least 5 years later.

Stroke

Ischemic stroke may also be associated with a decline in pituitary function. To date, only one series of 42 ischemic stroke patients revealed hypopituitarism in 14 (33%) while they were enrolled in rehabilitation programs (8). It is unclear if these results can be reproduced in larger trials. At this point, pituitary screening is not recommended in patients following a stroke, but should be considered in patients with symptoms of hypopituitarism.

Pituitary Apoplexy

Pituitary apoplexy is a rare condition characterized by an acute intrapituitary hemorrhage and a sudden loss of pituitary function. It may occur spontaneously or in the presence of a pituitary adenoma. Other predisposing factors include previous radiation, systemic anticoagulation, mechanical ventilation, and while in the postpartum period (Sheehan's syndrome). Clinically, patients experience a sudden, severe headache, visual field defects, and opthalmoplegia. Computed tomography (CT) or magnetic resonance imaging (MRI) of the head can reveal sellar hemorrhage, though MR imaging has been more reliable in several case series (9,10). If left untreated, patients may develop hypoglycemia, hypotension, and death. The recommended treatment includes empiric dexamethasone 2 mg every 6 hours to reduce cerebral edema and replacement for presumed secondary adrenal insufficiency. Surgery is reccomended in patients with visual field defects or severe opthalmoplegia. Hypopituitarism persists in the vast majority of patients. Additionally, one third of patients require desmopressin therapy for central diabetes insipidus (9).

Empty Sella

Occasionally, patients who undergo head MRI will incidentally have an empty sella turcica. These patients usually have normal pituitary function because of a rim of functional pituitary cells that line the sella. Unless these patients are symptomatic, checking serum prolactin, free thyroxine, and testosterone (in men) should be sufficient to evaluate pituitary function. Table 8.2 provides values for normal ranges of pituitary and related hormones.

Table 8.2

Normal Ranges of Pituitary and Related Hormones

	Men	Women	
GH	0–10	0–10	ng/mL
PRL	2–15	2–25	ng/mL
TSH	0.3–3.50	0.3–3.50	µU/mL
ACTH	20–100	20–100	pg/mL
LH	0.9–5.6	0.6–57	IU/L
FSH	1.5–14.3	1.1–124	mIU/mL
IGF-1	90–360	90–360	ng/mL
Free T4	0.8–1.8	0.8–1.8	ng/dL
Cortisol	2–24	2–24	µg/dL
Testosterone	260–1000	7–70	ng/dL
Estrogen	4–23	7–135	ng/dL
Progesterone	10–50	10–50	ng/dL
luteal phase		300–2500	ng/dL

Diagnostic Approach and Treatment

The evaluation of pituitary function involves checking plasma levels of pituitary hormones and their end products. If one is suspicious of pituitary dysfunction, it is reasonable to send a complete pituitary function panel, which includes checking TSH and free thyroxine, morning ACTH and cortisol, RL, FSH, LH, and insulin-like growth factor-1 (IGF-1), which is secreted by the liver in response to GH.

Treatment of hypopituitarism generally entails replacement with peripheral gland end products (Table 8.3). For example, ACTH deficiency is treated with corticosteroids (prednisone 7.5 mg daily or hydrocortisone 20 mg each morning 10 mg each evening) and TSH deficiency is treated with levothyroxine (1.6 µg/kg daily). Depending on the clinical situation, gonadotropin (FSH and LH) deficiency can be treated with either testosterone (Androgel® 5 g/day or Androderm® 5 mg/day) or estrogen (0.625 mg/day) with or without progesterone (medroxyprogesterone 2.5 mg/day). The use of growth hormone replacement therapy in adults is controversial, and not currently recommended (11).

SYNDROME OF INAPPROPRIATE ANTIDIURETIC HORMONE

The excessive production of antidiuretic hormone (ADH) by the posterior pituitary can lead to the syndrome of inappropriate antidiuretic hormone (SIADH) action. This syndrome is marked by retention of free water, high urine osmolality, urine sodium levels ranging from 40 to 70 mmol/liter, and hyponatremia. Common etiologies of SIADH include head trauma, meningitis, encephalitis, brain tumors, intracranial hemorrhage, pituitary or other brain surgery, certain medications (selective serotonin reuptake inhibitors [SSRIs], carbamazepine, among others), severe pain, and nausea. ADH may also be synthesized ectopically in lung tumors, gastrointestinal tumors, lymphomas, and pulmonary infections.

Treatment of SIADH involves free water restriction and addressing the underlying condition. Daily weights and total volume taken in and put out should be recorded. In severe cases, hypertonic saline can be used to raise the plasma sodium. This should only be done in a closely monitored setting, such as an ICU.

DIABETES INSIPIDUS

The loss of ADH production results in diabetes insipidus (DI). Patients are unable to produce concentrated urine and lose a substantial amount of free water. Generally, patients are able to compensate for renal losses by consuming fluids and they develop classic symptoms of polydipsia and polyuria. Urine output often exceeds 300 cc/hour and is dilute, with osmolality below 200 mOsm. The plasma sodium may be normal but can be elevated if a patient does

Table 8.3

Common Medications and Dosages

Medication	Usual Dose	Adverse Effects	Common drug interactions	Basis for Dose Adjustment
DDAVP	0.5–1 µg IV as needed 5–10 µg Inhaled BID 50–100 µg PO BID	Hyponatremia	NSAIDs – may enhance DDAVP activity	Urine Output, Na level
Levothyroxine	75–200 µg daily (1.6 µg / kg)	Hyperthyroidism by excessive dosage	Carbamazepine, phenytoin, barbituates – increase levothyroxine clearance	TSH; free T4 in pituitary patients
Methimazole	5–15 mg BID	agranulocytosis, elevated LFTs, rash	Decreased clearance of theophylline Decreased effectiveness of warfarin	TSH
Propylthiouracil (PTU)	50–200 mg TID	agranulocytosis, elevated LFTs, rash	Decreased effectiveness of warfarin	TSH
Paricalcitol	0.5–2 µg daily	hypercalcemia, hyperphosphate-mia, adynamic bone disease	Thiazide diuretics – hypercalcemia	PTH, Calcium
Cinacalcet	90–180 mg daily	hypocalcemia, adynamic bone disease	Ketoconazole – decreased clearance of cinacalcet	PTH, Calcium
Prednisone	7.5–10 mg daily	Cushing's syndrome, osteoporosis	Carbamazepine – increases corticosteroid clearance	Clinical hypoadrenalism
Hydrocortisone	10 mg each morning, 5 mg each evening	Cushing's syndrome, osteoporosis	Carbamazepine – increases corticosteroid clearance	Clinical hypoadrenalism
Fludrocortisone	0.1–0.3 mg daily	Hypokalemia, metabolic alkalosis, hypertension	Loop diuretics – hypokalemia	Blood pressure, electrolytes
Testosterone	5–10 g gel apply daily 5–10 mg patch apply daily	Decreased HDL, elevated LFTs, Hematocrit, acne, BPH	Resistance to curare based neuromuscular blockers	Testosterone level
Eplerenone	50 mg qd–50 mg BID	Hyperkalemia	Phenobarbitol, phenytoin – may reduce circulating eplerenone levels	Blood pressure, electrolytes
Spironolactone	25 mg–100 mg daily	Hyperkalemia, painful gynecomastia	ACE inhibitors, angiotensin receptor blockers – hyperkalemia	Blood pressure, electrolytes

not have access to water or his or her thirst mechanism is impaired. Common causes of DI include head trauma, pituitary, or other brain surgery, Sheehan's syndrome, neurosarcoid, and brain tumors. DI can also result if the cells of the renal collecting ducts do not respond to circulating ADH, a condition known as nephrogenic DI.

DI is treated with desmopressin (DDAVP), a synthetic analogue of ADH that preferentially targets the renal vasopressin receptors. DDAVP is available in oral, inhaled, and intravenous preparations. The dose should be titrated to maintain a normal urine output. Usually DDAVP is given twice per day. The starting dose is usually 100 µg oral, 10 µg inhaled, or 1 µg IV at bedtime. Dose adjustments should be made every 1–2 days, increasing or decreasing by 100 µg oral, 10 µg inhaled, or 1 µg IV at a time. Plasma sodium should be monitored to avoid hyponatremia.

PITUITARY TUMOR

Pituitary tumors are common incidental findings on brain imaging. Their overall prevalence is about 10% and increases with age (12). Most commonly, pituitary tumors are nonfunctional, benign adenomas. They can cause hypopituitarism by mass effect or secrete any of the pituitary hormones. Thus, a full pituitary function panel should be sent, as well as a dedicated pituitary MRI. The MRI can differentiate pituitary adenomas from other masses that may occupy the sella turcica, such as craniopharyngiomas or Rathke's cleft cysts.

Pituitary tumors can extend and compress the optic chiasm, leading to bitemporal visual field loss, or they can extend to the cavernous sinus and may cause dysfunction of cranial nerves III, IV, V_1, V_2, and VI. Either of these conditions would be an indication for surgery, except in the case of prolactinomas, where medical therapy can be effective.

Tumors that secrete active hormones such as GH, causing acromegaly, or ACTH, causing Cushing's disease, are considered functional pituitary tumors. These patients should be evaluated for surgical resection. Surgical treatment of functional tumors is not always curative, as it may be difficult to resect all the active tissue. These patients may require more than one operation or possibly γ-knife or whole brain radiation.

Prolactin-secreting tumors, or prolactinomas, are an exception to the above rule. The lactotroph cells of a prolactinoma remain under negative regulatory control by hypothalamic dopamine-secreting neurons. These tumors regress quickly with dopamine agonist therapy such as cabergoline or bromocriptine.

Patients who have surgery for a pituitary adenoma should be placed on a corticosteroid taper to reduce local inflammation and to prevent hypoadrenalism in case pituitary function is disrupted during the procedure. In the immediate postoperative period, patients should be monitored for SIADH or DI, which may develop days to weeks after surgery. All patients should have their pituitary function reassessed 6 weeks postoperatively.

THYROID DISEASE

The thyroid gland is located in the neck, posterior to the strap muscles and inferior to the thyroid cartilage. In response to TSH signaling by the pituitary, the thyroid synthesizes and secretes thyroid hormone or thyroxine (T4), which helps to regulate overall metabolism. T4 is converted to the physiologically active triiodothyronine (T3) or the inactive reverse triiodothyronine (rT3) in the peripheral tissues. In assessing thyroid function, plasma levels of TSH and free T4 should be measured. Most of the circulating T4 is protein-bound, and thus measuring total T4 and thyroid-binding globulin is an acceptable alternative to free T4. In most cases, T3 levels are not helpful in diagnosing thyroid disease, except when Graves' disease is suspected. Patients with neurologic disease tend to have similar rates of thyroid disorders as the general population, although an increase in subclinical hyperthyroidism has been reported in patients with Parkinson's disease (13).

Thyroid Nodules

Thyroid nodules are common incidental findings on neck imaging studies. Their overall prevalence has been reported as up to 50% in the general population and increases with age (14). A newly discovered nodule should be evaluated with a dedicated thyroid ultrasound and be assessed for function by checking a plasma TSH level. In the case of a patient with a thyroid nodule and suppressed TSH, a thyroid radionuclide scan should be performed to confirm the presence of a hyperfunctioning, or "hot" nodule. Hot nodules are treated by radioactive iodine ablation or by surgical resection. They are generally considered benign.

For patients who have nonsecreting thyroid nodules, the possibility of thyroid malignancy should be considered. Fine needle aspiration (FNA) biopsy should be performed on all patients with a nodule greater than 1 cm in size or if a smaller nodule has malignant features on ultrasound. Benign nodules are usually followed with yearly ultrasounds and may require repeat FNA biopsy if growth is noted.

The workup for patients with multiple nodules or multinodular goiter is similar to that of a solitary nodule. Plasma TSH and thyroid ultrasound should be performed. If possible, nodules larger than 1 cm in size or those with malignant features should be subject to FNA biopsy. Figure 8.1 provides a Thyroid Nodule Workup flow sheet.

Thyroid Cancer

Less than 7% of thyroid nodules are malignant. Risk factors for thyroid cancer include family history of thyroid cancer, radiation exposure, and the presence of a nodule in a male patient or a patient less than 20 or more than 70 years old. Regardless of histologic type, thyroid cancer is treated by thyroidectomy. This is often followed by radioactive iodine (RAI) therapy to ablate any remain-

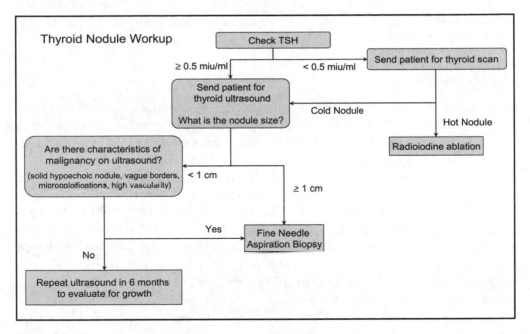

Figure 8.1. Thyroid nodule workup.

ing thyroid cancer tissue. In the case of medullary thyroid cancer, patients should be evaluated prior to surgery for the presence of a pheochromocytoma, which may be present as part of the multiple endocrine neoplasia 2 (MEN2) syndrome. After a thyroidectomy, these patients will require levothyroxine therapy. Replacement doses should be titrated to a goal TSH of 0.1 mU/liter.

Hyperthyroidism

A patient is considered hyperthyroid when an excessive amount of thyroxine is released in circulation, yielding typical clinical findings. Patients are warm, tachycardic, diaphoretic, hyperreflexic, and have a fine tremor. The metabolic rate is increased, and they often report a history of weight loss, hair loss, and loose bowel movements. TSH levels are low, with normal to elevated free T4 levels.

The common causes for hyperthyroidism are Graves' disease, in which auto-antibodies activate the TSH receptor, subacute thyroiditis, a hot nodule, toxic multinodular goiter, and surreptitious use of levothyroxine. A thyroid uptake and scan can help to differentiate these conditions if the diagnosis is not clear.

Hyperthyroid patients are at risk for atrial fibrillation and osteoporosis. Treatment for hyperthyroidism depends on the etiology. The options include medical therapy such as methimazole or propylthiouracil (PTU), radioactive iodine ablation, or surgical resection of the thyroid. Methimazole should be started at 10 mg twice a day. The maximum total daily dose is 30 mg. PTU should be started at 50 or 100 mg three times per day. Both should be titrated based on free T4 levels.

Hypothyroidism

In patients with less than the required thyroxine production, hypothyroidism ensues. These patients generally have cool, clammy skin and experience fatigue, constipation, cold intolerance, and weight gain. The TSH is elevated, usually above 10 mU/liter, with normal to low free T4 levels. Common causes include autoimmune thyroiditis or Hashimoto's disease, history of subacute thyroiditis, or treatment with radioactive iodine ablation for hyperthyroidism.

Hypothyroidism is treated by oral replacement levothyroxine. Patients should be started at 25 μg per day and titrated up every 2–3 days by 50 μg to a dose near 1.6 μg/kg per day. The dose can be adjusted every 2–4 months based on TSH with a goal range of 0.5–2.0 mIU/ml. Because of poor absorption, levothyroxine should be taken on an empty stomach, separate from food or other medications by at least 1 hour.

Table 8.4 provides an overview of common findings in hyper- and hypothyroidism.

Nonthyroidal Illness

The pituitary gland is quite sensitive to a patient's medical condition, and TSH levels often decrease during acute illness, even though the patient is clinically euthyroid. Free T4 levels remain normal. As a patient recovers, the TSH can become elevated. Thus, thyroid function tests can be difficult to interpret in the setting of acute illness or hospitalization. This phenomenon is known as nonthyroidal illness or, previously, the sick-euthyroid syndrome. If such a patient exhibits symptoms of hyper- or hypothyroidism, a complete thyroid panel (TSH, free T4, total T3) may be helpful, but these tests generally do not return to normal until months after acute illness. Treating this condition is controver-

Table 8.4

Signs and Symptoms of Hyperthyroidism and Hypothyroidism

Hyperthyroidism	Hypothyroidism
Weight loss	Weight gain
Heat intolerance	Cold intolerance
Brisk reflexes	Mental slowing
Fine tremor	Fatigue
Tachycardia	Bradycardia
Diarrhea	Constipation
Fine oily hair, soft skin	Dry skin and hair

sial and has not been shown to affect overall outcome (15). The best advice is to refrain from checking thyroid function tests in these types of patients.

PARATHYROID DISEASE

The parathyroid glands secrete parathyroid hormone (PTH), a peptide hormone that regulates calcium metabolism through its effects mainly on bone, causing liberation of calcium, and on the kidneys, inducing tubular calcium resorption and vitamin D activation. Primary hyperparathyroidism commonly results from increased secretion of PTH from a parathyroid adenoma or parathyroid hyperplasia. These patients are hypercalcemic and can develop kidney stones, osteoporosis or fractures, constipation, depression, muscle weakness, and fatigue. Hyperparathyroidism is a common cause for hypercalcemia, and PTH should be checked in patients with elevated serum calcium (normal ranges vary by laboratory). Levels of 25-hydroxy-vitamin D (normal > 32 ng/ml) should also be checked as the PTH can be elevated in states of vitamin D deficiency. A 24-hour urinary calcium should also be collected to discriminate hyperparathyroidism from familial hypercalcemic hypocalcuria, a rare benign condition with high serum calcium and PTH. Treatment for primary hyperparathyroidism is parathyroidectomy, which is indicated for symptomatic patients or young patients (<45 years old), as they may develop symptoms if left untreated.

Patients with renal disease can develop secondary hyperparathyroidism due to low circulating levels of activated vitamin D. Medical management with vitamin D analogues can lower PTH levels in these patients.

Hypoparathyroidism is rare and usually is the result of anterior neck surgery. Serum calcium is low, as is serum PTH. Treatment goals are symptomatic relief with calcium (1–2 g twice daily) and calcitriol (0.5–2 µg/day) supplementation.

DISEASES OF THE ADRENAL GLANDS

The adrenal glands produce epinephrine in the adrenal medulla and steroid hormones including cortisol, aldosterone, and adrenal androgens in the cortex. Cortisol is synthesized in response to ACTH as part of the stress response. Aldosterone release is regulated by angiotensin.

Excessive release of cortisol by the adrenals or excessive intake of exogenous corticosteroids leads to Cushing's syndrome, characterized by central obesity, thin extremities with proximal muscle weakness, facial plethora, moon facies, buffalo hump, easy bruising, depression, and impaired glucose tolerance. Cushing's syndrome is most commonly caused by an ACTH-secreting pituitary tumor or by ectopic production of ACTH, such as in lung cancer. Rarely, high cortisol levels originate from an adrenal source, either hyperplasia, an adrenal adenoma, or adrenal carcinoma. After establishing high cortisol levels by 24-hour urine free cortisol or midnight salivary cortisol testing, dexamethasone suppression testing may help identify the source of the high cortisol levels. Surgery is the usual treatment for Cushing's syndrome.

Excessive secretion of aldosterone, such as in Conn's syndrome, leads to hypertension as the major clinical characteristic. Because hypertension is so common, the overall prevalence of Conn's syndrome is unknown—many patients remain undiagnosed. Some estimate that up to 30% of hypertensive patients have Conn's syndrome. If hyperaldosteronism is suspected based on excessively high blood pressure, hypertension that is refractory to treatment, hypertension in young patients, or low serum potassium levels, a renin/aldosterone ratio (normal < 20) may be checked as the initial test. If positive, the diagnosis is confirmed by a salt challenge test in which aldosterone levels fail to suppress with administration of 10 g NaCl. Treatment is with eplerenone or spironolactone combined with other antihypertensives as needed. If patients fail medical therapy, adrenalectomy can be considered, but this is usually not necessary.

Adrenal Incidentaloma

Adrenal masses are common incidental findings on imaging studies. Autopsy and CT studies show a prevalence of 4–6% in the general population (16). When discovered, adrenal masses should be evaluated for functionality and malignant potential (Figure 8.2).

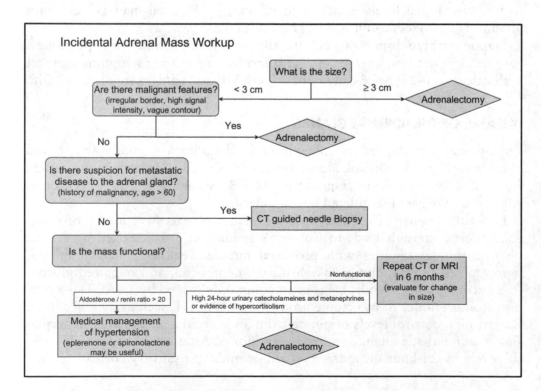

Figure 8.2. Incidental adrenal mass workup.

   Adrenal function screening includes sending plasma free metanerphines, serum renin/aldosterone ratio, and measuring the morning cortisol levels after giving 1 mg oral dexamethasone the night before. If any of these tests are positive, a more complete workup should be performed. In assessing for malignancy, size and the appearance on imaging are the most important factors. History of other cancer raises the suspicion for metastasic disease, and needle biopsy may be considered. For functional and malignant adrenal masses, surgical resection is indicated. Smaller, nonfunctional masses should be reevaluated by CT scan 6 months later.

Adrenal Insufficiency

The undersecretion of cortisol leads to adrenal insufficiency (AI). Patients experience symptoms of malaise, abdominal pain, and hypotension. AI may result from autoimmune, infectious, or hemorrhagic processes or from overly rapid tapering of a patient's corticosteroid dose. The diagnosis is made by ACTH stimulation testing. Failure of cortisol levels to reach 18 μg/dl 1 hour after administering recombinant ACTH is diagnostic for AI. Treatment is with corticosteroids, usually hydrocortisone at doses that depend on the clinical situation (the usual dose is 10 mg every morning and 5 mg every night). Therapy with fludrocortisone, a mineralocorticoid analogue, may also be considered.

   For patients on steroid therapy, the rate at which the steroids should be safely tapered depends largely on the duration of therapy and the dose. In general, steroids should be tapered by dose increments of 5–10% over weeks to months.

Patient Safety

1. Screening for hypopituitarism: For head trauma, intracranial hemorrhage or postop neurosurgical patients, pituitary function should be assessed 6–8 weeks after the event. For patients with brain irradiation, pituitary function should not be tested until at least 5 years postirradiation.
2. Conn's syndrome: Excessive secretion of aldosterone leads to hypertension. Because hypertension is so common, the overall prevalence of Conn's syndrome is unknown, but some estimate that up to 30% of hypertensive patients have it. It is important to screen for this condition in patients with excessively high blood pressure, hypertension that is refractory to treatment, hypertension in young patients, or in patients with low serum potassium levels.
3. Adrenal masses: When discovered, adrenal masses should be evaluated for functionality and malignant potential.
4. A safe steroid taper is important to avoid the development of adrenal insufficiency in patients on longstanding use of corticosteroids.
5. Medication safety: Table 8.3 outlines some common medications used to treat the endocrine conditions discussed in the text as well as their adverse effects and drug interactions.

Some Key Points for Patient Education

SIADH
- Limit fluid intake
- Do not correct sodium at a rate greater than 0.5 mmol/L per hour
- May liberalize fluids as the condition causing SIADH resolves

DI
- Have the patient take DDAVP
- The patient should weigh themselves daily. If their weight increases by 2–3 pounds in one day, cut back on the DDAVP dose
- Periodically check serum sodium levels, daily at first, then at greater intervals while sodium levels remain constant

Hypopituitarism
- Have the patient take their replacement hormones
- Periodically monitor hormone levels (every 2–6 months)

Hyperthyroidism
- If the patient is treated with methimazole or PTU, periodically (every 2–6 months) check thyroid function by TSH and free T4.
- If the patient is treated with radioactive iodine, they should be also continued on methimazole or PTU for several months to give the radioactive iodine time to work. They should also have periodic (every 2–6 months) thyroid function testing including TSH and free T4.
- The TSH may remain suppressed for months after treatment, even as the free T4 returns to normal and the patient is euthyroid

Hypothyroidism
- Have the patient take levothyroxine as directed, by itself with only water, separated from food, vitamins and other medications by at least 1 hour.
- Periodically monitor TSH levels (every 2–12 months).

Hyperparathyroidism
- Monitor patient for an indication for surgery (renal stone, excessively high calcium, osteoporosis, bone fracture)
- Follow calcium levels

Adrenal Insufficiency
- Have patient take corticosteroid replacement
- If the patient develops acute illness or requires surgery, have the patient triple the steroid dose for 3 days, and then return to usual dose

REFERENCES

1. Popovic V, Aimaretti G, Casanueva FF, Ghigo E. Hypopituitarism following traumatic brain injury. Front Horm Res 2005; 33:33–44.
2. Popovic V, Aimaretti G, Casanueva FF, Ghigo E. Hypopituitarism following traumatic brain injury (TBI): call for attention. J Endocrinol Invest 2005; 28(5 Suppl):61–64.

3. Dimopoulou I, Kouyialis AT, Tzanella M, et al. High incidence of neuroendocrine dysfunction in long-term survivors of aneurysmal subarachnoid hemorrhage. Stroke 2004; 35:2884–2889.

4. Nomikos P, Ladar C, Fahlbusch R, Buchfelder M. Impact of primary surgery on pituitary function in patients with nonfunctioning pituitary adenomas—a study on 721 patients. Acta Neurochirurgica 2004; 146:27–35.

5. Honegger J, Buchfelder M, Fahlbusch R. Surgical treatment of craniopharyngiomas: endocrinological results. J Neurosurg 1999; 90:251–257.

6. De Marinis L, Fusco A, Bianchi A, et al. Hypopituitarism findings in patients with primary brain tumors 1 year after neurosurgical treatment: preliminary report. J Endocrinol Invest 2006; 29(6):516–522.

7. Schneider HJ, Rovere S, Corneli G, et al. Endocrine dysfunction in patients operated on for non-pituitary intracranial tumors. Eur J Endocrinol 2006; 155(4):559–566.

8. Bondanelli M, Ambrosio MR, Onofri A, et al. Predictive value of circulating insulin-like growth factor i levels in ischemic stroke outcome. J Clin Endocrinol Metab 2006; 91:3928–3934.

9. Gruber A, Clayton J, Kumar S, Robertson I, Howlett TA, Mansell P. Pituitary apoplexy: a retrospective review of thirty patients—Is surgical intervention always necessary? Br J Neurosurg 2006; 20(6):379–385.

10. Randeva HS, Schoebel J, Byrne J, Esiri M, Adams CBT, Wass JAH. Classical pituitary apoplexy: clinical features, management and outcome. Clin Endocrinol 1999; 51:181–188.

11. Clayton P, Gleeson H, Monson J, Popovic V, Shalet SM, Christiansen JS. Growth hormone replacement throughout life: insights into age-related responses to treatment. Growth Horm IGF Res 2007.

12. Teramoto A, Hirakawa K, Sanno N, et al. Incidental pituitary lesions in 1,000 unselected autopsy specimens. Radiology 1994; 193:161.

13. Tandeter H, Levy A, Gutman G, Svartzman P. Subclinical thyroid disease in patients with parkinsons disease. Arch Gerentol Geriatr 2001; (33):295–300.

14. AACE/AME Task Force on Thyroid Nodules. Medical guidelines for clinical practice for the diagnosis and management of thyroid nodules. Endocr Pract 2006; 12(1):63–102.

15. De Groot LJ. Non-thyroidal illness syndrome is a manifestation of hypothalamic-pituitary dysfunction, and in view of current evidence, should be treated with appropriate replacement therapies. Crit Care Clin 2006; 22(1):57–86, vi.

16. Young WF. The incidentally discovered adrenal mass. N Engl J Med 2007; 355(6):601–610.

9 | Exercise

James H. Rimmer

As persons with neurologic disability age, the interaction between the natural aging process and the secondary conditions associated with the disability (e.g., weight gain, deconditioning) create a demanding physical environment (1). Tasks that could be accomplished in younger adulthood often become significantly more difficult in middle and later life. Climbing stairs, walking with a cane or walker, carrying packages, transferring from a wheelchair to a bed, commode, chair, or car, pushing a wheelchair up a ramp or over a curb, and standing for long periods require adequate levels of fitness (e.g., cardiorespiratory endurance, strength, flexibility, balance). Low physical fitness, in combination with impairments (e.g., loss of function, spasticity) and secondary conditions (e.g., obesity, osteoporosis, deconditioning) associated with the disability, reduces physical independence and limits opportunities to participate in many community events that require moderate to high levels of energy expenditure (community ambulation). For this reason, it is critical that clinicians put greater emphasis on advising patients how to safely and effectively participate in a physical fitness conditioning program to postpone or minimize the effects of deconditioning. In this chapter, the following neurologic conditions will be discussed: cerebral palsy, multiple sclerosis, spinal cord injury, stroke, and traumatic brain injury.

EXERCISE PRESCRIPTION

An exercise prescription for individuals with neurologic conditions should include the same four elements that are used with the general population: frequency, intensity, duration, and type. The only difference is that the amount (dose) and type of activity prescribed will differ based on the individual's condition, fitness level, and environmental circumstances (e.g., availability of adaptations necessary for performing exercise, need for more assistance or supervision). Frequency of exercise refers to the number of days a week that the exercise bout is engaged in. Intensity is the training threshold

115

associated with exercising at a certain percentage of maximum heart rate or peak oxygen consumption for cardiovascular exercise and percent overload for resistance (strength) exercise. Duration refers to the length of the exercise bout. Type or modality refers to the specific activities that are performed during the exercise bout.

Frequency

The American College of Sports Medicine (ACSM) and American Heart Association (AHA) (2) recommend regular, sustainable exercise 3–7 days a week. The precise dose of exercise will depend on the fitness (conditioning) level of the client, current health status, interest level in exercising several times a week, and the availability/accessibility of exercise equipment/programs in their home or community (e.g., fitness center with accessible equipment, transportation, home exercise equipment). Individuals with neurologic disability who use assistive aids to ambulate (e.g., wheelchairs) may be at a disadvantage in terms of exercising regularly outdoors compared to someone who is able to walk because of difficulty pushing their wheelchair for long periods, outdoor neighborhoods may have many uneven or damaged sidewalks or there may be no sidewalks, or roads and hills may be difficult to traverse. Indoor exercise settings may have limited or no access to adaptive exercise equipment and/or adaptive sports and recreation programs, and resources to purchase exercise equipment or transportation to get to and from an exercise facility may be unavailable (3).

Intensity

Exercise intensity is the most complex aspect of the exercise prescription. In order to improve fitness, heart rate must be increased to a certain percentage of maximum heart rate to allow for physiologic and musculoskeletal adaptations. Table 9.1 provides three different methods for computing exercise intensity based on the guidelines established by the ACSM (4). For individuals with neurologic disability, the third method using VO_{2peak} is the most accurate for setting the intensity level because predicted maximum heart rate (Table. 9.1, Equations 1 and 2) is lower in individuals with autonomic dysfunction and persons using β-blockers.

The key to any training program is to ensure that the exercise intensity matches the conditioning level of the client. Individuals with neurologic disability may require frequent adjustments to training intensity after a change in health status (e.g., multiple sclerosis [MS] exacerbation). Higher intensity training will generally require more supervision to prevent overuse injury and other potential health issues associated with greater training loads. For most individuals with a neurologic disability, duration of exercise is generally more important than intensity, particularly during the early stages of the program when the individual is adjusting to the workload.

Table 9.1

Training Intensity Guidelines

Heart Rate Formulas:[a]

1. % of heart rate max
   $220 - age \times$ % intensity (i.e., 50–90%)
2. Heart rate reserve
   Similar to above but takes into consideration resting heart rate (RHR)
   $(220 - age) - RHR \times 40/50-85\% + RHR$
3. Oxygen consumption (VO_{2peak})
   $VO_{2reserve}$ $(VO_{2peak} - VO_{2rest}) \times$ %intensity + VO_{2rest}

Example: VO_{2peak} = 25 ml/kg/min
$\quad\quad\quad\quad$ 25 – resting VO_2 (3.5 ml/kg/min) = 21.5 × 50% intensity (multiple by 0.50)
$\quad\quad\quad\quad$ = ~11 ml/kg/min + 3.5 (rest) or approximately 4 METs (1 MET – 3.5 ml/kg/min)

[a]Formula 3 is the most accurate method for individuals with neurologic disability since maximum heart rate may be compromised in individuals with autonomic dysfunction. If formula 1 or 2 is used, RPE should also be measured for a more accurate assessment of exertion.
Source: Ref 4.

Duration

The most current physical activity guidelines published by the ACSM and American Heart Association recommend 30 minutes of moderate-intensity aerobic physical activity (3–6 METs) 5 days a week or vigorous-intensity aerobic physical activity 3 days a week (>6 METs) (2). For individuals who are severely deconditioned, shorter, more frequent, less intense bouts of exercise may be equally effective (e.g., three 10-minute bouts spread across the day). While 30 minutes is the minimum recommendation for moderate-intensity physical activity, less daily physical activity is often beneficial for deconditioned clients who are starting an exercise program or are in the postacute phase of recovery. For older individuals with significant physical/cognitive impairments, several minutes a day of exercise may be a good starting point, gradually increasing to 30 minutes a day once a certain conditioning level is achieved. The rate of progression will depend on the client's age, conditioning level, and overall health status. For postacute patients, progression should begin with 15 minutes per day for the first 2 weeks, gradually increasing by 5 minutes per session per week for the next several weeks until the target duration is achieved.

Type (Modality)

Any activity that increases energy expenditure above rest safely and effectively can be used to enhance cardiorespiratory or musculoskeletal fitness. Both forms of exercise should be conducted weekly, and for many individuals with neurologic disability, flexibility and balance training should also be incorporated into the weekly training regimen. A variety of accessible pieces of exercise equipment should be considered. Two of the more popular cardiorespiratory machines that are wheelchair accessible are the NuStep™ and BioDex™ recumbent steppers. These machines allow wheelchair users to transfer onto the machine (height of seat is equivalent to seat height of wheelchair), and the seat is wide enough for maintaining comfort and safety. Several lines of strength equipment are also accessible depending on the functional needs of the individual. A listing of accessible exercise equipment can be found on the National Center on Physical Activity and Disability website at www.ncpad.org.

PATIENT ASSESSMENT

When developing an exercise prescription for individuals with neurologic disability, it is important to assess the functional limitations associated with each disability. There are many available instruments and techniques that can be used to evaluate each fitness component (cardiorespiratory endurance, strength, flexibility/ROM, and balance). This section provides the reader with key questions and physical examination findings when considering an exercise program for adults with neurologic disabilities.

1. What impairments and secondary conditions are associated with each neurologic disability?

Clinicians must consider certain impairments and secondary conditions associated with each neurologic disability when prescribing exercise for their patient population. For example, an individual with MS who has spastic paraparesis may have difficulty walking on a treadmill and may need a harness to protect them from falling. Secondary conditions such as fatigue, pain, and weight gain must also be considered since any of these conditions, if not considered, can limit a person's ability to exercise.

2. Is the condition progressive or nonprogressive?

Knowing the type and level of progression for some individuals (e.g., MS) is critical for providing a safe and effective program. Clinicians must provide an adequate dose of exercise that will be address fluctuations in the person's health status.

3. What muscle groups are still functional?

Nerve innervations of muscle groups still intact are critical for prescribing appropriate exercise to the target population. The clinician must be aware of innervated muscle groups and prescribe appropriate levels of exercise to accommodate any weakness (e.g., paresis) to targeted muscle groups. Depending on the disability, muscle groups may be functional, partially functional (paresis), or nonfunctional (paralysis). The clinician will need to identify which muscle groups fall into each category. There may also be some joint irregularity that needs to be considered in the exercise prescription. For example, individuals with cerebral palsy often have hip dislocations due to the strong pull of the adductor muscles. If there has been a history of hip displacement, the clinician should verify with the client's physician that it is safe to perform lower extremity strength and aerobic exercise.

4. Is there noticeable weakness on one side of the body (hemiplegia)?

Many individuals with neurologic disability will experience asymmetric weakness or paralysis on the right or left side. Certain adaptations or assistive aids can be used to allow the individual to maintain the hemiparetic side in alignment with the body while performing exercise routines. Gloves, straps/bands, or harnesses can be used to keep the trunk or legs in alignment during the exercise motion, as illustrated in Figure 9.1.

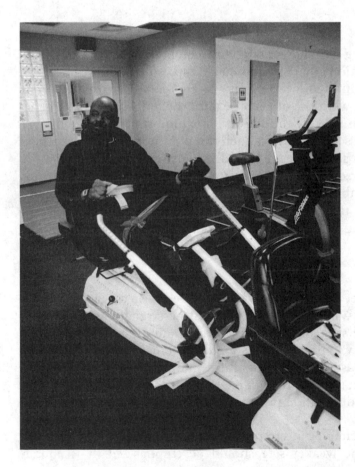

Figure 9.1. Participant with stroke exercising on recumbent stepper.

It may also be necessary to develop a separate resistance training program for the weakened side using isolateral machines (machines that allow different weight loads for the right or left sides of the body). Life Fitness™ offers a set of isolateral machines for upper and lower body exercise. Having hemiplegia may require active-assistive resistance exercise on the affected side while using standard exercises on the nonaffected side.

5. Is spasticity present?

Many individuals with neurologic disability present with some degree of spasticity. Flexibility training should always be combined with resistance training. It is important for the clinician to identify the "spastic" muscle groups and develop a long-range plan to increase range of motion. If the joint has been in a "fixed" position for many years or if the spasticity is severe, it may not be possible to fully extend the joint. Active-assistive stretching can be very beneficial for weak (paretic) or tight (spastic) muscle groups.

EXERCISE PRESCRIPTION GUIDELINES FOR SPECIFIC NEUROLOGIC DISABILITIES

Cerebral Palsy

Cardiorespiratory

Cardiorespiratory training for individuals with cerebral palsy must address specific movement limitations or neuromuscular impairments. Certain movement patterns can result in high levels of fatigue and energy expenditure and therefore may require a lower dose of exercise until the individual has a higher conditioning level and can tolerate the activity. It is important for the clinician to make sure that the prescribed physical activity does not produce excessive loads on certain joints. In some cases (e.g., individuals with crouch gait) walking may not be the preferred activity as excessive loads and shear forces already occurring during daily ambulatory activity may result in excessive overuse and injury. Smooth, rhythmic types of activities should be encouraged (e.g. swimming, non–weight-bearing exercise such as recumbent stepping or arm/leg cycling).

Strength and Flexibility

Many individuals with cerebral palsy have some level of spasticity in the hip and shoulder adductors. While these muscles must be strengthened, it is also important for them to be stretched in order to maintain an adequate balance of strength and flexibility. The hip and shoulder abductors should also be strengthened while emphasizing good alignment and technique (no hiking or overextension and moving through the full ROM). It is important to make sure there is no history of hip dislocation prior to initiating a lower extremity resistance training program.

In individuals with hemiplegia, strengthening the functional or partially functional muscles on the weaker side should be emphasized. It is equally important to attempt the smoothest motion possible; however, some "jerki-ness" may be unavoidable due to hyperactive stretch reflexes and a lack of reciprocal inhibition.

Falls are a recurrent problem for many ambulatory adults with cerebral palsy. In addition to specific exercises to improve static and dynamic balance, the conditioning program should also include strengthening the anterior chest, shoulder, and arm musculature to possibly protect the individual from serious injury occurring from a fall. In individuals with crouch gait, strengthening lower extremity musculature may also assist the person with improved gait and posture.

Multiple Sclerosis

Cardiorespiratory

Cardiorespiratory training for individuals with MS must consider the cur-rent health status of the individual. The exercise prescription should take into account the possibility of declining health status (e.g., exacerbation and pro-gression of the condition) as well as elevated external temperatures. Examples of endurance activities include cycling with legs and/or arms, swimming and aquatic exercise, walking, and lifestyle activities such as gardening and yard work that incorporate large muscle groups. The program should protect the client from excessive fatigue, a common secondary condition among persons with MS. Duration of exercise should initially start with a few minutes per day when the individual is not feeling well or has had an exacerbation and gradually progress to 30–60 minutes per day as the individual's medical condi-tion improves. Exercise can be interspersed throughout the day (e.g., in 10- to 15-minute intervals) for individuals presenting with high levels of postexercise fatigue.

Strength

Strength activities are critical for allowing individuals with MS to perform basic and instrumental activities of daily living (BADL and IADL). Strength can be improved using a number of different modalities, including weight machines, elastic bands, pulley systems, or lifting household items (e.g., one-gallon milk containers filled with water—one full container weighs 8 lb). The amount of resistance and number of repetitions will depend on the person's health status. In general, one to three sets of 10-to-12 repetitions are usually recommended for improving or maintaining strength. As strength increases, the amount of weight should be increased. Ideally, strength training should not be performed on consecutive days in order to allow the muscle groups being exercised to recover between sessions. Upper and lower body muscles should be included in the strength training program for all functional muscle groups. Muscles in the lower trunk (ankles, legs, and hips) are particularly important for helping to maintain mobility, and muscles in the upper trunk are important for perform-ing transfers, getting up from the floor, and lifting and carrying various items.

Flexibility

Individuals with MS may benefit from a routine of daily flexibility exercises, preferably in the morning, to assist with BADL and IADL. Flexibility exercises can also be incorporated during the day at work or home, or may be done as part of an exercise class during the warm-up and/or cool-down phases of the class. Stretching should include static and/or dynamic exercises. In dynamic stretching the muscle moves through the full range of motion of a joint. A static stretch is when the muscle is lengthened or stretched to the point where there is some mild discomfort or tension and the person is able to hold this stretch for 15–45 seconds. Static and dynamic flexibility are both important for maintaining joint integrity.

Balance

Another important training component for persons with MS is balance. Variations in balance are common in persons with different types of MS. Traditional static and dynamic balance exercises such as standing on one leg with eyes open and closed, walking on various uneven surfaces such as foam cushions or mats, and walking along narrow lines or surfaces should be encouraged on a daily basis. On days when balance is not good, the person can perform sitting balance exercises from a chair or on the floor.

MS Exacerbations

It may be necessary to temporarily stop the training program because of an exacerbation. These can occur frequently or infrequently depending on the amount of involvement. After an exacerbation, it will often be necessary to start out at a lower training intensity, frequency, and duration because of the complications that result from the exacerbation. Although the person may be unable to reach the same prior level of strength and endurance, it is important that he or she be reassured that strength levels can be improved. Clients who have exacerbations should understand that they begin with a "new slate" and that the goal is to always attain the highest level of strength and endurance possible.

Spinal Cord Injury

An exercise prescription for persons with spinal cord injury (SCI) must be based on the level of injury. There is a strong relationship between level of injury and the person's ability to increase workload and peak oxygen uptake. In general, persons with paraplegia will be able to generate higher levels of energy expenditure and have more exercise options available to them because of the greater availability in musculature compared to persons with tetraplegia. Persons with tetraplegia will require more adaptations to engage in various forms of exercise. The National Center on Physical Activity and Disability has produced two exercise videos for persons with paraplegia and tetraplegia. Each video contains cardiorespiratory, strength, and flexibility exercises and can be purchased from the following website: www.ncpad.org.

Cardiorespiratory

Given the variation in function among persons with SCI based on the level (tetra vs. para) and type (complete vs. incomplete) of injury, it is prudent to establish a cardiorespiratory training regimen (e.g., target heart rate) from a VO_{2peak} test. However, if VO_{2peak} is not available, rating of perceived exertion (RPE) along with heart rate can be used to monitor the intensity of the activity. Due to impaired sympathetic drive, persons with high-level complete SCI (i.e., tetraplegia) will only be able to achieve a maximum heart rate in the mid-120 beats per minute (bpm) range. Individuals with high-level paraplegia (above T6) will also have a blunted heart rate response to exercise due to autonomic dysfunction.

Aerobic training recommendations are generally the same as for the general population (5). In persons with paraplegia, cardiorespiratory exercise should be performed 3–7 days a week at an intensity level of 50–80% VO_{2peak}. Exercise frequency and duration should be carefully monitored to avoid overuse injury. Persons with low tetraplegia may be able to exercise using specialized gloves that allow the hand to be attached to an arm ergometer.

Various modes of exercise training exist. These include arm cranking, wheelchair propulsion, swimming, wheelchair sports, circuit training, exercise videos, and functional electrical stimulation (FES). Many persons with tetraplegia can train with these same modalities provided they have the necessary adaptations (e.g., specialized gloves, straps, harness) to use the equipment.

Strength

Resistance training is very important for persons with SCI. Upper body strength is crucial to successful independent living in performing transfers, IADL (pulling self into car), BADL (e.g., dressing—lifting one side of body to get pants leg on), and pressure relief. The training program will vary in persons with different levels of injury. In general, recommendations by ACSM should apply to persons with SCI.

Intensity: three sets of 8–12 reps
Duration: moderate to high intensity
Frequency: two sessions per week
Mode: free weights with appropriate supervision, weight machines, elastic bands

In general, starting resistance should be approximately 50% of one repetition maximum (1-RM) and progression should be based on the individual's level of conditioning. Resistance training should always be combined with an appropriate flexibility program. Balance training using a series of standard balance exercises can be added to the regimen. A variety of balance exercises can be found on the National Center on Physical Activity and Disability website (www.ncpad.org).

Stroke

Cardiorespiratory

Improving cardiorespiratory fitness in stroke survivors can reduce the physiologic burden of performing BADL and IADL, thus increasing the likelihood that individuals with stroke will be able to perform a greater volume of daily physical activity. Thirty to 60 minutes a day most days of the week is ideal, but if the individual has substantial barriers to participating in physical activity or has certain health limitations (3), a lower intensity, duration, and frequency of exercise is also beneficial since most stroke survivors are severely deconditioned. High-risk individuals with cardiopulmonary disease or increased risk of falls should exercise under the supervision of a qualified staff person, preferably trained in rehabilitation or clinical exercise physiology. Whenever possible, the intensity level of the exercise should be derived from a graded exercise test.

Examples of cardiovascular training modalities for stroke survivors include stationary cycling (recumbent and upright), over-ground supervised walking or walking on a treadmill (with or without harness support), elliptical cross-training, and recumbent stepping.

The National Center on Physical Activity and Disability has produced a home exercise video for persons with stroke that includes cardiorespiratory, strength and flexibility exercises. The video can be found at www.ncpad.org or by calling their toll-free number (800-900-8086). Other ideas for home exercise can be found on this website.

Strength

A general strength training prescription for persons with stroke should use a minimum of one set of 8–10 reps (two to three sets in clients with better health and fitness) with lighter weights and higher repetitions. The recommended frequency is 2–3 days a week. Blood pressure and RPE should be recorded at the completion of each set in clients with hypertension. Adaptive mitts or wrist cuffs (Figures 9.2) or other assistive devices may be necessary to ensure that the participant can safely hold or grasp the weight.

Flexibility

Flexibility exercises are useful for persons with stroke in allowing them greater range of motion while performing BADL or IADL. Participants should be taught a variety of stretching exercises targeting both the upper and lower trunk. Emphasis should be placed on any tight musculature, especially on the hemiparetic side, in persons with unilateral stroke. Stretching the hamstrings can be performed by having the person sitting in a chair and reaching down to touch his or her toes. Arm stretches can be performed by having the participant reach over the head and touch the opposite shoulder.

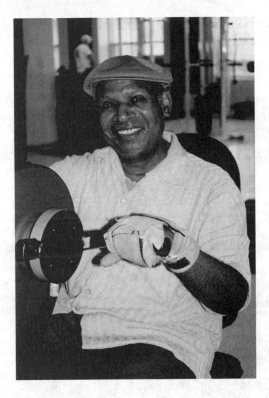

Figure 9.2. Commercial adaptive mitt to keep hand attached to exercise device.

Traumatic Brain Injury

Several studies have reported that people with traumatic brain injury (TBI) are more likely to be sedentary, have greater health problems, and experience substantially more barriers to physical activity participation compared to the general population (6). Deconditioning exacerbates the physical and cognitive limitations that many people with TBI experience, and persons with moderate to severe TBI may have a low tolerance for physical activity and become easily fatigued. Unfortunately, as physical activities are eliminated from their daily routine, the ability to perform equal or greater amounts of activity declines even further for this population. As a result of these limitations, people with TBI often find it difficult to function within their community.

Mental health problems, including depression and psychosocial issues (e.g., decreased self-esteem, limited social networking) can also prove to be considerable physical activity barriers for persons with TBI. Social isolation exacerbates such problems, and the challenges of community reentry (e.g., joining an exercise class) after a TBI are substantial. The exercise prescription will be largely dependent on the level of cognitive function. Some individuals may require full or partial supervision during exercise, while others may be able to participate independently. Duration and intensity are generally not as important for individuals with TBI as frequency of training. The critical feature of the program is to maintain some sense of regularity to a prescribed training regimen. Having the person exercise in a community setting such as a YMCA may be an effective way to enhance socialization.

Patient Safety

Patient safety is a key component of any exercise program. Adults with neurologic disabilities pose unique challenges and risks during exercise, and vigilance on the part of clinicians is warranted to minimize harm and maximize benefits. Tables 9.2 and 9.3 provide an overview of some patient safety principles.

Patient Education

Patients should be educated about the benefits and risks of exercising as well as principles of exercising safely within the limitations imposed by their neurologic disabilities. They should also be educated on exercise techniques and equipment that minimize the risk of injuries. Patients should be taught to avoid exercising to the point of fatigue, during an acute illness, or in extremes of temperature.

Exercise and Disability Resource Center

The National Center on Physical Activity and Disability (www.ncpad.org) provides information on exercise for people with disabilities. This information and resource center offers clinicians the latest information on fitness, recreation, and sports programs for people with disabilities. For clinicians who have questions related to a specific disability, information specialists are available during work hours to answer questions (800-900-8086). The Center also publishes a free monthly electronic newsletter. Clinicians or individuals with neurologic disability can subscribe to a listserv and receive this information for free by calling the hotline or by emailing staff at ncpad@uic.edu.

ACKNOWLEDGMENT

This work was supported by the National Institute on Disability and Rehabilitation Research, Rehabilitation Engineering Center on Recreational Technologies and Exercise Physiology for People with Disabilities, H133E070029.

Table 9.2

General Patient Safety Issues for Aerobic Training in Individuals with Neurologic Disability

- Vital signs (e.g., blood pressure, heart rate) must be in prescribed range based on patients' typical baseline measures. *Note*: Patients taking β-blockers and those with autonomic dysfunction can have a blunted heart rate response. In these instances consider using the rating of perceived exertion (RPE) scale.
- Blood pressure should be measured before exercise to ensure that it is in a typical range for the patient; every 10 minutes during exercise; and immediately following exercise.
- External temperature must be carefully monitored to avoid hyper- or hypothermia in persons with SCI and MS who may have thermoregulatory issues.
- Clients with balance difficulties who present a high risk of falls should use a sitting modality such as the recumbent stepper or stationary or recumbent cycle.
- When using a treadmill for training purposes, a body weight–supported harness is recommended for clients with balance difficulties.
- The participant should not feel overly fatigued or have any pain or discomfort after the exercise session.
- Avoid overuse injuries by varying exercise routine (e.g., cross-training with various types of equipment) and using equipment safely. Participant should have good posture and body mechanics while performing the exercise routine.
- Balance should be assessed before implementing standing activities (e.g., weight routine, aerobic dance class).
- In persons with SCI above T6, avoid autonomic dysreflexia by ensuring that bladder and bowel are voided prior to exercise and that there is no urinary outflow obstruction.

Table 9.3

General Patient Safety Issues for Strength Training in Individuals with Neurologic Disability

- Co-contraction may offset strength in tested muscle groups (agonists).
- Measure range of motion (ROM) in tested muscle groups to allow muscle group to move through available ROM.
- Test muscle groups unilaterally (may be more spasticity on one side).
- Focus on stability, coordination, ROM, and timing.
- Wide benches, low seats, and trunk and pelvic strapping will help support and protect the person from injury during the exercise routine.
- Machines are safer than free weights and provide greater "fluidity" to the movement.
- Use nonslip handgrips and gloves (if necessary).
- Avoid "hiking" the body on weak side.
- Avoid person holding breath while lifting weight (e.g., Valsalva maneuver)
- Use straps whenever necessary to keep body part in contact or alignment while lifting weight.

REFERENCES

1. Rimmer JH. Exercise and physical activity in persons aging with a physical disability. Phys Med Rehabil Clin N Am Feb 2005; 16(1):41–56.

2. Haskell WL, Lee I-Min, Pate RR, et al. Physical activity and public health: updated recommendation for adults from the American College of Sports Medicine and the American Heart Association. Med Sci Sports Exerc 2007; 39:1423–1434.

3. Rimmer JH. The conspicuous absence of people with disabilities in public fitness and recreation facilities: lack of interest or lack of access? Am J Health Promot 2005; 19:327–329.

4. American College of Sports Medicine. ACSM's Guidelines for Exercise Testing and Prescription, 7th ed. Baltimore: Lippincott Williams & Wilkins; 2006.

5. Jacobs P, Nash MS. Exercise recommendations for individuals with spinal cord injury. Sports Med 2004; 34:727–751.

6. Driver S, Rees K, O'Connor J, et al. Aquatics, health-promoting self-care behaviors and adults with brain injuries. Brain Inj 2006; 20:133–141.

10 | Fatigue

Brian D. Greenwald
David L. Ripley

Fatigue is a commonly reported symptom after traumatic brain injury (TBI), stroke, spinal cord injury (SCI), and in persons living with multiple sclerosis (MS). Fatigue compounds underlying impairments for all these neurologic disabilities. It can also lead to greater unemployment, handicap, and lower life satisfaction. Medical literature generally defines fatigue as overwhelming sense of tiredness, lack of energy, and feeling of exhaustion. Although there is no universally accepted definition for fatigue, there is a general distinction between central and peripheral fatigue.

Central fatigue results from dysfunction of the supratentorial structure involved in performing cognitive tasks. The inability to maintain focused attention is a key component of central fatigue since focused attention is necessary to incorporate the mental, physical, and sensory inputs involved in completing a task. Once focused attention is impaired, then integrating the various types of information needed to complete a task becomes more difficult and requires greater effort to complete.

Peripheral fatigue can be physical, metabolic, or peripheral in origin. This is most commonly expressed in musculoskeletal symptoms that impair mobility or in reduced exercise tolerance.

In persons with TBI and stroke, central fatigue predominates, whereas fatigue complaints are often mixed in SCI and MS. In evaluating patients with complaints of fatigue, differentiating between physical and cognitive fatigue is an initial step.

Fatigue is reported to be almost ubiquitous in individuals with neurologic disorders. Estimates of the range of the problem depend somewhat on the specific neurologic disorder in question and the study cited. Additionally, the definition of fatigue tends to vary from study to study, and this may account for some of the variability. Regardless, a general concept is that fatigue is an extremely common problem associated with neurologic disorders, is reported with significantly higher frequency than in the general population, and may significantly affect an individual's return to independent living.

One interesting concept regarding fatigue is that people with neurologic disorders report characteristic differences between what the general population describes as fatigue and what people with neurologic disorders describe as fatigue. One important concept is that the fatigue experienced by individuals with neurologic disorders does not respond to rest or sleep. This implies that the fatigue is characteristically different from what the average population describes as fatigue. This phenomenon becomes extremely important when performing research on the topic. In other words, the standard measures developed for fatigue in the general population may not accurately measure what individuals with neurologic disorders are experiencing as fatigue.

An excellent review article was published by de Groot, Phillips, and Eskes on fatigue associated with cerebrovascular accident. The frequency of fatigue reported after CVA ranges from 30 to 68% (1). Fatigue is reported both in the acute phase and the late phase after stroke. Ingles et al. found that fatigue problems, measured by the fatigue impact scale, were reported in 68% of subjects between 3 and 13 months after stroke, compared to 36% of age-matched control subjects (2). Two years poststroke 51% of survivors have elevated scores on the fatigue subscale of the Checklist Individual Strength compared to 12% of control subjects, and 50% report that fatigue is their main complaint. Of stroke survivors, 39.2% experience significant fatigue independent of reports of depression. In addition, the frequency of fatigue associated with clinically relevant depression was found to be 67% in individuals who had strokes at least 7 years earlier.

Fatigue is also a more commonly recognized problem following TBI. Additionally, prior studies suggest that the level of fatigue is not necessarily associated with severity or type of brain injury. In one study, as many as 70% of patients with mild TBI reported to have clinically significant levels of fatigue. For more severe brain injuries, 84% reported fatigue at a 6-week follow-up visit. The fatigue experienced by this population is also reported to occur chronically. In one study, subjects reported significantly more fatigue than control subjects at a mean of 44.3 months following their injury. Finally, patients also report that fatigue is one of the more troublesome complaints. In this study, 50% of subjects reported that fatigue was their most troublesome symptom after TBI.

Fatigue in SCI appears to be more related to the physical strength required to perform an activity. Individuals with SCI in general do not report the same types of cognitive fatigue that are reported in other diagnoses of central origin. However, physical fatigue remains a significant problem. In general, this seems to be more of an issue in the early recovery period after SCI. Patients report less fatigue as they become more accommodated to their condition and their physical endurance improves. Additionally, there seems to be a direct correlation between the level of injury and the reports of fatigue, as in general, individuals with higher levels of SCI report more significant problems with fatigue. Correlation with completeness of injury, or ASIA Classification Score, has not been studied.

Fatigue is also one of the more common complaints of patients with multiple sclerosis. Up to 70% of subjects reported significant fatigue, and, of those, 33–40% described it as problematic or severe. Fatigue may be characteristically different in patients with MS compared to other neurologic populations, as it is noted to be not relieved by rest or sleep. Additionally, fatigue in MS is often worsened by things that do not appear to worsen fatigue in other populations, such as stress or increases in temperature. Individuals with MS will frequently report that the energy required to perform various activities, both cognitive and physical, is often greater than what they believe the task should demand.

The goal of this chapter is to provide the reader with an overview of the etiology, assessment, and treatment of this common symptom in adults with neurologic disabilities.

ANATOMY AND PHYSIOLOGY

The basal ganglia has been implicated as the neuroanatomic site at which fatigue is generated after a neurologic injury. Injury to the dopaminergic pathways may disrupt or delay execution of motor tasks. Neuroimaging after TBI has revealed more dispersed cerebral activation than would be expected for a simple task, indicating that an increased level of cortical activation may be necessary. This may place the brain under a higher level of metabolic stress, which in turn may cause central fatigue.

In the MS population recent reports have indicated that fatigue is related to hypometabolism in certain brain areas and has also been related to axonal damage and brain atrophy. EEG has shown cortical desynchronization, which can be an indicator of cortical dysfunction in fatigued MS patients (3). Depression and physical fatigue have also been shown contribute to contribute to cognitive fatigue (4).

It is also important to differentiate between primary and secondary causes for fatigue. Primary fatigue is caused by the neurologic disorder, whereas secondary fatigue can be due to multiple factors such as anemia, lack of conditioning, depression, side effects of medications, infection, endocrine dysfunction, or sleep disturbance (Table 10.1).

PATIENT ASSESSMENT

In the assessment of fatigue, the clinician should attempt to differentiate between central and peripheral origins as well as primary versus secondary causes. Central fatigue questioning and examination typically focus on fatigue when attempting to perform cognitive tasks that require one or more steps. Peripheral fatigue questions focus on fatigue with physical activities such as walking or lifting. In assessing for secondary causes of fatigue, questioning about current medications, difficulties sleeping, and depression can yield useful information.

Table 10.1

Underlying Causes of Fatigue

- Infectious
- Sleep disorders
- Endocrine—hypothyroidism
    Anterior pituitary dysfunction
    Hypogonadism
    Growth hormone deficiency
    Adrenal insufficiency
- Infections
- Rheumatologic diseases
- Cardiac diseases
- Renal and liver diseases
- Pulmonary diseases
- Psychiatric—depression, anxiety
- Hematologic—anemia, cancer

Many medications can cause fatigue as a side effect. Examples are listed in Table 10.2. Onset of fatigue after starting a medication, checking serum levels of some medications, and review of medications for interactions should be a part of the evaluation of fatigue.

Evaluation for sleep disturbance is a core component in evaluating the etiology of fatigue. High rates of sleep disturbance have been associated with all

Table 10.2

Patient Assessment of Fatigue

- Mental fatigue: fatigue with cognitive tasks
- Physical fatigue: fatigue with walking, lifting, and other physical activities of daily living
- Assess for depression
- Sleep dysfunction—difficulty falling asleep, staying asleep, nightmares
- Infection: fever, chills, sweats, urinary symptoms
- Weight loss, loss of appetite; symptoms suggestive of underlying malignancy
- Pulmonary symptoms—shortness of breath, wheezing, productive cough
- Medication review for side effects and drug–drug interactions
- Drug classes associated with fatigue:
    o Antispasticity agents
    o Analgesics
    o Anticonvulsants
    o Antihistamines
    o Anti-inflammatories
    o Antipsychotics
    o Antidepressants
    o Muscle relaxants
    o Gastrointestinal drugs

neurologic disabilities, although for varying reasons. Management of sleep impairment through sleep hygiene, treatment of comorbid illness or through pharmacology can decrease fatigue. See Chapter 28 on sleep disorders for additional information.

Depression is often associated with disturbances in sleep, appetite, and concentration as well as fatigue. When one symptom predominates, management should be tailored to treat that symptom along with the depression. Examples include using Trazodone with sleep initiation with depression and using stimulants when fatigue or impaired concentration predominates.

Hematologic, infectious, endocrine, cardiac, rheumatologic, and metabolic causes of fatigue should be considered. A history and physical examination will help guide the workup, but laboratory testing for metabolic and endocrine function should be standard.

Anterior pituitary dysfunction has been documented after TBI, stroke, SCI, and MS. Endocrine dysfunction has been shown to be as high as 59% after TBI (5). Growth hormone deficiency and hypogonadism are associated with decreased bone mineral densities, aerobic capacity, muscle strength, lower quality of life, and cognitive impairments as well as fatigue (6). Basic screening for endocrine dysfunction should include a thyroid panel, A.M. cortisol, testosterone, follicle-stimulating hormone (FSH) and luteinizing hormone (LH) as appropriate, and insulin-like growth factor (IGF)-1 as a marker of growth hormone. This topic is further discussed elsewhere in this book. Understanding of the relationship between fatigue and neuroendocrine dysfunction is still evolving.

To understand the magnitude and impact of fatigue, several scales are available. Some of the more commonly used scales include the Fatigue Severity Scale (FSS) (Table 10.3), the Fatigue Impact Scale (FIS), and the Modified Fatigue Impact Scale (MFIS). The FSS has the patient answer nine different questions rating different components of fatigue 1 to 7 and then the score is averaged.

Table 10.3

Fatigue Severity Scale

Each statement is rated 1 to 7: 1 indicates strong disagreement and 7 indicates strong agreement.
1. My motivation is lower when I am fatigued.
2. Exercise brings on my fatigue.
3. I am easily fatigued.
4. Fatigue interferes with my physical functioning.
5. Fatigue causes frequent problems for me.
6. My fatigue prevents sustained physical functioning.
7. Fatigue interferes with carrying out certain duties and responsibilities.
8. Fatigue is among my three most disabling symptoms.
9. Fatigue interferes with my work, family, or social life.

Source: Ref. 12.

People with depression alone score about 4.5. But people with fatigue related to MS average about 6.5. The FIS is a 40-item questionnaire that separates functional categories into physical, cognitive, and psychosocial sections. Each question is rated 1 to 4. The MFIS is a 21-item derivative and has most frequently been used in the MS population.

TREATMENT

The treatment of fatigue can be broadly divided into pharmacologic and non-pharmacologic interventions. These are discussed below.

Medications for Fatigue

Several classes of medications have been demonstrated to be effective for the treatment of fatigue after neurologic disease or injury. Primary among these are the classic neurostimulants, other wakefulness-promoting agents, and antidepressants (discussed in greater detail elsewhere in this book). Many anecdotal reports exist for other medications for fatigue. However, as with most issues regarding the pharmacologic treatment of symptoms following neurologic disorders, there is scant objective research studying effects of these medications on fatigue. The information below is not intended to be a comprehensive list, but rather to offer some "broad" information about typical prescribing practices for this problem.

The classic neurostimulants are probably the most widely studied medications for fatigue following a multitude of disorders, including cancer, TBI, and stroke. In a comparison study with sertraline, methylphenidate was found to be more efficacious for daytime sleepiness on the Epworth Sleepiness scale (7). Other neurostimulants that have been used clinically include dextroamphetamine, pemoline, and mixed amphetamine-dextroamphetamine salts. Most of these medications have broad effects on increasing the activity of, or stimulating receptors of, endogenous adrenergic or cholinergic receptors. This has a general effect on the patient's subjective feeling of wakefulness and may also have other cognitive effects, such as improving attention and concentration.

Modafinil has been widely used as an agent to combat fatigue. Modafinil is an agent indicated for the treatment of narcolepsy and daytime somnolence. Although anecdotal reports suggest that it is helpful in treating fatigue, a controlled study by Jha et al. failed to show consistent patterns of relief of fatigue in a brain-injured population (8). However, this remains a widely used drug for the treatment of fatigue in stroke, TBI, and MS.

Dopaminergic medications, especially amantadine, have been utilized as medications for arousal following TBI, MS, and stroke. In the MS population, amantadine has garnered the most research attention and has been shown to be clinically effective in combating fatigue when compared to placebo (9).

Traditional antidepressant medications, especially selective serotonin reuptake inhibitors (SSRIs), have also been medications of interest. Paroxetine has been reported as an agent to combat fatigue following TBI, MS, and stroke. However, its use has not been strongly identified for the treatment of fatigue in the absence of depressive symptoms.

The tricyclic antidepressants, especially amitriptyline, have also been reported to be effective for fatigue, although the effects noted are more likely a result of improved sleep patterns and decreased vegetative symptoms of depression, rather than relief from primary effects of fatigue. Like Paroxetine, their use to treat fatigue in the absence of depression has not been formally assessed. Due to their propensity to cause increased confusion, use of tricyclic antidepressants in patients with cognitive impairment must be done carefully, and routine use in this population is not typically recommended.

Atomoxetine is an agent that has also been promoted as a medication for arousal. Although most clinicians would associate this medication with the traditional neurostimulant medications, it technically is more similar pharmacologically to the antidepressant drugs. While no study has been done to evaluate its effects as a medication for combating fatigue, anecdotal reports suggest that it may have a beneficial effect at higher doses (10).

Recent research has focused on endocrine abnormalities, especially growth hormone deficiency, as a potential cause for fatigue following TBI. However, the research has had mixed results. To date, a controlled study evaluating the effects of growth hormone replacement therapy on fatigue has not been completed.

Many herbal preparations have been promoted for use in fatigue. Among these are Ginkgo biloba, St. John's wort, and Panax ginseng. Caffeine, also potentially considered an herbal remedy due to its widespread over-the-counter use and presence in multiple beverages, has also been promoted as an agent to combat fatigue, both in its typical liquid form and as a tablet. Other herbal medications that have reported use in combating fatigue are covered in greater detail elsewhere in this book.

Exercise and Fatigue

Exercise training is a promising strategy for decreasing both physical and cognitive fatigue in persons with neurologic disorders. Aerobic exercise has been shown to improve cognition and mood in the general population. Cognitive functioning demonstrated improvement on neuropsychological tests for those individuals who were aerobically trained compared to those who received strength and flexibility training, as well as those who did not exercise. Although research examining the effects of aerobic exercise in individuals with TBI is limited, exercise has been shown to be effective in improving cognition and depression in individuals with cancer, MS, fibromyalgia, dementia, chronic fatigue syndrome, and chronic obstructive pulmonary disease. Aerobic training has been found to improve fitness and improve factors related to quality of life. In addition, studies have found aquatic therapy to result in strength gains.

Aerobic exercise training has also been shown to be associated with a higher quality of life in persons with MS (11). However, caution must be taken when prescribing physical activity to MS patients. Symptoms can temporarily be worsened on exposure to heat or during physical exercise. Exercise programs need to be designed to activate working muscles but avoid overload. Exercise evaluation and prescription must account for fatigue, spasticity, ataxia, and impaired coordination. Emphasis should be on maintenance of function with evaluation of decreasing general debility. Maximizing passive and active range of motion is critical to any muscular fitness program. Programs should be tailored to the variety of neurologic deficits seen in MS. The subject of exercise is covered in greater detail elsewhere in this book.

Cognitive behavioral therapy which is based on teaching patients how to manage thought and behaviors that contribute to depression as well as problem solving has been successful in decreasing fatigue.

Patient Safety

It is important to evaluate for secondary causes for fatigue. These can include:
1. Medication side effects
2. Depression
3. Endocrine dysfunction
4. Hematologic/oncologic
5. Infections.
6. Sleep dysfunction
7. Cardiac, pulmonary, rheumatologic, renal, and hepatic diseases

Patient Education

Patients should be educated on the underlying cause of the fatigue and its potential impact on the patient. The patient and the caregiver should be educated on coping strategies for fatigue:
1. Take frequent rests
2. Break up tasks
3. Don't do more than one task at a time.
4. Focus on completing tasks rather than on completing tasks quickly.
5. Know warning signs of fatigue-irritability, making mistakes.
6. Know side effects of medications.
7. Don't operate heavy equipment or drive when tired.

REFERENCES

1. De Groot MH, Phillips SJ, Eskes GA. Fatigue associated with stroke and other neurological conditions: implications for stroke rehabilitation. Arch Phys Med Rehabil 2003; 84:1714–1720.

2. Ingles JL, Eskes GA, Phillips SJ. Fatigue after stroke. Arch Phys Med Rehabil 1999; 80:173–178.

3. Zwarts MJ, Bleijenberg G, van Engelen BGM. Clinical neurophysiology of fatigue. Clin Neurophysiol 2008; 119:2–10.

4. Krupp LB, Christodoulou C. Fatigue in multiple sclerosis. Curr Neurol Neurosci Rep 2001; 1(3):294–298.

5. Bushnik T, Englander J, Katznelson L. Fatigue after TBI: association with neuroendocrine abnormalities. Brain Inj 2007; 21(6):559–566.

6. Kelly DF, McArthur DL, Levin H, et al. Neurobehavioral and quality of life changes associated with growth hormone insufficiency after complicated mild, moderate, or severe traumatic brain injury. J Neurotrauma 2006; 23(6):928–942.

7. Lee H, Kim SW, Kim JM, Shin IS, Yang SJ, Yoon JS. Comparing effects of methylphenidate, sertraline and placebo on neuropsychiatric sequelae in patients with traumatic brain injury. Hum Psychopharmacol 2005; 20(2):97–104.

8. Jha A, Weintraub A, Allshouse A, et al. A randomized trial of Modafinil for the treatment of fatigue and excessive daytime sleepiness in individuals with chronic traumatic brain injury. J Head Trauma Rehabil 2008; 23(1):52–63.

9. Pucci E, Branãs P, D'Amico R, Giuliani G, Solari A, Taus C. Amantadine for fatigue in multiple sclerosis. Cochrane Database Syst Rev 2007; (1):CD002818.

10. Ripley DL. Atomoxetine for individuals with traumatic brain injury. J Head Trauma Rehabil 2006; 21(1):85–88.

11. Motyl RW, Gosney JL. Effect of exercise training on quality of life in multiple sclerosis: a meta- analysis. Multiple Sclerosis 2008; 14:129–135.

12. Krupp LB, LaRocca NG, Muir-Nash J, Steinberg AD. The fatigue severity scale. Application to patients with multiple sclerosis and systemic lupus erythematosis. Arch Neurol 1989; 46:1121–1123.

11 | Gastrointestinal Diseases

Ashwani K. Singal
Naomi Betesh
Mark A. Korsten

The gastrointestinal (GI) system is under the control of GI hormones and autonomic and somatic nerves. The latter, in turn, are controlled by the higher neurologic centers. The GI system, therefore, is often altered in patients with neurologic diseases. Indeed, GI problems can be expected in patients suffering from upper motor neuron (UMN) lesions (dementia, stroke, traumatic brain injury, Parkinson's disease, spinal cord injury [SCI], and multiple sclerosis [MS]) and lower motor neuron (LMN) lesions (cauda equina injury, diabetic neuropathy, and other peripheral neuropathies) (1).

Management of GI problems in patients with neurologic diseases is complex and challenging. The occurrence of GI symptoms in these patients increases their debilitation and frustration. With the loss of ability to perceive sensations, the presentation of GI problems can be quite different from that in able-bodied (AB) individuals. Furthermore, significant cognitive dysfunction in patients with brain involvement is a barrier to patient education and with aging many of these patients will have age-related changes in the GI function as well. Collectively, these factors complicate the management of GI symptoms. In this chapter we will approach the management of GI problems in patients with neurologic diseases with the aim of helping physicians and staff working in rehabilitation units and nursing homes to identify and adequately address these problems.

Bowel problems have been reported to be present in 66% of adults living with SCI (1). The prevalence of GI dysfunction in patients with MS is 41–68%, with 36–43% complaining of constipation (2). Individuals with strokes often have chronic constipation or fecal incontinence. In one study, chronic constipation occurred in 30% of neurologically stable hemiplegic patients after stroke (3). The onset of constipation was independent of injured hemisphere and physical activity. In the Copenhagen Stroke Study, age, history of diabetes, lesion size, comorbidities, and stroke severity increased the risk of fecal incontinence. Individuals with traumatic brain injury also have a high incidence of fecal incontinence (3). In one study, using data from the Traumatic Brain Injury Model Systems National Database, the incidence of fecal incontinence was 68% at admission to an inpatient reha-bilitation, 12.4% at the time of discharge from rehabilitation units, and 5.2% at 1-year follow-up (4).

ANATOMY AND PHYSIOLOGY

The colon is a closed tube with the ileocecal valve and the internal anal sphinc-ter (IAS) at the proximal and distal ends, respectively. Coordinated colonic contractions help in the absorption of water, propagation of undigested food, and defecation. These contractions are accomplished by autonomic (parasym-pathetic and sympathetic) and somatic (sensory and motor) nerves innervating the colon (Figure 11.1).

These form the enteric nervous system (ENS) together with Auerbach's (between muscle layers of the colon) and Meissner's (submucosal) plexuses. The parasympathetic nerve supply (mediated via the vagus on the right side and S2–4 spinal segments on the left side) is the most important innervation for colonic motility and contractions. These, in turn are controlled and regulated by the higher centers in the brain and spinal cord.

Defecation is the process for expulsion of feces and is under voluntary con-trol. Continence is maintained by the sphincters (internal anal sphincter [IAS]

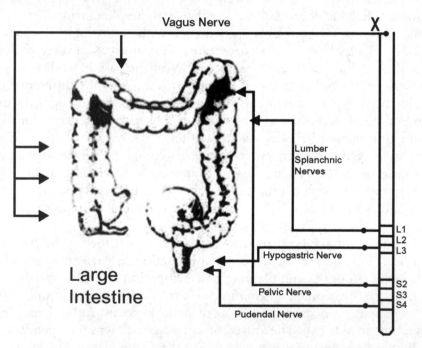

Figure 11.1. Extrinsic innervation of the large intestine. The vagus (X) nerve innervates the right colon while propulsive activity in the left colon is mediated by the parasympathetic (pel-vic) nerves. Sympathetic innervation (L1–3) via the splanchnic nerves and hypogastric nerves is inhibitory. The anal canal is innervated by voluntary efferent motor fibers to the external anal sphincter via the pudendal nerve from the sacral spinal cord (S2–4). (From Ref. 5.)

and external anal sphincter [EAS]) and puborectalis muscle. The IAS is a high-pressure zone maintained by sympathetic nerves and is inhibited by the stools entering the rectum. Voluntary relaxation of the EAS and puborectalis muscle combined with increased intra-abdominal pressure and continued peristalsis results in defecation.

Patients with neurologic diseases have impaired motility of the colon resulting in GI symptoms such as constipation (fewer than three bowel movements per week), DWE (constipation with prolonged bowel care time and abdominal bloating), and incontinence (1). Individuals with UMN lesions (above conus medularis or T10 vertebral segment) have a hyperreflexic bowel with spastic EAS and pelvic floor muscles. As the spinal reflexes remain intact, stool can be propelled by reflex activity such as digital rectal stimulation (DRS), mini-enemas, Valsalva maneuver, and abdominal belt. Overflow incontinence can occur due to an inability to perceive sensations of rectal fullness with feces. In contrast, in individuals with LMN (below conus medularis or T10 vertebral level), the bowel is areflexic. Both the colon and EAS are flaccid. With the loss of spinal reflexes, manual evacuation is frequently required. It is important to keep the stool firm as incontinence is a major and often an embarrassing feature due to the lax EAS. In addition, patients with neurogenic bowel are prone to complications, namely autonomic dysreflexia and fecal impaction (Table 11.1).

PATIENT ASSESSMENT

To improve the quality of life of individuals with neurologic bowel, an effective bowel management is essential. Good bowel care should achieve complete stool evacuation but avoid the hazard of incontinence. Before starting the bowel regimen, it is essential to obtain a complete history and perform a thorough physical examination (Table 11.2). In addition, laboratory evaluation should be carried out including complete blood count, basic metabolic panel, and serum amylase or lipase. Plain x-ray of the abdomen should be obtained to rule out fecal impaction.

TREATMENT

There is no fixed regimen for managing neurogenic bowel. Instead, it must be tailored to personal factors such as cognitive status, functional ability, and social support (1). It is important to determine whether the patient can learn and/or perform the bowel care on his own or needs assistance. Ideally, bowel care should be performed in the natural position and environment. This may require adaptation of the home environment to improve access to the toilet as well as use of special chairs and equipment to assist in transferring the patient. Left lateral position is used if the bowel care is given in the bed. If the patient is mobile during the day, it is better to schedule the regimen in the morning to prevent bowel accidents during the day. It is recommended to drink at least

Table 11.1

Gastrointestinal Problems in Patients with Neurologic Diseases

Oral cavity and esophagus
- Gastroesophageal reflux disease (GERD)
- Esophageal perforation
- Tartar and dental caries

Stomach
- Stress ulcers
- Peptic ulcers
- Acute gastric dilatation
- Incomplete gastric emptying and gastric stasis
- Superior mesenteric artery syndrome

Biliary tract and pancreas
- Acute pancreatitis
- Cholelithiasis

Small bowel
- Adynamic ileus
- Pseudo-obstruction

Neurogenic bowel
- Spastic or hyperreflexic bowel (UMN lesion)
- Flaccid or areflexic bowel (LMN lesion)

Complications of neurogenic bowel
- Fecal impaction
- Autonomic dysreflexia
- Sigmoid volvulus
- Pseudo-obstruction

UMN, upper motor neuron; LMN, lower motor neuron.

2–3 liters of fluids and ingest 10–15 g of fiber every day in the diet (5). This is particularly important in the elderly with poor dietary intake. Fiber helps to retain water, making the stool softer and more bulky.

Associated comorbidities, such as hypokalemia, hypercalcemia, thyroid function, and blood sugar, should be adequately controlled. Congestive heart failure, which is quite prevalent in the elderly, may cause bowel edema and exacerbate their symptoms. The physician treating these patients should avoid medications that can have a negative impact on the colonic motility. These include anticholinergics, tricyclic antidepressants, opiates, antiparkinsonian drugs, calcium channel blockers, iron, calcium, and aluminum containing antacids.

As patients with UMN lesions have intact spinal reflexes, measures that can stimulate these reflexes may be added to the above measures to achieve efficacy. These include digital rectal stimulation (DRS), abdominal belt or massage, Valsalva maneuver, leaning forward, and use of warm fluids before the bowel regimen. DRS should be gentle using a well-lubricated gloved finger, and Valsalva maneuver should be avoided in patients with cardiac disease (6).

Table 11.2

History and Physical Examination in Patients with Spinal Cord Injury

History taking
- Details of neurologic disease such as level and completeness of lesion, etiology of SCI, and duration of SCI
- Current dietary intake specifically regarding fluids and fiber
- Premorbid bowel habits
- Patient's occupation and social mobility
- Comorbidities liable to affect GI function such as diabetes mellitus, thyroid disease, celiac disease, irritable bowel syndrome, lactose intolerance, and inflammatory bowel disease
- Current medications, both prescribed as well as over the counter

Physical examination
- General physical examination should focus on vital signs, nutritional and hydration status, and pressure ulcers
- Careful examination of the abdomen for distension, visible peristalsis, presence of percutaneous gastrostomy tube or suprapubic catheter, quality of bowel sounds, tenderness, rigidity, palpable masses or fecoliths, or organomegaly
- Rectal examination should assess for fecal impaction, sphincter tone, masses, and stool guiac for occult blood
- Neurologic examination for cognitive status of the patient, extremity strength and transfer skills, fine motor skills, sensations, coordination and balance, and gait

Pharmacologic interventions are used if the above-mentioned general measures are ineffective. Of the various laxatives, oral agents such as docusate and lactulose are commonly used. Administration of laxatives may be timed based on the knowledge of onset of action of various laxatives (Table 11.3) and the time at which bowel movement is desired. Enemas are recommended for fecal impaction but are not routinely used.

In intractable cases, surgical options such as sacral posterior rhizotomy, sacral anterior nerve root stimulation, appendectomy, antegrade continent enema of Malone (MACE), and colostomy may be useful (5). Colostomy has been shown to produce improvement in the patient's symptoms and quality of life, prevention of fecal incontinence, simplification of bowel care, and better healing of pressure ulcers (5). Studying the transit time of the colon is useful in deciding the site of colostomy in these individuals. Apart from the technique and selection of proper site, timing of surgery is important for a positive outcome. Patients should be in otherwise good health and have an optimal nutritional status prior to surgery.

Whether these patients are at increased risk for colorectal cancer (CRC) is not clearly known. Indications for CRC screening in patients with neurologic diseases are similar to those in able-bodied individuals. These include all individuals greater than 50 years of age. However, in those with a family history of CRC, screening should be performed 10 years earlier than the age of diagnosis in the family member or at age 50, whichever is earlier. Repeat

Table 11.3

Pharmacological Agents Used in Bowel Care

Medication	Dose	Onset of action (hr)
Bulk laxatives		
• Docusate sodium	100–300 mg daily once or in divided doses	12–72
• Psyllium	1 tsp (3.6 g of fiber) 1–2 times a day	12–72
Stimulant laxatives		
• Senna	15–30 mg orally, maximum 60 mg/day	6–12
• Bisacodyl tablet	5–15 mg orally	6–12
• Bisacodyl suppository	10 mg per rectum	0.25–1
• Castor oil	15–60 ml daily	6–8
• Cascara	1–2 tablets daily (325 mg tablet)	6–8
Saline laxatives		
• Magnesium hydroxide	15–30 ml 1–2 times a day	0.5–6
• Sodium phosphate	45–90 ml once a day orally or 45 ml rectal enema	0.5–6
Hyperosmolar laxatives		
• Lactulose	15–60 ml 1–3 times a day	0.5–3
• Sorbitol 70%	15–60 ml 1–3 times a day	0.5–3
• Polyethylene glycol	17 g in 8 oz of water 12 times a day	0.5–3

colonoscopy is done after 10 years if the initial examination is normal. Testing for occult blood in the stool is not helpful since it may be positive due to a higher frequency of hemorrhoids and anal fissures in these patients. Instead, colonoscopy is the ideal tool for CRC screening in these individuals. However, limitations to the use of colonoscopy include: 1) colonic inertia—with long and redundant colon, 2) ineffective bowel preparation, 3) the possibility of inducing autonomic dysreflexia during colonoscopy, particularly in patients with cardiopulmonary disease. These features pose technical difficulties and can lead to incomplete examination with higher chances of missing lesions (7,8).

Dysphagia

Patients with dementia, multiple strokes, pseudo-bulbar palsy, Parkinson's disease, and motor neuron disease often lose innervation of the esophagus with weakness of the pharyngeal muscles and the upper esophageal sphincter. This results in difficulty in the transfer of the food bolus from the mouth to the pharynx and esophagus (oropharyngeal dysphagia) with subsequent nutritional deficiencies and morbidity.

Gastroesophageal Reflux Disease (GERD)

The cause of the increased prevalence of GERD in patients with neurologic diseases is multifactorial (9). Prolonged stays in bed in the supine position increase the risk of GERD. Increased abdominal pressure in patients with severe constipation adds to reflux of gastric contents. Moreover, some of the medications commonly used in patients with neurologic diseases such as antidepressants, benzodiazepines, opioids, and medications with anticholinergic side effects can aggravate GERD. The characteristic symptom of GERD in able-bodied individuals is heartburn. Due to loss of sensations, patients with neurologic illness above the T7 level may not report heartburn and present with atypical features such as water brash (an acidic taste in mouth) or with complications of GERD such as GI bleeding due to Barrett's ulcer or dysphagia due to peptic stricture. Once the disease is identified, patients are treated with proton pump inhibitors (PPIs). Esophago-gastro-duodenoscopic (EGD) examination is indicated if patients do not improve with PPIs or have complications of GERD.

Stress and Peptic Ulcers

During the acute phase of the neurologic illness or injury, the stomach is prone to ulceration due to either gastric ischemia or imbalance in autonomic innervation (parasympathetic excess). In one study, stress ulcers were seen in 75–100% of patients with head trauma on an EGD performed within 72 hours of the injury (10). Ulcers after a few days of the injury tend to be deeper. Patients at high risk for stress ulcers are those 1) with co-existent traumatic brain injury, 2) requiring mechanical ventilation, 3) in shock, and 4) with co-existent hepatic or renal failure. Mortality in patients with stress ulceration is high due to complications such as GI bleeding and perforation. The best strategy is prevention of stress ulcers using oral PPIs. Intravenous H2 receptor blockers are more cost-effective compared to intravenous PPIs in patients who are unable to take medications by the enteral route.

Biliary and Pancreatic Disease

A higher incidence of acute pancreatitis has been reported in patients with SCI. Autonomic imbalance with resultant hyperstimulation of the sphincter of Oddi is the postulated mechanism. Patients with neurologic diseases (lesions above T10) also have increased prevalence of gallstones due to impaired gall bladder motility and consequent bile stasis (1).

Superior Mesenteric Artery Syndrome (SMAS)

The SMA comes off the aorta and traverses the root of the mesentery of the small intestine over the duodenum in a ventral and caudal direction. The angle between the small bowel mesentery and the aorta is most acute when patients are supine.

SMAS is the result of intermittent functional obstruction of the third part of the duodenum between the superior mesenteric artery and the aorta. Patients present with persistent epigastric pain, postprandial fullness, nausea, and vomiting. The syndrome is rare in patients with SCI, but is more common in tetraplegics compared to paraplegics (1). The diagnosis is confirmed with a barium upper GI series, which shows dilatation of the proximal duodenum with a "cut-off" at the mid-3rd part of duodenum.

Treatment starts with a constellation of conservative measures such as eating small meals and replacement of fluids and electrolytes if needed. Meals should all be taken sitting upright as this helps the flow of food into the distal small bowel. If patients do not improve with conservative measures, duodenojejunostomy (anastamosis between 2nd part of duodenum and the jejunum) is an option.

Autonomic Dysreflexia

This is a potentially serious complication in patients with UMN lesions involving the spinal cord above the T6 spinal segment. It is the result of an exaggerated sympathetic response to certain stimuli (innocuous in AB individuals) such as bladder distension, catheterization, DRS, fecal impaction, and colonoscopy (11). Clinical features are sweating, goose flesh, palpitations, tachycardia, hypertension, and increased nasal secretions. If not diagnosed and treated in time, this can lead to fatal complications such as stroke, seizures, and subarachnoid hemorrhage. Once identified, this should be treated as a medical emergency. Autonomic dysreflexia is discussed in greater detail in a separate chapter in this volume.

Fecal Impaction

This should be suspected in patients who fail to have a bowel movement for more than 3 days. It can present with atypical features such as abdominal bloating, nausea, anorexia, vomiting, or acute confusional states. Delay in diagnosis and treatment can lead to rectal ulcerations with bleeding, intestinal obstruction, autonomic dysreflexia, and, rarely, colonic perforation (12). The treatment involves a combination of enemas, laxatives, and manual evacuation from the rectum. Prevention is the most cost-effective strategy and is achieved by the effective bowel regimens discussed above.

Acute Abdomen in Patients with Neurologic Diseases

General Approach
An acute abdomen in patients with neurologic disease could be due to conditions that are common in able-bodied individuals. However, certain problems are more frequent in these patients (Figure 11.2).

In able-bodied individuals, abdominal pain or distress is the most common complaint of an acute abdomen. Patients with neurologic diseases may

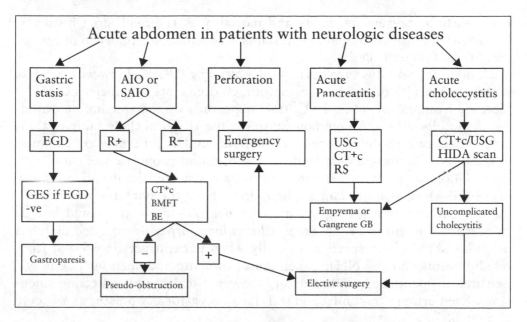

Figure 11.2. Algorithm for the workup of neurologically impaired patients with a suspected acute abdomen. USG, ultrasonogram; AIO, acute intestinal obstruction; SAIO, subacute intestinal obstruction; R+, response to conservative treatment; R-, no response to conservative treatment; EGD, esophagogastroduodenoscopy; GES, gastric emptying study; CT+c, contrast-enhanced CT scan; BMFT, barium meal follow through; BE, barium enema; RS, Ranson's scoring; MRC, magnetic resonance cholangiogram; HIDA, hepatic iminodiacetic acid.

be unable to perceive such pain (13). Instead, these individuals may present with other, less specific, symptoms of acute abdomen (ileus, nausea, vomiting, diarrhea, jaundice, hematemesis, and melena), atypical symptoms (anorexia, weight loss, confusion, and pallor), symptoms suggestive of infection (fever, confusion, and hypotension), or symptoms of autonomic dysreflexia (sweating, palpitations, and hypertension). Sometimes, the presentation is confined to abnormalities on abdominal examination (distension, visible peristalsis, hypo- or hyperactive bowel sounds) or laboratory values (leukocytosis, increased levels of amylase/lipase). Therefore, a high index of suspicion is required and development of any new symptom or abnormality needs a thorough workup.

In patients presenting with vomiting, the presence of stale food particles in the vomitus indicates gastric outlet obstruction or impaired gastric emptying. The presence of bile in the vomitus suggests that the problem is distal to the second portion of the duodenum (adynamic ileus, intestinal obstruction, and SMAS). Fecal impaction in these patients may present with similar features. Institutionalized elderly patients with neurologic diseases such as Parkinson's disease can present with bowel obstruction due to sigmoid volvulus. Pancreatitis and cholecystitis may present with only vomiting or fever of unknown origin. These individuals are prone to acalculous cholecystitis, and diagnosis must be made early to prevent morbidity and mortality. A thorough drug history is important because opiates, antidepressants, and anticholinergics can impair GI motility and present similarly.

Blood in the vomitus suggests upper GI bleeding (UGIB). However, patients with bright red blood per rectum, maroon-colored clots, and melena could be bleeding from anywhere in the GI tract depending on the amount and rapidity of the blood loss. A common cause for the UGIB in these individuals is peptic ulcer or stress ulceration. Hemorrhoids and anal fissures are common in these individuals and contribute to a substantial proportion of cases with lower GI bleeding (LGIB). A history of using nonsteroidal anti-inflammatory drugs (NSAIDs) is important as these drugs have the potential to cause GI bleeding. Acute diarrhea in patients with neurologic diseases could be due to overflow incontinence. However, *Clostridium difficile*-associated diarrhea or colitis should be suspected especially when patients are transferred from rehabilitation units or NHs. Other causes of acute abdomen include bowel ischemia, appendicitis, inflammatory bowel disease, and dissecting aneurysm. Even urinary tract infection (UTI) may occasionally present as an acute abdomen.

The physical examination should focus on evidence of dehydration, jaundice, and sepsis (tachycardia, hypotension, tachypnea, altered mental status). The abdomen should be examined for visible gastric (left to right in upper quadrant) or intestinal (step ladder) peristalsis, tenderness, rigidity, or masses. Auscultations of the abdomen should be done for bowel sounds and presence of "succussion splash," a splashing noise over the stomach when patient's abdomen is shaken vigorously from side to side. It is abnormal when heard 3–4 hours after a meal and indicates the presence of gastric stasis or gastric outlet obstruction. Rectal examination should be done to rule out fecal impaction, masses, and GI bleeding. In terms of laboratory analysis, a drop in hematocrit might indicate GI bleeding. Likewise, a leukocytosis might indicate an infectious process. Electrolyte abnormalities such as hypokalemia and hyponatremia are common in patients who are not eating adequately or who are having associated diarrhea or vomiting. Patients with continuous vomiting can develop a metabolic alkalosis. A metabolic acidosis with a high anion gap can occur in patients with sepsis. It may also be seen in patients with an intra-abdominal process complicated by gangrene or perforation. Amylase and lipase levels elevated more than three times the upper limit of normal indicate acute pancreatitis. Urine analysis and culture are ordered to exclude a UTI. Erect and supine films of abdomen are crucial. They should be evaluated for air–fluid levels (may indicate intestinal obstruction), free air under the diaphragm (may suggest perforation), or a dislodged percutaneous endoscopic gastrostomy (PEG) tube. A supine film may show the characteristic coffee bean sign of sigmoid volvulus as a result of closed loop obstruction of the sigmoid colon with grossly dilated bowel loops.

Radiographic interpretation may be challenging in patients with neurologic diseases as they frequently have retention of air and fecal matter.

Ultrasonography (USG) is a useful modality for imaging the gall bladder. However, USG has limitations for assessment of the pancreas, particularly in obese and individuals with abdominal distention. Contrast-enhanced computed tomography (CT) scan of the abdomen (if renal function is normal) is useful for assessment of the pancreas when USG is not helpful. However, renal function should be carefully checked before administering the contrast to these patients.

Patients with an acute abdomen are managed initially with conservative measures. Bowel rest is assured by keeping the patient nil by mouth. Appropriate IV fluids should be given. Electrolytes and acid–base status should be monitored. Pain medications are provided as needed. Opiates should be avoided in patients with intestinal obstruction, and NSAIDs should not be administered to those with GI bleeding. PPIs by the parenteral route are given for patients with acute upper GI bleeding and those with gastric outlet obstruction due to peptic ulcer disease. Nasogastric suction may be necessary when there is repetitive vomiting or when there is concern regarding a perforated viscus. Antibiotics are given to patients with acute cholecystitis, intestinal obstruction, perforation, and severe pancreatitis. It is imperative to draw relevant cultures before administration of antibiotics. The vital signs, the abdominal examination, the urinary output, and blood tests must be monitored on a regular basis.

Additional Workup

After the above general approach, additional workup is dependent upon the likely diagnosis (Figures 11.2 and 11.3). For example, if SMA syndrome is suspected, a UGI barium examination is done. A dislodged PEG tube is confirmed using gastrograffin. Patients with pancreatitis should be assessed for its severity using contrast-enhanced CT scan. Magnetic resonance cholangiopancreatography (MRCP) is done in those with evidence of biliary obstruction or dilated biliary channels on USG. However, MRCP is contraindicated in the presence of metal implants As in neurologically intact patients, stones in the common bile duct can be removed by endoscopic retrograde cholangiopancreatography (ERCP). A HIDA (hepatobiliary iminodiacetic acid) scan can diagnose acute cholecystitis with a sensitivity of 97% and specificity of 90% when suspicion for acute cholecystitis is high (14). Nonvisualization of the gall bladder suggests cystic duct obstruction and acute cholecystitis.

Specific management decisions also depend upon the cause of the acute abdomen. Intravenous metoclopramide or erythromycin is used for impaired gastric emptying. Patients with obstruction who have been decompressed should undergo evaluation to look for a stricture or tumor. If no cause is identified, patients are diagnosed as pseudo-obstruction. Intravenous neostigmine may be useful in this setting. A sigmoid volvulus can be detorsed by use of a flexible sigmoidoscope. Patients with an acute abdomen may require emergency surgery for unrelieved obstruction, perforated viscus, or a complicated cholecystitis (Fig. 11.2). When the cause of GI bleeding remains unknown despite endoscopic assessment, radionuclide study, angiography, or emergency laparotomy may be required.

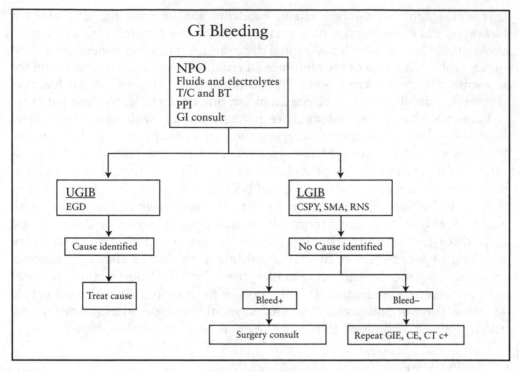

Figure 11.3. Algorithm for the workup of neurologically impaired patients with GI bleeding. NPO, nil per oral; T/C, type and cross-match; BT, blood transfusion; PPI, proton pump inhibitor; EGD, esophagogastrodudenoscopy; UGIB, upper GI bleeding; LGIB, lower GI bleeding; CSPY, colonoscopy; SMA, superior mesenteric angiography; RNS, radionuclide study; GIE, GI endoscopy; CE, capsule endoscopy; CTc+, contrast-enhanced CT scan.

PEG

If the GI tract is intact and functional, enteral nutrition can be provided through a PEG tube. Placement of PEG requires consent from the patient or from a health care proxy in patients with cognitive dysfunction. A normal coagulation profile should be assured, and 1 g of cefazolin should be administered about 30–60 minutes before the procedure. Once proper tube positioning is verified on flat film of the abdomen, PEG may be used for medications and feeding may be started within 24 hours. In patients at risk of aspiration (those with altered mental status), it may be safer to provide nutrition through a jejunostomy tube.

A dislodged PEG may be safely replaced if a fistulous tract has formed (usually 3–4 weeks). However, if the dislodgement occurs within the first 2 weeks of PEG placement, a GI consult should be requested, a NGT placed, and antibiotics administered. A plain x-ray of the abdomen should be taken to rule out perforation. If the patient is stable, a repeat PEG placement may be done after 7–10 days. This allows time for the original PEG site to heal.

Patient Safety

- Patients with acute spinal cord injury with or without traumatic brain injury are at high risk for stress ulcers and should be given prophylaxis using either oral proton pump inhibitors or intravenous H2 receptor antagonists.
- Patients with neurologic diseases are not able to perceive pain. Acute abdomen in these individuals invariably presents with atypical features, and its early identification requires a high index of suspicion.
- Medications that can adversely affect GI motility should be limited or eliminated.
- Digital rectal examination can trigger autonomic dysreflexia in adults with SCI.

Patient Education

- Patients and caregivers should be educated about neurogenic bowel and its treatment. This may require educational material in different formats—written, verbal, and visual (i.e., videotapes, dvds).
- Patients should be encouraged to consume plenty of fluids (2–3 liters per day) and adequate amounts of fiber (10–15 g).
- Patients should be educated to avoid medications that can worsen constipation.
- Patients and caregivers should be educated on the signs and symptoms associated with an acute abdomen to ensure timely care in the event of an emergency.

REFERENCES

1. Stiens SA, Singal AK, Korsten MA. The Gastrointestinal System After Spinal Cord Injury. In: V L, ed. Spinal Cord Medicine Principles and Practice. New York: Demos, 2003:321–349.
2. Krogh K, Christensen P, Laurberg S. Colorectal symptoms in patients with neurologic diseases. Acta Neurol Scand 2001; 103(6):335–343.
3. Nakayama H, Jorgensen HS, Pedersen PM, Raaschou HO, Olsen TS. Prevalence and risk factors of incontinence after stroke. The Copenhagen Stroke Study. Stroke 1997; 28(1):58–62.
4. Foxx-Orenstein A, Kolakowsky-Hayner S, Marwitz JH, et al. Incidence, risk factors, and outcomes of fecal incontinence after acute brain injury: findings from the Traumatic Brain Injury Model Systems national database. Arch Phys Med Rehabil 2003; 84(2):231–237.
5. Singal AK, Rosman AS, Bauman WA, Korsten MA. Recent concepts in the management of bowel problems after spinal cord injury. Adv Med Sci 2006; 51:15–22.
6. Korsten MA, Singal AK, Monga A, Chaparala G, Khan AM, Palmon R. Anorectal stimulation causes increased colonic motor activity in subjects with spinal cord injury. J Spinal Cord Med 2007; 30(1):31–35.

7. Korsten MA. Polyp detection rates are lower in persons with spinal cord injury: a prospective study. Unpublished data, 2007.
8. Singal AK, Shaw S, Galea M, Spungen AM, Bauman WA. Colonoscopy in persons with spinal cord injury: a prospective study on safety and efficacy of colon preparation [abstr]. J Spinal Cord Med 2007; 30:402.
9. Richter JE. Gastroesophageal reflux disease in the older patient: presentation, treatment, and complications. Am J Gastroenterol 2000; 95(2):368–373.
10. DePriest JL. Stress ulcer prophylaxis. Do critically ill patients need it? Postgrad Med 1995; 98(4):159–161, 165–166, 168.
11. Kewalramani LS. Neurogenic gastroduodenal ulceration and bleeding associated with spinal cord injuries. J Trauma 1979; 19(4):259–265.
12. Wrenn K. Fecal impaction. NEJM 1989; 321(10):658–662.
13. Mowrey K. The challenge of assessing and diagnosing acute abdomen in tetraplegics: a case study. J Neurosci Nurs 2007; 39(1):5–8.
14. Alobaidi M, Gupta R, Jafri SZ, Fink-Bennett DM. Curent trends in imaging evaluation of acute cholecystitis. Emerg Radiol 2004; 10(5):256–258.

12 Genitourinary System

Hyon Schneider
Adam Stein

Voiding disorders are common among patients with neurologic disorders such as spinal cord injury (SCI), multiple sclerosis (MS), brain injury (BI), stroke, and Parkinson's disease. Such voiding disorders are referred to as neurogenic bladder dysfunction. Abnormalities in bladder function can lead to incontinence and/or urinary retention. Voiding dysfunction often becomes a psychological and social burden for an individual that may create a poor self-image and avoidance of social interaction. Further, bladder dysfunction creates a physical burden by predisposing the affected individual to secondary medical complications. These medical complications include frequent urinary tract infections (UTIs), urinary tract stones, and kidney disease. It is critical, therefore, to strive for a bladder management strategy that preserves kidney function, minimizes stone disease and UTI, and provides a socially acceptable method of bladder drainage for the affected individual.

The cause and location of nervous system injury correlates with the type of bladder dysfunction experienced by the individual. Bladder disorders are nearly universal in patients with SCI. The estimated incidence of urologic disorders in patients with stroke on hospital admission ranges from 32 to 79% and upon discharge from 25 to 28% (1). In MS, bladder disorders are reported in 40–90% of patients (1). Urologic disorders in traumatic brain injury (TBI) can range from 32 to 70% depending on the location of the injury within the brain (1).

Renal failure, once the leading cause of death in SCI, is now an uncommon cause of death because of the use of clean intermittent catheterization in management of patients with neurogenic bladder as well as improved methods of urinary tract screening. Patients with neurogenic bladder often lack sensation and may not experience typical symptoms of UTI, stone disease, and hydronephrosis. Preventative screening for such conditions is of paramount importance in management of neurogenic bladder dysfunction.

The goal of this chapter is to provide an overview of the pertinent anatomy and physiology of neurogenic bladder, key points in its assessment and treatment as well as relevant information regarding patient safety and patient education.

ANATOMY AND PHYSIOLOGY

Anatomy

The urinary system is divided into upper and lower urinary tracts. The upper urinary tract consists of the kidneys and ureters. The lower urinary tract consists of the bladder (fundus, trigone, and neck of bladder), prostate gland, urethra, and the pelvic diaphragm. There are two sphincters in the lower tract. The internal sphincter lies at the neck of the bladder and is composed of smooth muscle that is not under voluntary control. This is the primary muscle for preventing the release of urine. Unlike the internal sphincter muscle, the external urethral sphincter is composed of skeletal muscle and is therefore under voluntary control. This muscle contracts to maintain continence, when the awareness of the need to void occurs, until an appropriate receptacle is identified.

The bladder is divided into three regions—fundus, trigone, and neck—and consists of four layers—the detrusor (smooth) muscle, a serous layer, a submucous layer, and a thin mucous layer continuous with the urethral lining.

Neuroanatomy

The neuroanatomy of normal voiding can be divided into the central and peripheral nervous system. The relevant central nervous system structures include the frontal lobe of the brain, the pontine micturition center (PMC), and the spinal cord. The peripheral nervous system consists of autonomic and somatic pathways to the relevant anatomic structures noted above. The frontal lobe maintains bladder continence by preventing bladder contraction until a socially acceptable time and place is available. This is accomplished by inhibitory signals sent from the frontal lobe to the detrusor muscle, preventing bladder contraction and deactivating signals to the PMC, which diminishes the urge to urinate. When urination is appropriate, the brain sends excitatory signals to the pons to allow voiding. The pontine micturition center (PMC) is a major relay center between the brain and the bladder. PMC stimulation is an excitatory response that results in efficient voiding by coordinating simultaneous bladder contraction and sphincter relaxation. The spinal cord contains efferent, afferent, and interneurons, which compose the ascending and descending pathways carrying signals to and from the relevant brain regions and peripheral structures. Afferent fibers from the urinary bladder and urethra project to interneurons at the dorsal horn in the sacral spinal cord.

Parasympathetic activity via pelvic splanchnic nerves from the sacral cord (S2–S4) results in bladder contraction and bladder neck relaxation, resulting in urination. Parasympathetic excitatory input to the bladder wall is mediated by acetylcholine (ACh) binding to the M3 muscarinic receptors (2), while inhibitory inputs to the external urethral sphincter are mediated by nitric oxide (3). Sympathetic stimulation results in the release of norepinephrine (NE) from the hypogastric nerves, leading to stimulation of β-adrenergic receptors on the bladder wall. This causes an inhibition of detrusor contraction, while NE-mediated stimulation of α-adrenergic receptors in the bladder neck and urethra is excitatory and favors storage of urine. The somatic pudendal nerve, also originating from sacral segments with their cell bodies at S2–S4, innervates the external urinary sphincter. Bladder filling leads to activation of stretch receptors and chemoreceptors located in the bladder wall, which can stimulate sacral reflex centers, resulting in an urge to void. Involuntary voiding is suppressed by a cascade of inhibitory signaling initiated by the brain.

Classification of Neurogenic Bladder

Classification of neurogenic bladder dysfunction is divided into upper or lower motor neuron types based on the site of the neurologic injury and its effect upon voiding.

Upper Motor Neuron

Upper motor neuron–type bladder dysfunction results from injuries or diseases located above the sacral segments. In this type of bladder dysfunction, patients will have detrusor hyperreflexia (overactive bladder, spastic bladder) as a result of an uninhibited and intact reflex pathway. Voiding is characterized by urgency with or without incontinence because of the loss of cortical tonic inhibition to the bladder. Detrusor hyperreflexia is characteristic of suprapontine lesions such as those associated with Parkinson's disease, stroke, and TBI. Additionally, detrusor hyperreflexia may be accompanied by detrusor sphincter dyssynergia (DSD). DSD is characterized by intermittent or sustained failure of relaxation of the urinary sphincter during a bladder contraction. Lesions that cause DSD are either located at the PMC or involve the supra-sacral spinal cord and are most typified by complete spinal lesions. Voiding in persons with upper motor neuron voiding dysfunction is characterized by varying degrees of urge incontinence, "stop-start" voiding, and, rarely, urinary retention.

Lower Motor Neuron

Lower motor neuron (LMN) bladder is associated with lesions affecting the conus medullaris, the cauda equina, and the S2–S4 peripheral nerves. Trauma, such as lumbar or sacral fractures, central spinal canal stenosis, tumors, peripheral neuropathies, and infections are common causes of lower motor neuron voiding dysfunction. In general, such lesions lead to variable loss of parasympathetic and somatic nerve function resulting in detrusor areflexia, bladder neck incompetence, and/or incompetence of the external urethral sphincter. The clinical picture is one of urinary retention with varying degrees of stress-type incontinence.

Urologic Manifestations in Specific Neurologic Conditions

SCI

The urinary dysfunction in SCI varies depending on the level of injury. An initial voiding dysfunction following SCI may be due to a spinal shock, with absent somatic reflexes and flaccid muscle paralysis at and below the level of injury. In spinal shock, the bladder is areflexic and acontractile. Spinal shock generally lasts 6–12 weeks in a complete supra-sacral spinal cord lesion but may last up to 1–2 years. Spinal shock may last only a few days in patients with incomplete supra-sacral lesions. In general, SCI above the sacral cord results in detrusor-sphincter dyssynergia resulting in an elevated bladder pressure. Detrusor hyperactivity with a lack of sensation and striated sphincter dyssynergia is observed for complete spinal cord lesions between the sacral spinal cord and the area of the sympathetic outflow. Smooth muscle sphincter dyssynergia is observed in addition for lesions at or above the T7 spinal cord level. Lower motor neuron lesions, SCI involving the sacral cord, result in an atonic external sphincter which is prone to urine leakage.

Stroke/TBI

Urinary dysfunction in both stroke and TBI patients varies based on the area of brain or brain stem involved. Initial voiding dysfunction may be due to a cerebral shock with an initial period of detrusor areflexia. With lesions above the pontine micturition center, the most common chronic urinary dysfunction is involuntary bladder contractions (detrusor hyperactivity). In patients with more isolated brain stem injuries involving areas below the pontine micturition center, detrusor striated sphincter dyssynergia may also occur. Patients with lesions in only the basal ganglia or thalamus have normal sphincter function and may gain urinary control. True urgency incontinence with reduced bladder sensation is associated with global underperfusion of the cerebral cortex, especially the right frontal areas (4). While the most common chronic voiding dysfunction following the acute phase is bladder hyperactivity resulting in low bladder capacity, a small percentage of stroke patients have persistent detrusor hypocontractility or areflexia. Similar to spinal shock, a cerebral shock can occur in the acute phase of stroke, causing patients to have urinary retention from detrusor areflexia. Identification of a long-term urinary dysfunction may take a few weeks or months.

Multiple Sclerosis

As in stroke patients, detrusor hyperactivity is the most common urodynamic abnormality in MS. In MS, voiding dysfunction can be summarized into three basic patterns: 1) detrusor hyperactivity with striated sphincter synergia (average 38%); 2) detrusor hyperactivity with striated sphincter dyssynergia (average 29%); and 3) detrusor areflexia (average 26%) (5). The most common voiding dysfunction in MS is storage failure secondary to detrusor hyperactivity. This is commonly complicated by striated sphincter dyssynergia, with varying effects on the ability to empty completely at acceptable pressures.

PATIENT ASSESSMENT

To competently assist the patient in developing a bladder management plan, a targeted history and physical exam is required. The history should include a description of the individual's neurologic condition and its consequences, including the individual's manual dexterity and functional status for activities of daily living and mobility. The examiner needs to elicit a description of the individual's urinary pattern, including the method of urinary drainage and whether any medical devices, such as catheters, are utilized. The individual should be asked if he or she is content with his or her bladder function. Physical exam should include a neurologic exam, with attention to sensorimotor function and hand dexterity. Examination of the reflexes and muscle tone is important to identify the presence of an upper or lower motor neuron syndrome. A rectal examination is critical and must include an assessment of perirectal sensation, the presence or absence of volitional rectal sphincter contraction, and an evaluation of sacral reflexes such as the anal wink and bulbocavernosus reflex. Such information will be useful in predicting the potential for regaining bladder control as well as classifying upper or lower motor neuron patterns. Measurements of voided and retained urine are extremely useful. Postvoid residual urine can be determined by catheterization or using a simple ultrasound machine. Measurement of the BUN and serum creatinine measure kidney function should be performed at least annually. Diagnostic testing often includes renal and bladder sonography to evaluate for the presence of vesicoureteral reflux or stones. Urodynamic testing is an important physiologic test that measures pressure within the bladder, during both storage and voiding (Table 12.1).

Table 12.1

Assessment of the Patient with a Neurogenic Bladder

History
1. History of neurologic injury or disease process
2. History of underlying kidney disease
3. Visual symptoms or history of impaired vision
4. Current method of urinary drainage and patient's level of satisfaction with the current method

Physical Examination
1. Neurologic examination to establish type of injury (i.e., upper motor neuron vs. lower motor neuron injury).
2. Hand dexterity
3. Vision
4. Rectal exam—perirectal sensation; volitional sphincter control; sacral reflexes (anal wink, bulbocavernosus reflex)
5. Postvoid residual

Diagnostic Tests
1. Renal function tests (BUN, creatinine)
2. Renal and bladder ultrasound
3. Urodynamic testing

TREATMENT

There are three important factors to consider when selecting a bladder management option for an individual with neurogenic bladder dysfunction. The option being considered must be physically feasible (good hand function or assistance available to perform the task), be socially acceptable, and minimize medical complications. While there are differences in the acute setting versus long-term bladder management, both share common goals (Table 12.2).

Acute (Inpatient) Setting

Preserving urinary tract integrity and ensuring adequate bladder drainage while the patient is medically stabilized after an acute neurologic event and ensuring preservation of renal function are the goals in the acute setting. Monitoring urine output and fluid intake with an indwelling Foley catheter is the simplest method until the patient is medically and neurologically stable. Once stability is achieved, clean intermittent catheterization (CIC) can be initiated every 4–6 hours with a urine collection goal of less than 500 ml per catheterization. The frequency of CIC can be adjusted based on total fluid intake and catheterized volumes. Patients with sufficient hand function should be taught how to perform self-CIC as early as possible if the physician believes that rapid restoration of normal voiding is unlikely. Patient education and understanding play a crucial role in ensuring compliance; it is important that the patient understands the rationale for performing CIC. The patient is observed for the return of voiding, which may occur either with or without voluntary control, depending on the severity of the neurologic condition. It is very useful to check the postvoid residual volume once urination returns to verify adequate bladder emptying. Ideally, postvoid residual urine should be less than 100 cc.

Long-Term (Outpatient) Setting

A long-term bladder management plan requires thoughtful consideration of the patient's gender, degree of hand function and mobility, motivation, and learning ability when normal controlled urination does not return. CIC is generally accepted as the best and safest long-term bladder management method short of controlled urination (6).

Table 12.2

Goals of Neurogenic Bladder Management

---

1. Ensure socially acceptable method of bladder drainage for reintegration into the community that minimizes reliance on the assistance of caregivers
2. Allow low-pressure storage of urine and efficient bladder emptying at low detrusor pressures
3. Avoid stretch injury of the bladder from repeated overdistension
4. Prevent renal deterioration by avoiding high intravesical pressures
5. Prevent recurrent urinary tract infections

Techniques and Catheter Options in Neurogenic Bladder Management

Clean Intermittent Catheterization

CIC is a technique used by patients who are able to perform self-catheterization. Prerequisites for CIC use include sufficient outflow resistance to maintain continence between catheterizations (that is, a competent sphincter mechanism), relatively low bladder pressures, adequate bladder capacity (>300 ml), and hand function sufficient to perform the procedure. For a patient who consumes an average of 2000 cc per day, CIC is typically performed four to six times daily with a goal to obtain 500 cc or less per catheterization by adjusting the frequency of CIC. Since CIC does not require a drainage bag, patients often find this technique more socially acceptable and convenient than using a condom-type or indwelling catheter. Maintaining continence between catheterizations often requires medications, most notably anticholinergic agents, such as oxybutinin hydrochloride or tolteradine tartrate.

The most common problems with CIC are UTI, urethral trauma, and incontinence between catheterizations. Introduction of foreign bodies such as hair or lint can provide a nidus for bladder stone formation. Appropriate patients should be taught CIC; health care providers should confirm patients' skill and understanding of the procedure. Catheters can be washed and reused after proper cleaning. Studies have shown no significant increase in urinary complications when proper clean technique is practiced (7). A detailed explanation and instructions with diagrams are available for patients through a website: http://www.umm.edu/ency/article/003972.htm.

Timed Voiding

Timed voiding, also known as bladder training, refers to "scheduled" urination for persons with overactive bladder. In timed voiding, individuals adopt a schedule of regular bladder emptying (e.g., every 3–4 hours). At such intervals, the affected individual attempts to urinate. Techniques such as supra-pubic tapping to initiate a bladder contraction may be used to trigger voiding at the appropriate intervals. Timed voiding for long-term bladder management can be optimized by a daily intake and output diary to adjust for variable daily fluid intake. For an average 2000 cc daily total fluid intake, steady fluid consumption is encouraged since a steady rate of urine production is easier to manage than fluctuating volumes throughout the day.

Valsalva or Credé Maneuver

The Valsalva and Credé maneuvers are techniques to facilitate bladder emptying by indirectly increasing intravesical pressure. The Valsalva maneuver accomplishes this by using the abdominal muscles, while the Credé maneuver applies direct manual pressure to the supra-pubic area. These maneuvers are most useful in lower motor neuron injuries where the increased abdominal pressure allows urination to occur by exceeding the resistance of the weakened sphincter mechanism, often to complete, or near complete, bladder emptying.

Reflex Voiding

Reflex voiding requires intact sacral reflexes, as is seen in persons with Upper Motor Neuron (UMN) injuries. In such individuals, voiding occurs at inappropriately low bladder volumes and may occur without voluntary control. Men with UMN injuries and impaired hand function may opt to utilize a condom-type device which connects via tubing to a receptacle such as a leg bag. A new catheter is applied each day after bathing. In persons with lesions above the pontine micturition center, coordinated relaxation of the sphincter mechanism is present, and voiding is generally efficient, even if uncontrolled. In individuals with spinal lesions, on the other hand, coordination between the bladder and sphincter is often absent, which may result in inefficient high-pressure voiding. Such individuals may opt for use of a condom catheter but must be followed regularly for early detection of hydronephrosis or renal deterioration. Patients often favor the noninvasive nature of the condom catheter in comparison to an indwelling catheter. Penile skin breakdown, inadvertent dislodging of the catheter, interference with sexual activity, and unpleasant odor emanating from the collection bag are negative aspects of reflex voiding. There is no useful external urinary collection device for women with substantially overactive bladders. Detailed patient information is available at the following website: http://www. healthtouch.com/bin/EContent_HT/cnoteShowLfts.asp?fname=02528&title= HOW+TO+CARE+FOR+YOUR+CONDOM+CATHETER+&cid=HTHLTH.

Indwelling Catheters

An indwelling catheter can be either a Foley-type catheter inserted through the urethra or a supra-pubic cystostomy tube placed through the abdominal wall directly into the bladder. Such catheters then connect via tubing to a receptacle such as a leg bag or bedside bag. A long-term indwelling catheter may be utilized for patients who are unable to perform CIC as well as for those who are unable to successfully maintain or for those who disdain a condom-type catheter. Indwelling catheters are most commonly recommended for women with impaired hand function who are unable to perform CIC and who are otherwise unable to achieve continence. Complications from Foley catheters have been well documented, including UTI, epididymitis and prostatitis, urethral strictures, traumatic hypospadias, urethral incompetence in women, urethritis, bladder calculi, and development of a small, poorly compliant bladder (8). Complications of supra-pubic cystostomy tubes are similar to Foley catheters without the risk of epididymitis, prostatitis, and hypospadias. Supra-pubic catheters enhance the ease of sexual activity. Urinary colonization by bacteria is universal, as it is with any type of catheter. Recurrent chronic inflammation of the bladder wall as a result of UTI and indwelling catheters contribute to an increased risk of bladder cancer (9).

Medications to Treat Neurogenic Bladder (see Table 12.3)

Medications utilized to mollify the effects of neurogenic bladder include cholinergic and anticholinergic agents, -blockers, spasmolytics (oral and injected), tricyclic antidepressants, and desmopressin acetate (DDAVP).

Table 12.3

Medications for Neurogenic Bladder

Anticholinergics
Hyoscyamine:
- Short acting (Anaspaz, Levsin/SL, and NuLev) 0.125–0.25 mg every 4 hours
- Long acting (Levbid, Levsinex) 0.375-0.75 mg every 12 hours

Oxybutynin:
- Short acting (Ditropan) 5–10 mg two to three times daily
- Long acting (Ditropan XL) 5–30 mg daily
- Transdermal (Oxytrol) 3.9-mg patch, changed every third day

Has antispasmodic effect in addition to anticholinergic effect.

Tolterodine:
- Short acting (Detrol) 1–2 mg twice daily
- Long acting (Detrol LA) 2–4 mg daily.
- Differs from other anticholinergic types in that it has selectivity for urinary bladder over salivary glands; exhibits high specificity for muscarinic receptors

Darifenacin (Enablex) 7.5–15 mg daily
Solifenacin (VESIcare) 2–10 mg daily
Trospium:
- Short acting (Sanctura) 20 mg twice a day
- Long acting (Sanctura XR) 60 mg once every morning

α_1- *blockers*
Tamsulosin (Flomax) 0.4–0.8 mg once daily.
Terazosin (Hytrin) 1–10 mg once daily.
Doxazosin:
- Short acting (Cardura) 1–8 mg daily.
- Long acting (Cardura XL) 4–8 mg once daily
Prazosin (Minipress) 10–20 mg a day

Cholinergic medications
Bethanecol (Urecholine) 25–100 mg three to four times per day

Tricyclic antidepressants (TCAs)
Amitriptyline (Elavil) 25–150 mg at bedtime
Imipramine (Tofranil) 10–25 mg two to four times daily

Bethanechol (Duvoid, Urecholine) is used in the treatment of areflexic or underactive bladder. It functions as a muscarinic cholinergic receptor agonist. The most common side effects include diarrhea, bradycardia, excess salivation, and tearing. It should not be used in patients who may have any degree of bladder outlet obstruction, either anatomic, such as an enlarged prostate, or functional, as in DSD. In such a scenario it may lead to an increased intravesical pressure.

Anticholinergic agents are used in the treatment of hyperreflexic bladder or urge incontinence by inhibiting involuntary bladder contractions. They work as muscarinic cholinergic receptor antagonists to prevent uninhibited bladder contractions in patients with or without IC use. In addition, they may be helpful in patients with indwelling and supra-pubic catheters to prevent loss of capacity of the bladder. Potential adverse effects of all anticholinergic agents include dry mouth, blurred vision, palpitations, drowsiness, constipation, and facial flushing. When anticholinergic agents are used, acute urinary retention may occur. At times, as in persons seeking to perform self-IC with severe spinal cord injury, urinary retention may indeed be the desired effect. Anticholinergics are contraindicated if patients have documented narrow-angle glaucoma, urinary retention, bowel obstruction, ulcerative colitis, myasthenia gravis, and severe heart disease. Because of the potential for drowsiness, these agents may impair the patient's ability to perform certain activities, such as driving or operating heavy machinery. Anticholinergic drugs should not be taken in combination with alcohol, sedatives, or hypnotic drugs.

α-Blockers are used for smooth muscle inhibition at the bladder neck and in the prostate. These medications can help to open the bladder neck, especially with the reflex voiding management method. The main side effects are orthostatic hypotension, dizziness, rhinitis, and retrograde ejaculation. These medications are often given in the evening once the individual is recumbent to reduce the possibility of orthostasis in persons at risk. Because of its specificity, tamsulosin may be preferential to the other agents in terms of minimizing adverse effects—in particular, orthostatic hypotension.

Tricyclic antidepressants (TCAs) inhibit reuptake of norepinephrine and serotonin at presynaptic neurons. TCAs have both peripheral α-adrenergic and central anticholinergic properties, facilitating urine storage by decreasing bladder contractility and increasing outlet resistance. Hence, TCAs such as amitriptyline and imipramine have been used in the treatment of hyperreflexic bladder with incontinence and may have multiple benefits when used in patients with depression or chronic neuropathic pain. The most common side effects are dry mouth, excessive drowsiness, constipation, blurred vision, and tachycardia. Care should be taken if used in the elderly. Nortryptyline may have fewer anticholinergic side effects than amitryptyline or imipramine, but that may limit its use for persons with neurogenic bladder.

Antispasmodic medications for bladder spasticity with detrusor-sphincter dyssynergia include muscle relaxants such as Baclofen, Valium, and botulinum toxin. These medications potentially relax both the urinary bladder, by exerting a direct spasmolytic action on the smooth muscle of the bladder, and the striated external sphincter. While a seemingly attractive class of medications to improve symptoms of neurogenic bladder dysfunction, their clinical utility has been relatively minimal in clinical practice. Antispasmodics have been reported to increase the bladder capacity and decrease urge incontinence. These drugs may impair the patient's ability to perform activities requiring mental alertness and physical coordination. Drinking alcohol and using sedatives in combination with these antispasmodic drugs is contraindicated.

DDAVP is a synthetic antidiuretic hormone, which increases the resorption of water in the collecting tubules of the kidneys. Its function in neurogenic bladder patients is to decrease voiding frequency and/or incontinence by decreasing urine production. One study demonstrated the efficacy of DDAVP as an alternative therapy in the management of SCI patients with neurogenic bladder dysfunction unresponsive to conventional therapy (10). DDAVP can be administered parentally or as an intranasal preparation. However, intranasal delivery can be compromised by a variety of factors that can make nasal insufflations ineffective or inappropriate. These include poor intranasal absorption, nasal congestion and blockage, nasal discharge, atrophy of nasal mucosa, and severe atrophic rhinitis. DDAVP is contraindicated in patients with moderate to severe renal impairment (Cr clearance < 50 ml/min), and the potential for electrolyte abnormalities requires monitoring of serum chemistry.

SURGICAL OPTIONS IN NEUROGENIC BLADDER MANAGEMENT

For patients with neurogenic bladder who have failed medical management, surgical options may be considered. A surgical intervention is considered only after a thorough medical workup of the lower urinary tract and anatomic, physiologic, and functional evaluations have been carried out.

Surgical Interventions for Outlet Obstruction

Neurourologically, complete or partial outlet obstruction may be caused by hyperreflexic internal or external sphincter. For patients with hyperreflexic external sphincter, causing either undesired urinary retention or severe detrusor-sphincter dyssynergia, an external sphincteromy (transurethral resection of the external sphincter [TURES]) may be considered. This procedure allows urinary outflow with detrusor contraction to an external collecting device; therefore, it is only considered for men. Candidates for external sphincterotomy must have adequate detrusor contractions to allow for bladder emptying. Further, the procedure results in total incontinence, so it should not be considered for anyone who has any control of voiding. It is an ablative procedure and, therefore, irreversible.

For individuals with bladder neck obstruction refractory to medical therapy, a transurethral resection of the bladder neck (TURBN) may be performed to relieve obstruction. Bladder neck obstruction can be a result of hypertrophy, which may be seen in association with external sphincter dyssynergia. In TURBN surgery, the bladder neck tissue is incised or resected cystoscopically. In older male patients who may also have coincident benign prostatic hypertrophy, transurethral resection of prostate (TURP) is commonly done to excise hypertrophic prostate to relieve outflow obstruction. As is the case with TURES, the functional result is the use of a condom catheter for urine collection.

Surgical Intervention for Incompetent External Sphincter

To help prevent substantial urine incontinence associated with overfilling of the bladder or elevated intra-abdominal pressure caused by sphincter incompetence, a fascial sling can be constructed to support the weakened sphincter. This is done by utilizing strips of fascia, either from the tensor fascia lata or rectus abdominus muscles, to create a sling around the bladder neck. This sling serves as an external compressive support mechanism to "tighten" the sphincter. Once in place, the individual can utilize CIC in conjuction with the sling. Further, a commercially available artificial sphincter may be inserted that may be manually opened and closed for voiding and storage, respectively. There is a relatively high occurrence of erosion of this device through insensate skin; therefore, patient selection is of paramount importance.

Surgical Options for Detrusor Hyperreflexia

Bladder augmentation, also known as augmentation cystoplasty, is a reconstructive surgery to increase the storage capacity of the bladder, usually to allow CIC without incontinence between catheterizations. The procedure involves anastomosis of tissue grafts taken from a section of the ileum, colon, stomach, or other substitute that are sewn into an incised hyperreflexic bladder. The new bladder is characterized by increased capacity and decreased spasticity based on the inclusion of minimally contractile intestinal tissue. Augmentation cystoplasty is considered for persons who remain incontinent despite anticholinergic therapy and who can perform self-CIC. Various metabolic derangements and changes in bowel habits are common, though transient, complications of the procedure (11). An alternative surgical technique is a detrusor myomectomy, also known as autoaugmention, where excision of the detrusor submucosa creates a weakened muscle with a resultant intentional diverticulum to increase bladder capacity and decrease contractility (12).

Urinary Diversion Surgery

Urinary diversion procedures are recommended for patients with urethral anatomical pathology, such as stricture, fistula, peri-urethral abscess, or for SCI patients unable to self-catheterize or with intractable incontinence that impairs the treatment and prevention of significant pressure ulcers. A suprapubic catheter is the simplest method of urinary diversion. A catheter is inserted into the bladder through an incision in the abdomen a few inches below the umbilicus. This is a method of bladder management often utilized in male tetraplegics.

The Mitrofanoff procedure typically utilizes the appendix to create a continent catheterizable stoma between the abdominal wall and the bladder. The aperture is most commonly placed in the umbilicus, allowing persons to self-catheterize through the umbilicus rather than opening lower extremity garments which may substantially ease the procedure.

Other urinary diversions, also referred to as cutaneous conduits, surgically couple the ureters to an intestinal segment that is externalized through the anterior abdominal wall. This allows urine to drain into an external collecting device but is, in contrast to the Mitrofanoff, an incontinent diversion.

Functional Electrical Stimulation for Bladder Control

Functional electrical stimulation (FES) of the detrusor muscle to initiate voiding on command using an external controller is possible through an implantation of a bladder neuroprosthesis (VoCare System) (13). It is an implantable FES system for patients with complete SCI above the sacral spinal cord segments and requires intact peripheral innervation to the bladder. Stimulating electrodes are placed on the anterior roots of appropriate sacral nerves, and selective sacral dorsal rhizotomies are performed to eliminate the afferent pathway of the voiding reflex. This is an extensive surgical procedure, which will permanently damage dorsal nerve roots, and patients will lose reflex erectile function. On the other hand, advantages of this procedure include voiding on demand, increased bladder capacity, elimination of incontinence, improved bladder emptying, and reduced UTIs.

Medical Complications of Neurogenic Bladder

The treatment and prevention of medical complications are crucial parts of neurogenic bladder management. Urologic complications such as UTI (cystitis, pyelonephritis, and prostatitis), stone disease of the kidneys and bladder, vesico-ureteral reflux, renal failure, skin problems, bladder cancer, and urethral strictures and trauma have been significantly reduced since the implementation of improved screening techniques and the use of CIC. However, the task of minimizing such complications continues to be a major challenge in the management of patients affected by neurogenic bladder. Vesicoureteral reflux, renal failure, and stones will be discussed in the next section. UTIs are discussed further in Chapter 21.

Vesicoureteral Reflux and Renal Failure
In neurogenic bladder patients, vesicoureteral reflux may result from high detrusor pressures, which are typically related to severe DSD (6). Vesicoureteral reflux can lead to pyelonephritis and renal deterioration and failure, especially in the presence of recurrent infections (14). In patients with neurogenic bladder, most deaths from renal complications are a consequence of reflux. The occurrence of renal failure in patients with neurogenic bladder has substantially decreased over the last half century as a result of improvements in bladder management.

Urinary Stone Disease
Patients with longstanding neurogenic bladder are predisposed to the development of urinary stone disease, especially in the presence of vesicoureteral reflux

and recurrent infections (15). Other risk factors for urinary stone formation include hypercalcemia, advanced age, complete spinal injury, history of prior stones, sepsis, and use of indwelling catheters.

Stones can be found in any part of urinary system, including the kidneys, ureters, bladder, and, less likely, the urethra. Struvite stones (magnesium based) and calcium oxalate stones account for 90% of calculi in patients with neurogenic bladder (16). Struvite stones are consistently associated with urinary infections, specifically the urease-producing bacteria, most commonly *Proteus*. Other urease-producing bacteria include *Ureaplasma, Staphylococcus, Klebsiella, Providencia*, and *Pseudomonas. Escherichia coli* does not produce urease and is not associated with struvite stone formation. The prophylactic use of acetohydroxamic acid can help reduce the incidence of these stones (16). Struvite stones are radiolucent, whereas calcium oxalate stones are radiopaque. Calcium stones are very common and may result from hypercalciuria associated with bone hyperresorption.

The incidence of kidney stone formation is highest in patients with indwelling catheters. Small renal calculi, which are smaller than 1 cm and asymptomatic, can be followed without definitive treatment, but 50% will become symptomatic over 5 years. Half of these will require removal procedures. Enlarging calculi in the renal pelvis require treatments such as extracorporeal shock wave lithotripsy (ESWL) to avoid obstruction of the kidney. Ureteral stones can potentially obstruct urine drainage from the entire kidney and cause pyelonephritis and renal deterioration.

Bladder stones also occur because of UTI and bacterial colonization, obstruction of the urinary tract, or urinary retention from either a neurologic cause or an enlarged prostate gland or indwelling catheters. Diet and the amount of fluid intake also appear to be important factors in the development of bladder stones. People prone to forming calcium oxalate stones should limit or avoid foods high in oxalate (Table 12.4).

Table 12.4

High-Oxalate Foods

- Rhubarb,
- Spinach,
- Beets
- Swiss chard
- Wheat germ
- Soybean crackers
- Peanuts
- Okra
- Chocolate
- Black Indian tea
- Sweet potatoes

Bladder stones are significantly associated with indwelling catheters: 2.3% of intermittent catheter users had bladder stones in the first month, whereas 8.8% of indwelling catheter users developed bladder stones in their first month (7).

Cancer

Bladder cancer is associated with chronic indwelling catheters (17). The risk of bladder cancer has been related to the duration of chronic indwelling catheter use and attributed to chronic irritation and infection of the bladder leading to dysplastic change and squamous metaplasia (17,18). Squamous cell carcinoma is the most common type of bladder cancer seen in this population. Squamous cell cancer of the bladder is very aggressive and is often metastatic at diagnosis with an associated poor prognosis. Typical symptoms associated with bladder cancer are gross or microscopic hematuria or recurrent urinary tract infections (17). Screening cystosopic evaluations are recommended after 5–10 years of indwelling catheter use, then every other year.

Patient Safety

1. Urinary distension may trigger Autonomic Dyreflexia (AD).
2. Bethanechol should not be used in patients who may have any degree of bladder outlet obstruction, since it may lead to an increased intravesical pressure.
3. Anticholinergics are contraindicated in patients with documented narrow-angle glaucoma, urinary retention, bowel obstruction, ulcerative colitis, myasthenia gravis, and severe heart disease.
4. α-Blockers can cause orthostatic hypotension. Consider giving the medication in the evening once the individual is recumbent to reduce the possibility of orthostasis in persons at risk.
5. Tricyclic antidepressants, anticholinergics, and antispasmodics have the potential for causing drowsiness. They may impair the patient's ability to perform certain activities, such as driving or operating heavy machinery. Additionally they should not be taken in combination with alcohol, sedatives, or hypnotic drugs.
6. Screening cystosopic evaluations are recommended after 5–10 years of indwelling catheter use, then every other year.

Patient Education

1. Patients and their caregivers should be educated at an appropriate level of understanding on basic principles of neurogenic bladder, goals of management, and recommended management techniques.

2. Proper technique of CIC should be taught to minimize the risk of trauma to the urethra, introduction of foreign bodies, and UTIs.
3. Patients and their caregivers should be educated on the medications prescribed for neurogenic bladder—name, dosage, administration schedules, common side effects, significant adverse effects, and drug–drug interactions. Since many of the commonly used medications have the potential for cognitive impairment, patients should be counseled on refraining from activities such as driving or operating heavy machinery or drinking alcohol.
4. Patients with indwelling catheters should receive education on catheter care, which includes at least monthly catheter changes and the cleansing of collection bags.
5. Patients should be educated on common presenting signs and symptoms of urinary tract infections.

REFERENCES

1. Wein AJ, Kavoussi LR, Novick AC, Partin AW, Peters CA. Campbell–Walsh Urology, 9th ed. Philadelphia: Saunders, 2007; 3(59):12–20.
2. Matsui M, Motomura D, Fujikawa T, et al. Mice lacking M2 and M3 muscarinic acetylcholine receptors are devoid of cholinergic smooth muscle contractions but still viable. J Neurosci 2002; 22:10627–10632.
3. Andersson KE, Arner A. Urinary bladder contraction and relaxation: physiology and pathophysiology, Physiol Rev 2004; 84:935–986.
4. Griffiths D. Clinical studies of cerebral and urinary tract function in elderly people with urinary incontinence. Behav Brain Res 1998; 15:151–155.
5. Chancellor MB, Blaivas JG. Multiple sclerosis. Prob Urol 1993; 7:15–33.
6. Weld KJ, Graney MJ, Dmochowski RR. Differences in bladder compliance with time and association of bladder management with compliance in spinal cord injured patients. J Urol 2000; 163:1228–1233.
7. Braddom RL. Physical Medicine and Rehabilitation, 3rd ed. Philadelphia: Saunders, 2007.
8. Weld KJ, Wall BM, Mangold TA, et al. Influences on renal function in chronic spinal cord injured patients. J Urol 2000; 164(5):1490–1493.
9. Hess MJ, Zhan EH, Foo DK, et al. Bladder cancer in patients with spinal cord injury. J Spinal Cord Med 2003; 26:335–338.
10. Chancellar MB, Rivas DA, Staas WE Jr. DDAVP in the urological management of the difficult neurogenic bladder in spinal cord injury. J Am Paraplegia Soc 1994; 17(4):165–167.
11. Queek ML, Ginsberg DA. Long-term urodynamics followup of bladder augmentation for neurogenic bladder. J Urol 2003; 169:95–198.
12. Appell RA. Surgery for the treatment on overactive bladder. Urology 1998; 51:27–29.
13. Jezernik S, Craggs M, Grill WM, et al. Electrical stimulation for the treatment of bladder dysfunction: current status and future possibilities. Neural Res. 2002; 24:413–430.
14. Hackler RH, Katz PG. Management of common problems in spinal cord injured patients. Am Urol Assoc Update Ser 1991; 10(6):42–47.
15. Hall MK, Hackler RH, Zampieri TA, et al. Renal calculi in spinal cord-injured patients: association with reflux, bladder stones, and Foley catheter drainage. Urology 1989; 34:126–128.
16. Griffith DP, Khonsari F, Skurnick JH, et al. A randomized trial of acetohydroxamic acid for the treatment and prevention of infection-induced urinary stones in spinal cord injury patients. J Urol 1988; 140(2):318–324.
17. Kaufmann JM, Fam B, Jacobs SC, et al. Bladder cancer and squamous metaplasia in spinal cord injury patients. J Urol 1977; 118:967–971.
18. Goble NM, Clarke TJ, Hammonds JC. Histological changes in the urinary bladder secondary to urethral catheterization. Br J Urol 1989; 63:354–357.

13 | Headache

Gregory A. Elder

Headache is a common complaint among both neurologically intact and neurologically disabled populations, including patients with spinal cord injury (SCI), multiple sclerosis (MS), traumatic brain injury (TBI), and stroke. The overall prevalence of migraine is estimated to be approximately 15% in the general population in North America, and tension-type headache is even more prevalent.

Headache is common in the setting of acute stroke and one of the central features of the postconcussion syndrome. In general, the headache syndromes encountered in neurologically injured patient populations are similar to those found in the neurologically intact, with their diagnosis and management based on headache type rather than underlying neurologic disability, although some special considerations are discussed below.

ANATOMY AND PHYSIOLOGY

Pain-sensitive structures in the head include the skin, subcutaneous tissue, muscles, and the periosteum of the skull. The extracranial and intracranial blood vessels and cranial nerves are also pain sensitive. In general, pain originating in supratentorial structures is referred to the anterior two thirds of the head, while pain from the infratentorial compartment is referred to the back of the head and neck. However, it is important to recognize that the eyes, ears, nasal cavities, and paranasal sinuses are also pain-sensitive structures and that irritation of cervical nerve roots can cause pain referred to the back of the head. While a primary vascular etiology has long been postulated in migraine, its pathophysiologic basis remains incompletely understood. Likewise, although the pain of tension-type headaches has often been attributed to muscle contraction, there is little evidence for abnormal muscle contraction in tension-type headaches, and its pathophysiologic basis remains largely unexplained as well.

Primary headaches refer to headaches without an organic basis, while secondary headaches refer to those with an identifiable organic cause such as an intracranial mass lesion, bleeding, or central nervous system (CNS) infection. Most patients will have a primary headache disorder, with migraine and tension-type headaches being by far the most common. The clinical features of the major headache types are summarized in Table 13.1 (1).

Classic migraine, also called neurologic migraine or migraine with aura, is readily recognized by its aura, which is followed by a throbbing headache. The headache of common migraine is similar in quality but lacks the aura present in neurologic migraine. By contrast, tension-type headaches are usually described as being dull, aching, or having a pressure quality and may persist with only mild fluctuations for extended periods of time.

Among the causes of secondary headaches, the headache of raised intracranial pressure has no specific characteristics but is often described as aching and deep-seated. The headache of low intracranial pressure is most easily recognized by its sensitivity to positional changes. Subarachnoid hemorrhage is sudden in onset, intense, and is classically described by the patient as the "worst headache of my life." Headaches caused by meningeal inflammation are often associated with fever, neck stiffness, and signs of meningeal irritation. Temporal arteritis should be suspected in anyone with a new-onset headache over the age of 50, and its recognition is important due to the potential for visual loss.

Primary and secondary headaches must also be distinguished from pain in surrounding structures. Headaches associated with sinusitis are typically described as pressurelike or dull, and bending over intensifies the pain. When the maxillary or frontal sinuses are affected, there is often pain over the sinus. Pain from disease in the ethmoid or sphenoid sinuses is usually localized deep in the midline behind the root of the nose, although occasionally the pain may be referred to the vertex of the skull. Sinusitis-related pain is also typically accompanied by nasal congestion. Headaches that accompany disease of the ligaments, muscles, and apophyseal joints in the cervical spine are usually referred to the occiput and back of the neck. Patients with temporomandibular joint syndrome may complain of headache, although the pain is more typically found in front of the ear with radiation toward the jaw, temple, or neck. Closed angle glaucoma can also produce unilateral headaches of typically short duration and is most common in patients over age 50.

Headache is one of the core symptoms of the postconcussion syndrome, with as many as 90% of patients with TBI having some degree of headache. Fortunately most TBI-related headaches resolve spontaneously, and only when they persist longer than 3 months are they called chronic. Chronic headaches seem to be more common with mild TBI and most often resemble tension-type headaches, although migraines are seen as well. In TBI patients with chronic headaches, it is first of all important to consider secondary etiologies including chronic subdural hematomas, low-pressure headaches from cerebrospinal fluid (CSF) leaks, or occult injuries to the neck.

SCI patients may have headaches due to associated TBI or cervical spine injuries. Headaches are also common in the setting of acute stroke. Less is known about how often these headaches persist into the rehabilitation phase. Headaches in MS patients are typically tension-type headaches or migraine and do not appear to be, in general, more frequent in MS patients than in the general population, although there is some suggestion that headaches may be more frequent in patients treated with interferon-β.

PATIENT ASSESSMENT

History and Physical Exam

A good history is the single most important element in establishing a headache diagnosis. As in other pain syndromes, the history should focus on factors such as location, quality/quantity, aggravating/relieving factors, time course, and associated features with questions directed toward elements that allow the separation of primary from secondary causes of headache and the differentiation among the primary headache subtypes. Key questions in the history are listed in Table 13.2.

All patients should receive a general physical examination including vital signs, general appearance, and examination of the head, eyes, ears, nose, throat, teeth, and cervical spine. The arteries in the neck as well as the temporal arteries should be palpated. A funduscopic exam as well as a functional neurologic examine should also be performed. If indicated, signs of meningeal irritation should be sought by checking for Kernig and Brudzinski signs. The majority of patients presenting with headache will have a normal examination. A major focus of the history and physical exam is to identify warning signs or red flags that should prompt further investigation for a secondary headache etiology and in particular the need for neuroimaging. A summary of the major red flags in the headache history and exam are listed in Table 13.3.

Neuroimaging and Additional Laboratory Tests

Additional investigations are driven by the history and in particular by any red flags that become apparent. The major decision with most patients is whether to obtain neuroimaging (magnetic resonance imaging or computed tomography scan). Routine imaging is clearly not cost effective. Unfortunately, there are no controlled trials that allow a definitive judgment to be made as to when it is beneficial, and as a result the decision is left to clinical judgment. In general it can be agreed that neuroimaging is usually not warranted in patients with migraine and a normal neurologic examination (2). The presence of any of the red flags described in Table 13.3 should prompt neuroimaging as well as possibly other investigations. Neuroimaging should also be considered in patients with a new onset of headache after age 40. CSF examination must be considered when there is any suspicion of CNS infection and should be obtained when subarachnoid hemorrhage is a consideration but imaging is negative. Blood tests are typically not informative in the headache workup except that an elevated sedimentation rate is key in the diagnosis of temporal arteritis.

Table 13.1

Common Varieties of Headache

Type	Quality	Location	Duration	Frequency	Associated features
Migraine with aura (neurologic or classic migraine)	May begin as a dull pain but progresses to a throbbing/pulsatile pain, moderate to severe in intensity, aggravated by physical activity, often interferes with activities	Unilateral or bilateral, often frontotemporal	4–24 hr	Irregular intervals, recurs over weeks to months	Aura preceding headache, most often visual (enlarged blind spot, scintillating scotoma, flashing zigzag lines) but can be associated with focal neurologic symptoms/signs, nausea/vomiting, photophobia, phonophobia
Migraine without aura (common migraine)	Same as above	Same as above	Same as above	Same as above	Nausea/vomiting, photophobia, phonophobia, no aura
Tension-type headaches	Dull, pressure, tightness, aching quality, sometimes described as bandlike pressure around the head, usually not throbbing, mild–moderate intensity, not aggravated by routine physical activity, often does not interfere with activities	Bilateral, may have occipitonuchal, temporal, or frontal predominance	Variable but may persist with only mild fluctuations for days, weeks, or months	Variable but may recur over weeks, months, or years	Depression, absence of nausea/vomiting, photophobia, phonophobia
Cluster headaches	Sudden onset, sharp, non-throbbing, severe	Always unilateral orbital, supraorbital, or orbitotemporal	15 min to 3 hr	Nightly or daily for weeks to months	Usually nocturnal, may awaken patient from sleep, rhinorrhea, conjunctival injection, lacrimation, ptosis, miosis during the episode

	Quality	Location	Time Course	Periodicity	Associated Features
Raised intracranial pressure (brain tumor, other intracranial mass, pseudotumor cerebri)	Variable but most often aching, deep-seated, usually nonthrobbing variable intensity, may be worse in the morning, physical activity, changes in head position/lying down may provoke or aggravate pain	May be generalized or localized	Minutes to hours	Variable but often daily	Vomiting, focal neurologic symptoms/signs, papilledema
Low intracranial pressure headaches, (e.g., postlumbar puncture)	Steady	Occipitonuchal/frontal	Variable	Begins within minutes after arising from a recumbent position	Relieved by lying down
Subarachnoid hemorrhage	Sudden in onset, severe, "worst headache of my life"	Generalized, may be accentuated bifrontal or bioccipital	Hours to days	Most often single episode	May be transient loss of consciousness, neck stiffness, and vomiting, sometimes focal neurologic symptoms/signs, and subhyaloid hemorrhages, blood on CT scan or LP
Meningeal irritation (infection)	Often acute in onset, severe, deep-seated, constant, steady	Generalized but may be worse in neck	Evolves over minutes to hours	Single or multiple episodes	Fever, neck stiffness, signs of meningeal irritation
Temporal arteritis	Often throbbing initially but evolving to a more persistent achy pain sometimes with superimposed sharp, stabbing pains	Usually temporal, unilateral or bilateral, often localized to the site of the temporal arteries	Persists to some degree throughout the day, particularly severe at night	Untreated may last for many months	Over age 50, tender and thickened temporal arteries, sedimentation rate greatly elevated >50 mm/hr), elevated C-reactive protein, can progress to visual loss if not treated

Table 13.2

Questions in the Headache History

- Location of pain (unilateral, bilateral, frontal, temporal)
- Quality of the pain (throbbing, aching, pressure)
- Severity (what does the patient do during a headache, does the headache usually interfere with normal activities, how often are headaches severe, how often are they mild)
- Presence of an aura (visual, presence of focal neurologic symptoms)
- Associated symptoms during the headache (nausea, vomiting, photophobia, phonophobia)
- Precipitating/relieving factors (stress, alcohol, specific foods, lack of sleep, effect of activity, medications)
- Number of days with headache per month
- Age at onset of headaches
- Family history of migraine
- Response to any previous treatment
- Medications both prescription and over-the-counter
- Recent medical or dental procedures (e.g., lumbar puncture, tooth extraction, ENT procedures)
- Relationship to menstrual cycle in women
- History of head trauma
- When did the headaches start in relationship to any neurologic disability?
- How often are analgesics or other headache medications taken?
- Has there been any recent change in the character of the headaches or their pattern?

Table 13.3

Danger Signs or Red Flags in the History and Physical

- Papilledema (presence of an intracranial mass lesion, benign intracranial hypertension, encephalitis, or meningitis)
- Focal neurologic signs/change in mental status (intracranial mass lesion, other focal neurologic disease)
- Headache beginning after age 50 (temporal arteritis)
- Sudden onset, "the worst headache of my life" (subarachnoid hemorrhage)
- New onset headache in a patient with cancer or HIV infection (metastasis, opportunistic infection)
- Headaches precipitated by positional changes such as Valsalva, bending, or coughing (raised intracranial pressure or posterior fossa lesion)
- Newonset headache, progressive headache, or escalating medication requirements, change in pattern of headache in a patient with a primary headache disorder (secondary cause in a patient with primary headache syndrome)
- Neck stiffness and meningismus (meningeal inflammation)
- Fever (CNS or sinus infection)

TREATMENT

General Principles of Treatment

The treatment of secondary headaches is directed at the specific etiology. Therapy of primary headaches involves both pharmacologic and nonpharmacologic treatments. While pharmacologic approaches are important, nonpharmacologic approaches should be considered wherever possible.

Migraine

Treatment of migraine may be divided into therapy of the acute headache or preventive approaches aimed at reducing the frequency of headaches (3). Acute treatment is often divided into those therapies that are symptomatic being aimed at treatment of the pain (i.e., analgesics) versus abortive therapies directed at the underlying pathophysiology (e.g., triptans).

Acute Treatment of Migraine

The most commonly used agents are analgesics and triptans. Simple analgesics include aspirin, acetaminophen, and nonsteriodal anti-inflammatory drugs (NSAIDs) such as naproxen or ibuprofen. Symptomatic therapy with simple analgesics is appropriate for patients who have generally mild and infrequent headaches (e.g., one or two headaches per month). An NSAID is generally the preferred agent, although individual patients may find one NSAID better than another. Stronger analgesics such as opiates and combination medications, particularly those that contain barbiturates, should generally be avoided.

For patients with more frequent headaches or moderate–severe headaches, some attempt at abortive therapies is often warranted. The triptans are serotonin 1b/1d agonists. In contrast to analgesics, they are regarded as specific therapies in that they are thought to target the pathophysiologic basis of migraine. Available triptans include sumatriptan, zolmitriptan, naratriptan, rizatriptan, almotriptan, eletriptan, and frovatriptan. Multiple randomized controlled trials have demonstrated triptans to be effective therapies for treating acute migraine. However, relatively few trials have compared the various triptans with one another, and there are no data to indicate that one is more efficacious than another, making the question of which to choose more a matter of personal preference. The main difference between the triptans is their speed of onset of action, with naratriptan and frovatriptan having a slower onset of action than the others. There are also differences in the routes of administration available. Sumatriptan, zolmitriptan, and rizatriptan are available as a nasal spray in addition to oral forms and offer advantages when a nonoral route of administration is preferred in patients whose migraines present with significant nausea and vomiting. Zolmitriptan and rizatriptan are also available as self-dissolving tablets that can be administered on the tongue. Sumitriptan is available in a rapidly acting subcutaneous injectible form and as a suppository, both of which can be used in patients with severe headaches and/or significant nausea and vomiting. Triptans are most effective when administered at the first sign of a headache, and a single larger dose tends to be more effective than repeated small doses. Dosing schedules for sumitriptan and zomitriptan can be found in Table 13.4. A proprietary formulation of sumatriptan combined with naproxen also exists (Trexima), and recent randomized controlled trials have found this combination to be more effective than either agent alone. Prior to the introduction of triptans, ergot derivatives alone or in combination with caffeine were a mainstay of abortive therapy for migraine. Although effective, these agents have a generally less advantageous safety profile.

Triptans have proven to be safe and effective. However, they are difficult to use in certain neurologically disabled patients. It is generally recommended that triptans be avoided in older patients and not be used in patients with prior ischemic stroke, coronary or peripheral vascular disease, or uncontrolled hypertension due to their vaso-constrictive properties. They should also be used cautiously in SCI patients where the risk of autonomic dysreflexia is significant. For higher-risk patients triptans should if possible be administered for the first time under medical supervision. Triptans are also not optimal for patients with frequent headaches, and it is generally recommended that they not be used to treat more than four headaches per month. Triptans should not be given to patients with complicated migraine syndromes such as hemiplegic migraine, basilar migraine, or a prior history of migraine-associated infarction. The U.S. Food and Drug Administraion (FDA) has also issued an advisory warning of the possible risk of serotonin syndrome in patients receiving triptans and selective serotonin reuptake inhibitors (SSRIs) or selective serotonin/norepinephrine reuptake inhibitors (SNRIs). While the risk appears low, patients receiving both classes of medications should be warned about and monitored for symptoms of the serotonin syndrome.

Preventive Therapy for Migraine

The goals of preventive therapy are to reduce headache frequency, severity, and duration, thus reducing the disability associated with migraine. Preventive therapy may also improve responsiveness to acute treatments. Preventive treatment should be considered in patients with more than four headaches per month, if the headaches last longer than 12 hours, or if they cause significant disability. Other considerations are patient preference, as well as contraindications to or failure of or adverse reactions to standard acute therapies. Prophylactic therapy should also be considered in patients with complicated migraine syndromes such as hemiplegic migraine and in patients with a previous migraine-associated infarction to prevent further neurologic damage.

Medications that have proven effective in clinical trials include propranolol, metoprolol, timolol, amitriptyline, topiramate, and valproate. Of these, propranolol, timolol, valproate, and topiramate have been approved by the FDA for migraine prophylaxis. However, metoprolol, nadolol, and atenolol are also commonly used. A number of tricyclic antidepressants, including amitriptyline, nortriptyline, doxepin, and protriptyline, are also used for migraine prophylaxis, with amitriptyline having the most support in clinical trails.

Among the alternatives, no single medication or class of agents has emerged as the clear choice. As such, which agent to use is sometimes based on the presence of comorbid conditions such as depression or hypertension. Tricyclics offer the advantage that in patients with depression, they may treat the depression as well, while β-blockers may make the depression worse. By contrast, a β-blocker might be preferable in patients with hypertension. In cognitively impaired patients, nortriptyline is often recommended over amitriptyline due to its fewer anticholinergic side effects. Among the anticonvulsants, both topiramate and valproate have proven useful. However, topiramate has more cognitive side effects than valproate and thus may not be as advantageous in patients with significant cognitive impairment. Women of childbearing age must be warned of the teratogenic risks of valproate.

Regardless of the drug chosen, the common adage of start low and go slow applies. However, it should be realized that a given medication must be given an adequate trial both in terms of dosage and length of treatment. Most clinical trials suggest that efficacy is often first noted only after 4 weeks of therapy and may not be maximal until an adequate dose is reached after several months of therapy. If headaches are well controlled, drugs may be slowly decreased and patients will often continue to experience benefits on lower doses.

Other drugs that are in use for migraine prophylaxis include calcium channel blockers such as verapamil or nifedipine, angiotensin-converting enzyme (ACE) inhibitors such as lisinopril, and the angiotensin II receptor blocker (ARB) candesartan. While these agents may be effective, they lack the strong clinical trial–based evidence available for the medications discussed above. SSRIs have in general proven ineffective, although venlafaxine, a SNRI, has been shown to be effective in double-blind placebo-controlled trials. Gabapentin has also been used for preventive therapy. However, its efficacy is not as well established as the other approved anticonvulsants. Methysergide is an ergot derivative that has been used in the past in patients with refractory migraine. It is not, however, currently marketed in the United States and has rare but serious complications that have limited its use.

Migraine headaches that are temporally related to menstruation represent a special class of migraine. These headaches are often sensitive to NSAIDs, which are the treatment of choice for both acute therapy as well as prophylaxis of menstrual migraine. Naproxen 500 mg twice daily during the perimenstrual period is a commonly suggested regimen.

Other Agents for Migraine Prophylaxis

A number of other agents have been suggested as having utility for migraine prophylaxis, including an extract of the *Petasites hybridus* root known as butterbur, the herbal remedy feverfew, coenzyme Q10, and riboflavin. About the most that can be said for these agents is that their efficacy has not been established beyond a reasonable doubt. Despite some initially encouraging results,

Table 13.4

Common Medications Used in the Treatment of Migraine Headaches

Drug	Class	Indication	Oral dose	Side effects	Contraindications/Drug interactions
Naproxen	Nonsteroidal anti-inflammatory	Acute	500 mg, may repeat in 1–2 hr	Gastrointestinal disturbance, nausea, drowsiness, dizziness, edema, tinnitus	May cause increased risk of cardiovascular thrombotic events, myocardial infarction, stroke, gastrointestinal bleeding, and ulceration
Ibuprofen	Nonsteriodal anti-inflammatory	Acute	200 mg, may repeat in 1–2 hr	Gastrointestinal disturbance, nausea, drowsiness, dizziness	Same as naproxen
Sumitriptan	Triptan	Acute	25–100 mg, may repeat in 2 hr, no more than 200 mg/day[a]	Numbness, paresthesias, burning sensation, flushing, weakness, neck pain/stiffness	Contraindicated in patients with uncontrolled hypertension, previous myocardial infarction or stroke, monoamine oxidase inhibitor use within 2 weeks, use with caution in older patients or with history of seizures
Zolmitriptan	Triptan	Acute	2.5–5 mg, may repeat in 2 hr, no more than 10 mg/day[b]	Similar to sumitriptan	Similar to sumitriptan
Propranolol	β-Blocker	Preventive	Initial: 10 mg BID Maintenance: up to 240 mg/day[c]	Drowsiness, fatigue, depression, nausea, dizziness, insomnia, cognitive disturbance, hallucinations, cardiac (bradycardia, orthostatic hypotension, heart failure), exercise intolerance, impotence	Use with caution in patients with asthma, chronic obstructive pulmonary disease, diabetes mellitus, renal or hepatic dysfunction, cardiac conduction disturbances, or sinus bradycardia
Timolol	β-Blocker	Preventive	Initial: 5 mg BID Maintenance: up to 60 mg/day	Similar to propranolol	Similar to propranolol

Drug	Class	Use	Dosage	Side effects	Contraindications/cautions
Amitriptyline	Tricyclic antidepressant	Preventive	Initial: 10 mg QHS Maintenance: up to 150 mg/day	Sedation, dry mouth, blurred vision, constipation, urinary retention, cardiovascular (tachycardia, palpitations, orthostatic hypotension), weight gain, cognitive impairment	Contraindicated if monoamine oxidase inhibitors used within 14 days or acute recovery period following myocardial infarction, use with caution with history of seizures, glaucoma, hyperthyroidism, or liver dysfunction
Nortriptyline	Tricyclic antidepressant	Preventive	Initial: 10 mg QHS Maintenance: up to 75 mg/day	Similar to amitriptyline but less sedating, fewer anticholinergic side effects, fewer cognitive side effects	Similar to amitriptyline
Divalproex sodium	Anticonvulsant	Preventive	Initial: 250 mg BID Maintenance: up to 1500 mg/day[d]	Nausea/vomiting, tremor, diarrhea, alopecia, blurred vision, weight gain, hyperandrogenism in females, teratogenic, rarely hepatitis and pancreatitis	Should not be given during pregnancy, contraindicated in patients with history of hepatic dysfunction or pancreatitis as well as hematologic disorders, may affect levels of other anticonvulsants
Topiramate	Anticonvulsant	Preventive	Initial: 25 mg QHS Maintenance: up to 200 mg/day	Paresthesias, fatigue, anorexia, gastrointestinal distress, weight loss, taste perversion, sedation, insomnia, cognitive impairment, psychomotor slowing	Caution with renal or hepatic disease, withdraw slowly, may affect levels of other anticonvulsants

[a]Sumitriptan is also available as a nasal spray, a preparation for subcutaneous injection and a suppository.
[b]Zolmitriptan is also available as a disintegrating tablet that can be dissolved on the tongue and a nasal spray.
[c]Also available in a long-acting form.
[d]Also available in extended-release form.

several recent double-blind placebo-controlled trials have found no evidence that injections of botulinum toxin type A offer any benefit over placebo in prophylaxis of migraine.

Tension-Type Headache

Simple analgesics, such as aspirin, acetaminophen, or NSAIDs, may be useful in patients with infrequent headaches, but are generally not of benefit in patients with more frequent headaches and carry the risk of converting a simple tension-type headache into a more difficult to treat medication overuse headache. Tricyclic antidepressants are the best established pharmacologic treatment for tension-type headache. Patients with tension-type headaches should always be screened for depression, and, if present, a trial with a tricyclic antidepressant is warranted, although patients may respond to a tricyclic even if depression is not present. As noted above, in cognitively impaired patients, nortriptyline is often recommended over amitriptyline due to its fewer anticholinergic side effects. There is otherwise little evidence for any effective pharmacologic therapy of tension-type headache. In particular, the other drugs used for acute or preventive therapy in migraine have little impact on tension-type headache. Nonpharmacologic therapies should be especially considered. Interestingly, despite the implication of muscle tension as a pathophysiologic mechanism in tension-type headaches, botulinum toxin is not effective for the treatment of tension-type headache.

Nonpharmacologic Management of Headache

Nonpharmacological measures should always be considered and can often increase the effectiveness of pharmacologic approaches (4). Some specific examples of nonpharmacologic approaches are listed in Table 13.5. Which therapy is recommended will depend on local circumstances. However, all patients can benefit from education and attention to at least some behavioral modification. While some patients may identify foods such as hot dogs or red wine as spe-

Table 13.5

Nonpharmacologic Treatments for Headache

- Education
- Avoid headache triggers
- Stop smoking
- Improve sleep hygiene
- Daily exercise
- Biofeedback
- Other forms of relaxation therapy
- Cognitive behavioral therapy (coping strategies)
- Acupuncture

cific triggers, sleep disturbance and stress are in general much more important precipitating factors. Limiting caffeinated beverages and cessation of smoking may also be helpful.

Special Varieties of Headaches

Chronic Daily Headaches

Chronic daily headaches (CDH) are typically defined as headaches that occur on most days of the month for more than 3 months consecutively in the absence of organic pathology. Thus, CDH is not a primary headache type, but a syndrome. Both migraine and tension-type headaches can transform into CDH. When the result of transformed migraine, the headaches often become more tension type or mixed. CDH is often but not always associated with medication over use. Treatment of both transformed migraine and chronic tension-type headaches is similar to the treatment of chronic migraine and tension-type headache described above.

A distinct type of CDH is referred to as new-onset daily persistent headache. This headache can appear in patients without a significant prior headache history. The headaches most often resemble chronic tension-type headaches, and the patients are often able to describe exactly when the headache began. Headaches of this type should always prompt a search for a secondary etiology, including neuroimaging. Management is similar to other forms of CDH.

Medication Overuse Headache

Medication overuse is a common cause or contributing factor to the development of CDH. There is debate as to whether these headaches represent rebound headaches associated with repeated analgesic withdrawals or whether repeated analgesic exposure induces tolerance. It could also be argued that frequent medication use is a consequence of chronic headache. Whatever its basis, medication overuse headaches may occur in patients with both tension-type headaches and migraine. All classes of analgesics have been implicated, but combination drugs containing ergotamine, caffeine, butalbital, and codeine seem to be particularly problematic, although over-the-counter medications including acetaminophen and NSAIDs can be problematic as well. The diagnosis should be suspected in patients who have frequent or daily headaches and who use medications almost daily. The only effective treatment involves withdrawal of the offending medications, although this is often difficult. Prevention is important, and in general patients should be advised to limit the use of acute medications to no more than 10 days per month.

Cluster Headache

Cluster headaches are sudden in onset, severe, unilateral, and of relatively short duration. Their name comes from the fact that they that tend to recur in clusters lasting weeks to months with sometimes long symptom-free intervals in between. Cluster headaches, while distinctive in their presentation, are an uncommon headache type accounting for probably no more than 0.1% of all headaches in a primary care setting. Acute management involves inhalation of 100% oxygen at 6 liters/min for 20 minutes by a nonrebreathing mask. Triptans, octreotide, and dihydroergotamine have also been used for acute therapy. Lithium, verapamil, divalproex sodium, and prednisone have all been used for prophylaxis.

Chronic paroxysmal hemicrania is a term used to refer to headaches that resemble cluster headaches, being characterized by brief (15–20 minutes) intense focal attacks of pain in the eye, forehead, or sometimes the temple or periaural area that occur multiple times per day. They differ in not having the tendency to cluster. Like cluster, chronic paroxysmal hemicrania is a rare disorder, and the diagnosis should not be made until structural lesions have been ruled out. The headaches are, however, exquisitely responsive to indomethacin.

Patient Safety

1. Clinicians should be vigilant for potentially dangerous headaches with one or more of the following presentations: 1) focal neurologic signs, 2) change in mental status, 3) new-onset headaches in patients with a history of cancer or HIV, 4) headaches precipitated by positional changes, 5) "worst headache of my life" presentation, and 6) headaches with fever and neck stiffness.
2. Triptans should be avoided in patients with prior history of stroke, coronary artery disease, peripheral vascular disease, or uncontrolled hypertension.
3. Caution and close monitoring should be used in prescribing triptans to patients receiving SSRIs or SNRIs due to the possibility of the development of serotonin syndrome.

Patient Education

1. Educating the patient and his or her family is an important aspect of treatment. In particular, it is important to explain the nature of the condition and encourage patients to participate in their own management.
2. The rationale for treatments, dosing schedules, and the likely side effects of any treatment should be discussed.
3. Patient expectations should be addressed, and realistic expectations should be established regarding treatment results, in particular discussing the length of time it may take to achieve results.
4. Preventive therapy for migraine, for example, requires a sustained commitment on the part of the patient to achieve benefits.

5. Patients should also be encouraged to keep a headache diary, recording when headaches occur, their intensity, the degree to which the headaches interfere with functioning, and any special circumstances that might have precipitated the headache. Samples of headache diaries can be found on the website of the American Council for Headache Education (http://www.achenet.org), and educational materials for patients are available on this site as well as the website of the National Headache Foundation (www.headaches.org).

6. Patient should be encouraged to limit caffeinated beverages, avoid triggers (hot dogs, red wine, etc.), and stop smoking.

7. Patients should be educated as to proper sleep hygiene and stress management techniques.

REFERENCES

1. Headache Classification Subcomittee of the International Headache Society. The International Classification of Headache Disorders, 2nd ed. Cephalgia 2004; 24(Suppl):9–160.
2. Frishberg BM, Rosenberg JH, Matchar DB, et al. and the US Headache Consortium Participants. Evidence-based guidelines migraine headache: neuroimaging in patients with nonacute headache. Available from: http://www.aan.com/professionals/practice/guideline/index.cfm.
3. Silberstein SD. Practice parameter: evidence based guidelines for migraine headache (an evidence based review): report of the Quality Standards Subcommittee of the American Academy of Neurology. Neurology 2000; 55:754–762.
4. Rains JC, Penzien PB, McCory DC, et al. Behavioral headache treatment: history, review of the empirical literature, and methodological critique. Headache 2005; 45:S92–S109.

14 | Nutrition and Spinal Cord Injury

Carol Braunschweig
Kristen Tomey
HuiFang Liang

According to the "Healthy People 2010" report, individuals with disabilities not only have higher rates of obesity but also have lower rates for diagnosis and treatment for nutrition-related chronic diseases than nondisabled persons (http://www.healthypeople.gov/Document/HTML/Volume1/06Disability.htm). This report emphasized the tremendous need to establish health promotion programs designed to prevent the development of secondary conditions and eliminate the health disparities that exist between people with and without disabilities in the United States.

Nutritional care for individuals with neurologic conditions is complex and dependent on the type and degree of impairment in each individual. Examples of nutritional care issues that may arise from various neurologic impairments include impaired cognitive ability for feeding, dysphagia, and limited or inability to obtain and prepare food. Additionally, frequently their impairments prevent full employment, further limiting access to optimal nutrition. The nutritional issues most prominent in this population include inadequate nutrition leading to malnutrition and obesity associated with excess food intake.

This chapter will focus the discussion of these issues using spinal cord injury (SCI) as a model, however, most of the material presented can be applied to other neurologic impairments including stroke, multiple sclerosis (MS), Parkinson's disease, and traumatic brain injury (TBI). Compared to able-bodied (AB) populations, individuals with SCI have increased morbidity and mortality from cardiovascular disease (CVD), hypertension, and insulin resistance and type 2 diabetes. The cornerstone of prevention and treatment of these conditions is nutrition.

Methods for the assessment of obesity, malnutrition, energy and fluid needs, treatments, and key concepts for patient education in SCI populations will be presented(1). Expanding our understanding of their unique nutritional issues is an important component for optimizing their health care and is pivotal to developing effective prevention and intervention programs.

185

PATIENT ASSESSMENT

Body Mass Index

The goal of a nutritional assessment is to determine nutritional status, which can include both excessive nutrition (obesity) and malnutrition (undernutrition). The body mass index (BMI; weight in kilograms/height in square meters) is used to categorize an individual's weight status and provides a simple measure of the relation between height and weight that correlates with percentage body fat in young and middle-aged adults (2). The four categories identified by the National Institutes of Health are:

1. Underweight   BMI < 18.5
2. Normal weight   BMI 18.5–24.9
3. Overweight   BMI 25–29.9
4. Obese   BMI ≥ 30

Very few studies have assessed the prevalence of obesity or underweight in SCI populations, and of these, ethnic and gender issues generally were not examined. We recently assessed the BMI of 185 paraplegic men recruited from out patient clinics at an urban rehabilitation hospital. Overall their mean BMI was 26.2 ± 6.5; 57% had a BMI ≥ 25 and 18.9% had a BMI ≥ 30, indicating a smaller overweight and obesity prevalence than has been reported for the general population (67% overweight and 33% obese) (3).

Assessment of Height

Because standing is not feasible in individuals with SCI, self-reported preinjury height should be used to determine their BMI. Recalled height has been found to be the most accurate method of obtaining height, although they tend to be overestimated, and individuals with complete SCI tended to overestimate more than individuals with incomplete SCI (4).

The primary assumption of BMI is that it is an independent index of body fat. It assumes that after adjusting for body weight-for-stature, all individuals with the same BMI will have the same fatness, regardless of their age, gender, ethnicity, or disease history. Many investigations have demonstrated that this assumption is not correct for various populations. For example, it is widely recognized that body fat increases with age, is greater in females than in males, and differs among ethnic groups (Asian Indians and Chinese have greater percentage of fat at any BMI). Individuals with SCI have greater fat mass per kilogram body weight than able-bodied populations due to loss of bone mineral density and muscle mass after injury; the higher and more complete the injury level, the greater the loss in lean and gain in fat mass (5). To address these concerns Peiffer et al. suggested calculating desirable body weight for paraplegics 10–15 pounds below the Metropolitan Life Insurance ideal body weight for a given height and frame size (6). This adjustment was only based on the initial weight loss without considering the body composition shift and bone mineral loss that occur in long-term SCI; therefore, it has not been widely accepted. David Gater recently estimated that more than two thirds of the SCI population are obese (7) based on a review of studies that had reported BMI and percentage of adiposity assessed via several methods (e.g., dual energy x-ray absorptiometry, hydrostatic weighing). He found among the seven studies that were conducted in paraplegic participants that those with BMIs within the normal range (18.5–24.9 kg/m^2) had corresponding percentages of total adipose that ranged from 23 to 33.8%, indicating that these individuals did not necessarily have a corresponding "normal" or "healthy" level of adiposity.

In the general population ideal body weight is determined as described in Table 14.1. These formulas are used to determine protein needs and help determine the adjusted ideal body weight in obese individuals.

Obesity Classification Using Waist Circumference

Centrally located adipose as assessed by waist circumference (WC) was first associated with heightened risk for obesity-related disease risks approximately 50 years ago. Since that time numerous studies have confirmed the effect of excessive central fat distribution on increased risks for CVD and type 2 diabetes. The National Institutes of Health (NIH) and World Health Organization (WHO) recommend waist circumference (measured midway between the lower rib and the iliac crest) cut-points for central obesity classification at ≥88 cm for women and ≥102 cm for men (8).

Despite limited data in SCI populations, the conventional wisdom has been that they have higher prevalence for abdominal obesity, which predisposes them to increased risks for diabetes and CVD compared to the general population. We recently reported that paraplegic men ($n = 185$) with a mean age of 39 years (range 20–59 years) recruited from outpatient clinics in a urban rehabilitation hospital had significantly higher mean waist circumferences (0.98 m vs. 0.94 m, $p < 0.001$) and significantly higher prevalence for central obesity (35% vs. 23%, $p = 0.01$)) than age- and race-matched participants included in the 1999–2002 National Health Examination Survey (3). A larger waist circumferences and greater prevalence of central obesity in SCI. Individuals may contribute to their greater risk for diabetes, insulin resistance, and cardiovascular disease.

Assessment of waist circumference is relatively easy, inexpensive, and practical. It is recommended that this measurement become part of the routine component of the medical examination. The waist circumference should be obtained

Table 14.1

Estimation of Ideal Body Weight

Women	Men
Allow 100 lb (45.5 kg) for the first 5 ft (152 cm) of height plus 5 lb (2.3 kg) for each additional inch 92.5)	Allow 106 lb (48 kg) for first 5 ft (152 cm) of height plus 6 lb (2.7 kg) for each additional inch (2.5 cm)

with the patient in the supine position, as standing is not possible and sitting posture varies dependent on level and completeness of injury. Recumbent and standing measures of waist circumference are highly comparable.

Malnutrition

SCI individuals often experience initial weight losses in the early rehabilitation phase. Cox et al. observed an average weight loss of 5.3 kg for paraplegics and 9.1 kg for tetraplegics within first month postinjury. The initial weight losses may be due to hypermetabolic rate and losses of muscle mass and may be inevitable despite adequate nutrition support. In our sample of 185 urban men with paraplegia, 7.5% were classified as underweight using the standard cut-point of BMI < 18.5. This is over eight times higher than the 0.9% underweight prevalence reported among men in the general population. As previously stated, however, because of their higher percentage of body fat for a given BMI, it is likely that the cut-point used is too high to reflect true risk for underweight and resulted in overreporting of underweight in this population. When we reevaluated participants for underweight using a cut-point for underweight that was 10% less than the standard underweight cut-point (i.e., BMI < 16.7), the prevalence dropped to 2%, still over two times greater than the general population, but substantially reduced compared to the unadjusted findings.

Assessment of Malnutrition

Over 25 years ago Baker et al. devised the subjective global assessment (SGA) for categorizing individuals as normal, moderately malnourished, or severely malnourished based on clinical judgment rather than biochemical or other objective measures (Table 14.2) (9). Based upon the patient's history regarding weight loss, dietary intake, gastrointestinal symptoms, functional capacity, and physical signs of malnutrition, including loss of subcutaneous fat or muscle mass and the presence of edema or ascites, patients are classified as normally nourished (N), moderately malnourished (M), or severely malnourished (S). It has been shown to predict various nutrition-associated complications including infections, use of antibiotics, length of hospital stay, and improvements in biochemical markers of nutritional status (e.g., albumin, transferrin) (10–12). This tool has not been validated specifically for individuals with SCI; however, it likely is better suited for this population than other methods that use specific cut-points for "normal" classification that did not consider differences in their body composition postinjury.

TREATMENT

The goals of "Healthy People 2010" are to promote the health of people with disabilities, prevent secondary conditions, and eliminate disparities between people with and without disabilities in the U.S. population (USDDS). However, there are no specific recommendations for dietary guidelines or vitamin and

Table 14. 2

Nutrition Assessment with Subjective Global Assessment

---

1. Anthropometry
   Height:
   Current weight:
   Usual weight:
   Ideal weight:
   BMI:

2. Clinical Methods for Nutritional Status Assessment—Applying Subjective Global Assessment*
   a. Weight change   Results
      Maximum body weight
      Weight 6 months ago
      Overall weight loss in past 6 month
      Percent weight loss in past 6 months
      Change in past 2 weeks: increase, no change, decrease
   b. Dietary intake change (relative to normal): yes or no

      If yes, duration (no. of weeks) =
      If yes, type: increased intake, suboptimal solid diet,
          full liquid diet, hypocaloric liquids, starvation
   c. Gastrointestinal symptoms (lasting >2 weeks)
      None, or nausea, vomiting, diarrhea, anorexia (list all)
   d. Functional capacity:
      No dysfunction or dysfunctional
      If dysfunctional, duration (no. of weeks)
      If dysfunctional, type: working suboptimally, ambulatory,
          bedridden
   e. Physical (for each trait specify: normal, mild, moderate,
          severe)
      Loss of subcutaneous fat (triceps, chest)
      Muscle wasting (quadriceps, deltoids)
      Ankle edema
      Sacral edema
      Ascites

*Subjective Global Assessment Rating
   A = well nourished,
   B = moderately malnourished
   C = severely malnourished

Classification :
1. Normal
   - No weight loss or <5% (~1–2 lb) weight loss (disregard if the patient is edematous or has ascites)
     and/or
   - No abnormal dietary intake and/or
   - No history or <2 weeks of anorexia, nausea, vomiting, or diarrhea

2. Moderate Malnutrition
   - Weight loss of 5–10% of usual body weight in the past 6 months (disregard if the patient is edematous
     or has ascites) and/or

- Abnormal dietary intake for 1 month and/or
- History of anorexia, nausea, vomiting, or diarrhea for short periods

3. Severe Malnutrition
- Weight loss of >10% of upper body weight (UBW) in the <6 months (disregard if the patient is edematous or has ascites) and/or
- Inadequate dietary intake for >1 month and/or
- History of anorexia, nausea, vomiting, or diarrhea for >1 month
- Visual somatic wasting

mineral supplements that are uniquely tailored for SCI or for the wheelchair-using population.

The USDA Food Guide Pyramid is a schematic that provides dietary guidance on what types and amounts of foods and beverages to consume for optimal health. The pyramid is based upon a conceptual grouping of foods and beverages into five categories: breads, vegetables, fruits, dairy, meat/alternatives, and items that should be used sparingly; each of the categories includes standard serving sizes that provide the basis for advice on how much to consume. The 2005 *Dietary Guidelines for Americans* (http://www.health.gov/dietaryguidelines/dga2005/document/html/executivesummary.htm) is a set of dietary recommendations focused on dietary patterns rather than individual foods. These guidelines should be used for optimal dietary intake in populations with SCI. They include:
- Consume adequate nutrients within caloric needs.
- Maintain body weight in a healthy range.
- Engage in regular physical activity; at least 30 minutes of moderate intense physical activity most days of the week.
- Consume 2 cups of fruit and 2.5 cups of vegetables per day, three servings per day of non- or low-fat milk or equivalent products.
- Keep total fat intake between 20–35% of calories, with most fats from polyunsaturated and monounsaturated fats and <10% of total calories from saturated fat.
- Keep sodium consumption to <2300 mg/day.

Energy and Protein Requirements

Total daily energy expenditure, defined as the amount of energy expended by an individual in one day, is made up of three components: 1) resting energy expenditure, 2) physical activity, and 3) the thermic effect of food. Total energy expenditure and resting energy expenditure, measured by either the indirect or direct method, have been found to be lower in people with SCI. The lower resting energy expenditure is thought to be due to a greater percentage of fat and lower fat-free mass for a similar BMI as well as decreased sympathetic nervous system activity among individuals with SCI compared to able-bodied populations. Basal energy expenditure can be estimated using the Harris Benedict equation. For adult males:

$$\text{BEE (kcal/day)} = 66 + (13.7 \times \text{wt in kg}) + (5 \times \text{ht in cm}) - (6.8 \times \text{age})$$

For adult females:

$$\text{BEE (kcal/kcal)} = 655 + (9.6 \times \text{wt in kg})$$
$$+ (1.7 \times \text{ht in cm}) - (4.7 \times \text{age})$$

These energy needs should be multiplied by activity factors (1.2 for bed rest/ minimally active, 1.3 for moderately active, and 1.5 for repletion or very active individuals) to determine daily needs.

Protein needs are estimated at 0.8–1.0 g/kg ideal body weight (IBW). The IBW is a theoretical estimate described in Table 14.1. Protein needs in obese individuals (individuals with BMI > 30) are based on an adjusted ideal body weight. The adjusted ideal body weight is calculated using the following formula:

$$\text{Adjusted ideal body weight} = (\text{actual weight} - \text{ideal body weight})$$
$$\times 0.25 + \text{ideal body weight}$$

Fiber and Fluid Recommendations

Many individuals with SCI have impaired bowel function due to a neurogenic bowel. Adding bran to diets of 11 inpatients with injury levels that ranged from C4 to T12 to increase fiber to 31 g/day resulted in significantly increased mean colonic transit time, suggesting that dietary fiber does not have the same effect on bowel function as in able-bodied individuals, in whom fiber reduces mouth–anus transit time. In general a diet high in fiber (25–35 g/day) from mixed sources (fresh fruits and vegetables, nuts, whole grains, legumes) is recommended for individuals with SCI to assist with bowel motility.

Optimal fluid intake is also recommended to assist in bowel motility as well as assist in the prevention of urinary tract infections, particularly in patients who empty their bladder by intermittent catheterization. Bacteria increase in the urine when it remains in the bladder for a prolonged amount of time (more than 4–6 hours). Consumption of adequate fluids to keep the urine volume between 300 and 400 cc (1–1½ cup) and emptying the bladder at least once every 6 hours are important protective measures. Fluid requirements can be estimated using guidelines provided in Table 14.3.

Consumption of cranberry juice produces hippuric acid in the urine, which acidifies the urine and prevents bacteria from sticking to the walls of the bladder and has been shown to have positive effects on urinary tract infections. It should be noted that for a significant effect, individuals should consume 100% cranberry juice and not "juice cocktail" as this is not concentrated enough with cranberries.

Table 14.3

Estimates of Fluid Needs

Weight (kg)	Fluid
Up to 10	100 ml/kg/day
10–20	1000 ml + 50 ml for each kg over 10 kg
>20	1500 ml + 20 ml for each kg over 20 kg

Enteral Nutrition

Some adults with significant neurologic disabilities may require enteral nutrition delivered via a feeding tube at some point in their care. The initiation of enteral nutrition is recommended for the malnourished patient who is expected to be unable to eat for longer than 5–7 days and in the normally nourished patient expected to be unable to eat more than 7–9 days.

Once the decision to use enteral feeding has been made, several issues need to be determined: 1) the type of formula to be given (calories/ml and nutrient composition), 2) the method of feeding (bolus vs. continuous vs. nocturnal feedings), and 3) the route of administration (tip of tube placed in the stomach or small bowel).

Enteral formulas can range in energy density from 1 to 2 kcal/ml. They also range in nutrient complexity from those requiring very little digestion (elemental) to those requiring complete digestion. Standard formulas are high in carbohydrate (~50%), low in fat (~30%), and low in fiber (<2–3 g). The type selected will be based on the patient's clinical profile. Most individuals with SCI will not have impaired digestion or absorption, and thus a 1 kcal/ml polymeric formula is typically used. For patients requiring fluid restriction, a 1.5 or 2.0 kcal/ml formula should be used.

The general rule for the method of feeding is to use the method least restrictive to the patient. Thus, bolus feedings given over 45 minutes or nocturnal feedings are preferred to continuous (given over 24 hours) feeding. The general rule for tube placement is to place it as high in the gastrointestinal tract as possible to maximize "natural digestion and absorption," minimizing intolerance.

Patient Safety

1. It is important for clinicians to be vigilant about the nutritional state of the adult with a neurologic disability. These individuals are often very frail and live within a narrow margin of good health. An acute change in their medical condition–especially one that is associated with a hospitalization—can adversely affect their nutritional intake, predisposing them to malnutrition. Clinicians should assess patients' risk for malnutrition in both inpatient and outpatient settings and, if detected, address it early and appropriately.
2. Obesity is a significant problem in adults with neurologic disabilities. It is associated with increased health risks, such as for hypertension, coronary artery disease, and diabetes. Clinicians should routinely screen weight and BMI in this population and initiate treatment.

Patient Education

Any change in dietary habits takes time. Effective nutrition education involves behaviorally oriented counseling to help patients acquire the skills, motivation, and support needed to alter their daily eating patterns and food preparation practices.

Examples of behaviorally oriented counseling interventions include: 1) teaching self-monitoring, training to overcome common barriers to selecting a healthy diet, 2) helping patients to set their own goals, 3) providing guidance in shopping and food preparation, 4) role playing, and 5) arranging for intratreatment social support. The "5-A behavioral counseling" framework consists of the following:

1. Assess dietary practices and related risk factors.
2. Advise to change dietary practices.
3. Agree on individual diet change goals.
4. Assist to change dietary practices or address motivational barriers.
5. Arrange regular follow-up and support or refer to more intensive behavioral nutritional counseling (e.g., medical nutrition therapy) if needed.

Healthy eating involves variety and moderation. The largest effect of dietary counseling has been observed with more intensive interventions (multiple sessions lasting 30 minutes or longer). These longer, more intense sessions are typically conducted by a registered dietitian and should target patients unable to shop/cook for themselves and/or their caregivers who are involved in these activities.

For those who are not able to make frequent trips to the grocery store, frozen and canned vegetables as well as dried fruit may be good options. The registered dietitian can also provide assistance in how to eat healthfully on a limited budget and provide information on sources for federal and state food assistance.

Effective use of clinic visits from the physician should include the "30-second nutritional sound bite," which provides specific suggestions to achieve the nutritional goals followed by referral to the dietitian. Specific 30-second sound bite examples for increasing variation include:

1. Consume three colors at every meal (white does not count).
2. Change soda consumption to water or juice.
3. Messages that encourage portion control to improve moderation:
   a. Limit serving of meat to the size of a deck of cards
   b. 1 cup = the size of a fist
   c. 3 oz = the palm (not including thumb and fingers)
   d. 1 teaspoon = size of one dime (typically one portion of butter)
   e. 1 oz = thumb size (one serving of cheese)

REFERENCES

1. Ho CH, Wuermser LA, Priebe MM, Chiodo AE, Scelza WM, Kirshblum SC. Spinal cord injury medicine. 1. Epidemiology and classification. Arch Phys Med Rehabil 2007; 88: S49–54.
2. Willett WC, Dietz WH, Colditz GA. Guidelines for healthy weight. N Engl J Med 1999; 341:427–434.
3. Liang H, Chen D, Wang Y, Rimmer JH, Braunschweig CL. Different risk factor patterns for metabolic syndrome in men with spinal cord injury compared with able-bodied men despite similar prevalence rates. Arch Phys Med Rehabil 2007; 88:1198–1204.
4. Garshick E, Ashba J, Tun CG, Lieberman SL, Brown R. Assessment of stature in spinal cord injury. J Spinal Cord Med 1997; 20:36–42.
5. Nuhlicek DN, Spurr GB, Barboriak JJ, Rooney CB, el Ghatit AZ, Bongard RD. Body composition of patients with spinal cord injury. Eur J Clin Nutr 1988; 42:765–773.
6. Peiffer SC, Blust P, Leyson JF. Nutritional assessment of the spinal cord injured patient. J Am Diet Assoc 1981; 78:501–505.
7. Gater DR, Jr. Obesity after spinal cord injury. Phys Med Rehabil Clin N Am 2007; 18: 333–351, vii.
8. Executive summary of the clinical guidelines on the identification, evaluation, and treatment of overweight and obesity in adults. Arch Intern Med 1998; 158:1855–1867.
9. Baker JP, Detsky AS, Whitwell J, Langer B, Jeejeebhoy KN. A comparison of the predictive value of nutritional assessment techniques. Hum Nutr Clin Nutr 1982; 36:233–241.
10. Jeejeebhoy KN, Baker JP, Wolman SL, et al. Critical evaluation of the role of clinical assessment and body composition studies in patients with malnutrition and after total parenteral nutrition. Am J Clin Nutr 1982; 35:1117–1127.
11. Detsky AS, Baker JP, O'Rourke K, et al. Predicting nutrition-associated complications for patients undergoing gastrointestinal surgery. JPEN J Parenter Enteral Nutr 1987; 11: 440–446.
12. Ulander K, Grahn G, Jeppsson B. Subjective assessment of nutritional status—validity and reliability of a modified Detsky index in a Swedish setting. Clin Nutr 1993; 12:15–19.

15 | Obstetric and Gynecologic Care of the Adult Woman with a Neurologic Disability

Dorothy A. Miller

This chapter addresses obstetric and gynecologic (OB/GYN) issues common to women with spinal cord injury (SCI), traumatic brain injury (TBI), multiple sclerosis (MS), and stroke (CVA). These four diseases affect a large number of women. The incidence of SCI among American women of childbearing age is 3000 per annum (1). The overall incidence of TBI in Americans is estimated at 1.5 million annually, many of these people are female. MS affects up to 350,000 American men and women and is at least twice as common in women, especially those between 20 and 40 years of age (2). While CVA is relatively rare in younger women, its prevalence increases with age and women are now living longer than ever before. All of these women require sound gynecologic care. However, women with a neurologic disability face both attitudinal and structural barriers to consistent high-quality (OB/GYN) care; they rarely receive regular breast and pelvic exams. In turn, they are screened less frequently for gynecologic and breast malignancies. This chapter presents common clinical pearls coincident to the OB/GYN care of women with neurologic disability while highlighting a few disease-specific considerations. Pertinent items to address in a women's health history and physical exam are presented, and the potential obstetric emergency of autonomic dysreflexia is reviewed. Special concerns relevant to contraception, menstrual hygiene, and sexually transmitted diseases are discussed, and the current literature on pregnancy and SCI, TBI, MS, and CVA is reviewed. Issues related to pregnancy among patients with these four diagnoses are also addressed in this chapter. However, a comprehensive discussion of labor and delivery care is beyond the scope of this text.

According to the Center for Research on Women and Disabilities, between 1992 and 1996 31% of disabled women were refused care by a physician secondary to their disability (3,12). This and other studies noted the additional trend that the more severe the patient's functional limitation, the less likely she was to receive regular gynecologic care. Women with neurologic disabilities who are able to see a provider often face both structural and attitudinal barriers to optimal OB/GYN care (13). This situation culminates in a whole population of women who may receive suboptimal care compared with their able-bodied counterparts. Table 15.1 lists key care barriers alluded to above.

For reasons listed above, disabled women rarely receive regular breast and pelvic exams (1). Breast and pelvic exams along with breast mammography represent the mainstay of women's health cancer screening. Suggested health consequences of this phenomenon among these women would include an increased incidence of sexually transmitted diseases (STDs) and some malignancies including breast, endometrial, ovarian, and cervical cancer (11). An exhaustive search for current incidence of these diagnoses among women with disabilities relative to able-bodied women was unsuccessful at the writing of this chapter: information regarding gynecologic healthcare and screening in women with disabilities is scarce. The relative rarity of screening gynecologic and breast examinations performed in women with physical disabilities can be associated with an increase in morbidity secondary to delay in screening and diagnosis in this suboptimally served population (4,12).

PATIENT ASSESSMENT

There are several key questions to ask women with neurologic disabilities during the medical interview as well as important considerations in performing the physical examination. Table 15.2 outlines some of them.

Autonomic Dysreflexia: A Potential Obstetric Emergency

Women with SCI at or above the T6 neurologic level are at highest risk for autonomic dysreflexia (AD). This entity has been reported to occur among MS patients as well (14). Whereas AD is described in greater detail elsewhere in this book, it is important to mention that it is a potentially life-threatening complication during the pregnancy of women with these neurologic diseases.

The physiologic changes pregnant women with neurologic disease at T6 or above undergo certainly necessitate due diligence on the part of their doctors to monitor for and treat this serious complication. Three such changes include bladder stasis secondary to a growing fetus, constipation, and the increase

Table 15.1

Obstacles to Optimal OB/GYN Care

- Lack of patient knowledge and education
- Inaccessible facilities (lavatory, changing/exam rooms, hallways)
- Lack of appropriate equipment (height-adjustable exam tables, scales, transfer boards, Hoyer lift, wheelchair-accessible mammography machine)
- Lack of trained support staff (safe transfer techniques, accessibility issues, clinic visit planning)
- Inadequate healthcare provider education (disability-related comorbidities, alternative positioning for exam, altered focus during physical examination)

Table 15.2

Key Items and Questions to be Considered During Examination of Women with Neurologic Disabilities

Pertinent History
- Latex allergy
- Menstrual hygiene difficulties
- Change in spasticity, bladder, or self-care during menses
- History of autonomic dysreflexia in patient with SCI
- History of relapse triggers in MS
- Patient and/or caregiver ability to perform self–breast exam
- Sexual activity (actual and desired)
- Current form of birth control
- Comprehensive medication review
- Bladder and bowel management
- Childbearing plans
- Prior pregnancy history

Considerations in the Health Exam of Women with Neurologic Disabilities
- Perform breast exam prior to pelvic exam to reduce need for repositioning.
- Instruct patient to perform bowel care prior to office visit to avoid fecal incontinence.
- Instruct patient to empty bladder prior to exam to minimize risks of incontinence and AD.
- Warm speculum prior to use to decrease spasticity during exam.
- Have specialized transfer equipment readily available in exam room.
- Pad exam table and its stirrups well. Table should be wheelchair accessible (e.g., Powermatic examination table [Hausmann Industries, Northvale, NJ]).
- Ensure exam table has handrails or provide an extra assistant for fall prevention during examination.
- Use narrow blade insertion for patients with upper motor neuron (UMN) disease.
- Use larger, wider speculum for patients with lower motor disease and subsequent relaxed pelvic musculature.

in risk for decubitus ulcers with pregnancy-related weight gain. At regular clinic visits, patients should be educated about the signs and symptoms of AD. Patients should be screened for symptoms prior to pelvic exam, and pre-exam blood pressure should be taken.

If a patient should become symptomatic in the midst of a pelvic exam, the speculum should be removed and the following steps should be taken:

1. Sit the patient upright and remove restrictive clothing.
2. If the patient has an indwelling Foley catheter, check it for kinking or blockage. If it does not flush, it should be changed.
3. If the patient has neurogenic bladder and uses intermittent catheterization for management, then the patient should be catheterized.
4. Check the skin for pressure ulcers. If there is an area of skin breakdown, the patient should be positioned so she is not leaning on this area.

If these interventions do not offer symptomatic relief and lower the blood pressure, the rectum should be inspected for blockage or other potentially irritating source of dysreflexia. Pharmacologic treatment of AD includes the use of topical nitro-paste and nifedipine.

Gynecologic Issues: Infection, Menses, and Contraception

Women with neurologic disease are sexually active. Given the neurologic impairment in these patients, their providers should be alert for STDs presenting with generalized symptomatology over localized complaints. Fever, fatigue, increase in pain often elsewhere in the body, change in bladder or bowel habits, and increase in spasticity are all clues to gynecologic pathology. Decreased mobility, especially among wheelchair users, renders these patients prone to vaginal yeast infection. They also often have increased perineal moisture and more frequent antibiotic use—often for urinary tract infections (UTIs). Treatment for yeast infection is the same as in able-bodied women.

Many SCI patients complain of increased spasticity with menses and menopause. For unknown reasons, menopausal women with SCI may be more prone to AD. Within the SCI population, no relationship has been found between with level or etiology of injury and onset ages of menarche and menopause (1). However, functional differences due to the neurologic level of injury do affect the patient's ability to maintain perineal hygiene during menses. Tetraplegic women in particular struggle with this issue, but it is an issue among female MS, CVA, and TBI patients as well. The presence of spasticity, contractures, impaired trunk balance, mobility, and altered hand function, combined with chronic bladder instrumentation, creates a challenging hygienic environment during menstruation for these patients. Menstrual hygiene needs to be discussed with patients and caregivers, as poor hygiene can result in unnecessary morbidity. Clinicians should identify problems in this area and reinforce good hygienic habits with both patients and caregivers. When necessary, hormonal contraception may be offered to modulate menstrual flow. In severe cases, the provider may consider endometrial ablation.

For a detailed discussion of sexuality in adults with neurologic disability, the reader is referred to Chapter 27. With regard to family planning in particular, both able-bodied and neurologically impaired women have the same contraceptive options. When considering a nonhormonal form of contraception, the patient and her healthcare provider should take several factors into consideration. Impaired uterine and vaginal sensation along with spasticity increases the risk of complications such as infection and rupture in IUD users. Diaphragm use is accompanied by an increase in uterine cervical abrasion risk secondary to decreased pelvic sensation. The patient's level of manual dexterity also needs to be taken into account when deciding on a contraceptive method that requires the physical placement of a barrier method of birth control. For patients considering hormonal strategies, tobacco use increases the risk for thromboembolism in neurologically impaired women, as in the able-bodied population; this risk is likely amplified in more sedentary individuals such as women with neurologic disability. With thoughtful consideration, patient education, and proper monitoring, safe and effective contraception and family planning is possible.

Pregnancy and Neurologic Disease: Brief Literature Review and General Considerations

All women with chronic neurologic disease who are considering conceiving a child should undergo a review of their medication regimen; the practitioner should screen chronic medications for potential teratogenicity, associated nutritional deficiencies, and additional potential effects on maternal and fetal health over the course of pregnancy. TBI and CVA patients often take seizure medications, which commonly predispose to folate deficiency. The importance of folate supplementation in the prevention of neural tube defects has been well studied. Folic acid supplementation beginning prior to conception should be encouraged.

There is very little literature on obstetric issues among women with CVA or TBI. In 2004, Coppage et al. performed a descriptive, retrospective, non-standardized study on a small sample of women with a history of CVA due to varied etiologies. The authors found a zero percent maternal CVA recurrence risk with pregnancy. Approximately one third of newborns produced during this study were small for gestational age. The authors combined their data with that from two prior larger cohort studies—one evaluating ischemic CVA patients and the other thrombophilia patients (6,7). The combined data yielded an overall risk of recurrent CVA in pregnancy of 1% when the patient cohort had suffered predominantly "ischemic" CVA and 20% when most patients had a diagnosis of thrombophilia. Anticoagulation recommendations for these women are not well defined at this juncture. In Coppage's original study, 91% of women delivered at term.

There are slightly more data on SCI and pregnancy than for TBI and CVA. There is believed to be a trend toward premature and low-birthweight infants among women with SCI; however, the data to date are not definitive (9). Most SCI women who conceive do so approximately 5 years postinjury. One study cited roughly equal conception rates among paraplegic and tetraplegic subjects (8). For SCI women attempting to conceive, basal body temperature fluctuation is not a reliable indicator of ovulation secondary to postinjury changes in body temperature regulation.

Pregnant women with decreased mobility, neurogenic bladder, and bowel are at risk for several medical complications over the course of pregnancy: these include UTI, skin breakdown, fecal impaction or obstruction, deep vein thrombosis, and progressive functional impairment. If their disease includes an element of neuromuscular restrictive airway disease, they may also suffer respiratory decline over the course of pregnancy. SCI women fall comprehensively within these categories, but the medical considerations that follow are generalizable to women with TBI, CVA, and MS as well.

As in the able-bodied population, the risk for urinary stasis and subsequent UTI increases throughout pregnancy. This trend is exacerbated in patients with the aforementioned comorbidities. Patients with frequent bladder instrumentation are at a higher risk for UTI. However, prophylactic urinary tract infection treatment is not recommended secondary to concerns over microbial resistance and potential teratogenic affects of antibiotics often used for genitourinary infection. Bladder management, such as intermittent catheterization frequency, often changes over the course of pregnancy.

In order to avoid infection and AD, both patient and clinician should remain vigilant for changes and adapt bladder management as needed. The provider should inquire about changes in bowel habits at every visit and modify the patient's bowel program as needed; care should be taken to adapt the patient's bowel regimen to counter the constipating effects of oral iron supplementation. Weight gained during pregnancy places these patients' skin at greater risk for breakdown and may also be accompanied by a functional decline over the course of the pregnancy. Transfers and wheelchair propulsion often become more difficult as body mass increases. The healthcare provider needs to reassess the patient's seating during pregnancy, including a formal referral for pressure mapping. The patient should rent a tilt-in-space wheelchair toward the last trimester to aid in pressure relief; the physician should assess the patient's skin at least every 3–4 weeks. The patient and relevant caregiver should be reeducated in daily skin checks and regular pressure reliefs at every visit.

Patients with restrictive airway disease secondary to their neurologic diagnosis should practice regular incentive spirometry and undergo assessment by an anesthesiologist with possible pulmonary function testing prior to delivery. Referral to a high-risk obstetrician and anesthesiologist is encouraged. Providers should also maintain a high suspicion for deep vein thrombosis among pregnant women with neurologic disability and screen with ultrasound when necessary.

Unlike in CVA, TBI, and SCI, there has been much medical study of the effect of pregnancy on MS. The PRIMS (Pregnancy in Multiple Sclerosis) trial was the first large-scale prospective study on MS and pregnancy (10). It included 227 pregnant women with MS who carried their pregnancies to term, giving birth to live infants. The mean maternal age at conception was 30 years. They hailed from 12 European countries and were followed by Vukusic et al. from pregnancy to 2 years postpartum. The cohorts' MS relapse rate decreased significantly during pregnancy, a trend especially marked in the last trimester. Patients' disability did not worsen over the course of pregnancy. At 3 months postpartum, the mothers' MS relapse rate returned roughly to that of the prepregnancy year.

Screening for Breast Cancer, Cervical Cancer, and Sexually Transmitted Diseases

Cancer and STD screening recommendations are the same in able-bodied women as in women with a neurologic disease. Nulliparous women with a family history of breast cancer are considered at high risk for this disease. They should undergo mammography every 1–2 years starting at 40–49 years of age. All other women should begin the same screening at age 50–69 years. Cervical cancer screening consists of a PAP smear once sexually active, followed by additional smears every 3 years thereafter unless the women has multiple or new sexual partners. Pelvic exams and provider-performed manual breast exams should be performed annually. Patients should be educated in self–breast exam technique. If impaired manual dexterity precludes patient performance of monthly self–breast exam, then the patient caregiver should be trained to perform this screening.

It can be argued that pelvic exams, cancer, and STD screening are even more important in women with neurologic disease than in able-bodied women secondary to decreased pelvic sensation and subsequent decrease in patient ability to report symptoms commonly associated with gynecologic pathology. Initiating a therapeutic dialogue and providing a thoughtfully tailored exam are the provider's responsibility. In addition to the standard H&P, additional items to consider in the history and physical exam are as follows.

Patient Safety

1. As mentioned above, AD is a potential obstetric emergency and clinicians should monitor and treat it once it is identified.
2. Given the possible limited pelvic sensation, it is arguably more important that women with neurologic disabilities receive screening for cervical cancer and STDs.
3. Commonly used drugs by women with neurologic disabilities can have a teratogenic potential. Table 15.3 lists some of them as well as the U.S. Food and Drug Administration classification system for potential fetal risk.

Table 15.3

Teratogenic Medications Commonly Used by Women with Neurologic Disabilities

---

CLASS A: Folate, Colace, Senna, Dulcolax
CLASS B: Ditropan
CLASS C: Ritalin, Provigil, Baclofen, Tizanidine, Hytrin, Levoquin, Bactrim
  • All common MS immunosuppressive therapies are generally teratogenic. The following medications used in MS are contraindicated in pregnancy (all either C or D) associated with adverse fetal effects: azathioprine, cladribine, corticosteroids, cyclophosphamides, cyclosporine, glatiramir, interferons-1β and -1α, methotraxate, mitoxantrone, and natalizumab.

(Continued)

Table 15.3 (*Continued*)

CLASS D:

- Carbamazepine—dysmorphic facial features, heart defects, spina bifida, and intrauterine growth retardation (IUGR)
- Phenytoin—fetal hydantoin syndrome, neuroblastoma, and coagulation defects.
- Phenobarbitol—Cardiac defects, vitamin K depletion with hemorrhagic newborn disease, maternal folic acid deficiency, spina bifida, neonatal drug withdrawal.
- Aspirin—IUGR, premature closure of ductus arteriosus, pulmonary hypertension, talipes foot abnormality

U.S. FDA Pregnancy Category Definitions (Source, "Micromedex" 2008).

Controlled studies in women fail to demonstrate a risk to the fetus in the first trimester (and there is no evidence of a risk in later trimesters), and the possibility of fetal harm appears remote.

Either animal reproduction studies have not demonstrated a fetal risk but there are no controlled studies in pregnant women or animal reproduction studies have shown adverse effect (other than a decrease in fertility) that was not confirmed in controlled studies in women in the first trimester (and there is no evidence of a risk in later trimesters).

Either studies in animals have revealed adverse effects on the fetus (teratogenic or embryocidal or other) and there are no controlled studies in women or studies in women and animals are not available. Drugs should be given only if the potential benefit justifies the potential risk to the fetus.

There is positive evidence of human fetal risk, but the benefits from use in pregnant women may be acceptable despite the risk (e.g., if the drug is needed in a life-threatening situation or for a serious disease for which safer drugs cannot be used or are ineffective).

Studies in animals or human beings have demonstrated fetal abnormalities or there is evidence of fetal risk based on human experience or both, and the risk of the use of the drug in pregnant women clearly outweighs any possible benefit. The drug is contraindicated in women who are or may become pregnant.

Patient Education

Patients should be educated on the following:

1. Self–breast exam (Table 15.4).
2. Importance of screening for breast and cervical cancer as well as STDs.
3. Methods of contraception (Table 15.5).
4. Pregnant women should be educated on:
    a. AD—its clinical presentation as well as methods to reduce its occurrence.
    b. Monitoring for skin breakdown and importance of good bowel and bladder care during pregnancy.
    c. Avoidance of medications with teratogenic potential during pregnancy.
    d. Wheelchair cushion checks during pregnancy to prevent skin breakdown due to weight gain.
    e. Incentive spirometry during pregnancy.

Table 15.4

Self-Breast Exam: Five-Step Approach*

1. Look at your breasts in the mirror with your shoulders straight and your arms on your hips. Check that they are their usual size, shape, and color. Notify your doctor if you see any redness, rash, skin dimples or bulges, a nipple that is "inverted" (pushed in rather than sticking out).
2. Raise your arms and look for the same changes
3. Gently squeeze each nipple between your finger and thumb and check for nipple discharge. Note the color of discharge, if present, and tell your doctor.
4. Lie down on your back with one arm positioned over your head. If you are examining your right breast, place your right hand over your head and examine the right breast with your left hand. When feeling the breast tissue, keep your 1st three fingertips flat and together. Perform gentle circular movements beginning at the nipple and moving in larger and larger circles until you reach the outer edge of the breast. Examine the whole breast; this region includes the whole area from your collarbone, sternum, upper abdomen, to armpit. Examine each area starting with a very soft touch, increasing the pressure until you can feel your ribs.
5. Perform same exercise listed in (4) but while seated. With consistent monthly exams, you will become familiar with the way your breasts normally look and feel. Report any changes to your doctor for further evaluation.

* Perform once each month several days after your period ends; if you are postmenopausal, choose the same date each month for exam; if you are unable to perform self–breast exam, have your doctor train a trusted caregiver.

Table 15.5

Contraception Advice for Women with Neurologic Disease

- Women with neurologic diseases are at risk for experiencing numbness or lack of sensation in the sexual organs as well as in other areas of the body. It is important to consider these factors when choosing the form of contraception that is best for you. There are many different forms of contraception available; women with neurologic diagnoses have the same choices as able-bodied women.
- In general, there are a few main types of contraception available: barrier method, hormonal techniques, and the intrauterine device (IUD). The "barrier" forms of contraception physically block the sperm and egg from meeting and therefore fertilization from occurring. Barrier methods include the male condom, spermicides, cervical cap, diaphragm, and Lea's shield. Weakness and numbness in the arms and hands can influence successful and safe placement of barrier methods of contraception. Additionally, changed or lack of sensation in the vagina and cervix from your neurologic disease may place you at a higher risk for damaging the delicate tissue making up these structures when barrier contraception is used. These methods of birth control only work when they are placed consistently and correctly. It is also important to keep in mind that several of these products contain latex. If you or your partner is latex-allergic, do not choose a form of contraception that contains this substance. Some but not all barrier forms of contraception may protect you from sexually transmitted diseases (STDs); latex condoms are the most effective against

(Continued)

Table 15.5 (*Continued*)

    STDs but are slightly less effective in pregnancy protection then other forms of contraception, even with optimal use.

- The IUD is a small metal bit that is attached to the uterine wall and causes a local inflammatory reaction there. This change in the uterus prevents fetal implantation and therefore pregnancy. Patients with abnormal sensation are at a higher risk for infection and uterine rupture with the IUD than able-bodied women. Be aware!

- The third main type of contraception is hormonal; these extra hormones taken by the woman prevent female ovulation. They also change the climate of the woman's cervical mucus to decrease the chances of fertilization from occurring should egg and sperm meet. Birth control pills, hormonal injections, vaginal rings, and transdermal patches are all examples of this form of contraception. Just as in able-bodied women, those with neurologic impairments are at risk for blood clot formation with hormonal contraception use; this risk increases with physical inactivity and tobacco use. Keep in mind that hormonal contraceptives do not protect you from sexually transmitted diseases.

- Talk to your doctor about your options! More information on contraception can be found at the American College of Obstetricians and Gynecologists (ACOG) website: www.acog.org/publications/patient_education. Look specifically for ACOG pamphlets AP159 and AP022.

REFERENCES

1. Richman S. Gynecologic care of women with physical disabilities. Obstet Gynecol Survey 2007; 62(7):421–423.
2. Whitaker JN. Effects of pregnancy and delivery on disease activity in multiple sclerosis. N Engl J Med 1998; 339(5):339–340.
3. Burns AS, Jackson AB. Gynecologic and reproductive issues in women with spinal cord injury. Phys Med Rehabil Clin North Am 2001; 12(1):183–201.
4. Nosek MA, Howland C, Rintala DH. National Study of Women with Physical Disabilities: final report. Sexual Disabil 2001; 19(1):5–39.
5. Welner S. Screening issues in gyenocologic malignancies for women with disabilities: critical considerations. J Women's Health 1998; 7(3):281–285.
6. Coppage K, Hinton AC, Moldenhauer J. Maternal and perinatal outcome in women with a history of stroke. Am J Obstet Gynecol 2004; 190:1331–1334.
7. Lamy C, Hamon JB, Coste J. Ischemic stroke in young women. Neurology 2000; 55:269–274.
8. Soriano D, Carp H, Seidman DS. Management and outcome of pregnancy in women with thrombophylic disorders and past cerebrovascular events. Acta Obstet Gynecol Scand 2002; 81:204–207.
9. Jackson A, Wadley V. A multicenter study of women's self-reported health after spinal cord injury. Arch Phys Med Rehab 1999; 80:1420–1428.
10. Vukusic S, Hutchinson M, Hours M. Pregnancy and multiple sclerosis (The PRIMS Study): clinical predictors of post-partum relapse. Brain 2004; 127:1353–1360.
11. Welner S. Screening issues in gynecologic malignancies for woman with disabilities: critical considerations. J Women's Health 1998; 7(3):281–285.
12. Nosek MA, Howland BA. Breast and cervical cancer screening among women with physical disabilities. Arch Phys Med Rehabil 1997; 78:S39–S44.
13. Mele N, Archer J, Pusch BD. Access to breast cancer screening services for women with disabilities. J Obstet Gynecol Neonatal Nurs 2005; 34:453–464.
14. Bateman AM, Goldish GD. Autonomic dysreflexia in multiple sclerosis. J Spinal Cord Med 2002; 25:40–42.

16 | Management of Osteoporosis and Fractures in Adults with Neurologic Disabilities

Julie T. Lin

Osteoporosis is the most common metabolic bone disease and affects millions worldwide. Osteoporosis can manifest as fractures, which can result in devastating complications, even death, at its worst. While osteoporosis is increasingly prevalent in the general population, special populations such as those with neurologic disabilities due to spinal cord injury, multiple sclerosis (MS), traumatic brain injury (TBI), and cerebrovascular accident (CVA) possess drastically increased risk for bone loss and fracture. Adults with neurologic disabilities such as spinal cord injury (SCI) and CVA are special groups who are at extremely high risk for developing osteoporosis and fractures. Osteoporosis occurs in almost every SCI patient (1) and preferentially affects trabecular bone. Bone loss occurs acutely, with demineralization stabilizing between 16 months (2) and 24 months following SCI (3). Demineralization occurs in sublesional areas and primarily in weight-bearing skeletal sites such as the distal femur and proximal tibia (3). The incidence of lower extremity fractures has been cited as ranging from 1 to 34% (1).

Patients who have sustained motor paralysis due to central nervous system and peripheral nervous system injuries are at increased risk for osteoporosis and low bone mineral density (BMD) due to disuse. Due to limited mobility, there are decreases in osteoblast-mediated bone formation and increases in osteoclast-mediated bone resorption. There is typically more involved bone loss on the side of paresis, while bone density in the nonparetic limbs may increase due to increased use. The degree of bone loss appears to be inversely correlated to preservation of mobility and function. In one study involving women with hemiplegia, patients who had low ability to perform activities of daily living (ADL) were found to have greater decreases in BMD than those with high ability to perform ADL. For the low-ADL group, the BMD rate of change on the paretic side of the femoral neck was −9.6% over 3 months (4). Bone density in the paretic lower limb can decrease by more than 10% in less than 1 year, with smaller decreases being typical for the nonparetic lower limb (5). The affected hip areas are particularly vulnerable to bone loss, demonstrated by reduced hip BMD. This is of particular

205

importance because hip fractures are recognized for their association with increased morbidity and mortality.

The goal of this chapter is to provide an overview of osteoporosis in adults with the neurologic disabilities mentioned above. This includes pertinent anatomy, physiology, patient assessment, and treatment. Much of the work in this area has focused on SCI, so this will be used as a model, but many of the principles could also apply to the other diagnoses. Since osteoporosis can be associated with fractures, a small section on fractures is also included.

ANATOMY AND PHYSIOLOGY

Bone is a living organ and is constantly in the process of formation and resorption. Osteoblasts are responsible for bone formation, while osteoclasts are responsible for bone resorption. This delicate balance is disrupted in conditions that impair one's mobility and one's ability to perform weight-bearing exercise. As a result, there is typically significantly increased osteoclastic activity, unbalanced by osteoblastic activity.

In neurologic diseases such as spinal cord injury, there is a lack of bone formation coupled by a devastating increase in bone resorption. This may be quantified using markers of bone formation and resorption, which demonstrates the striking imbalance of bone homeostasis. In a study by Reiter et al. (6), markers of bone resorption such as N-terminal telopeptide of type I collagen (urinary NTX), increased more markedly in long-term SCI patients. The bone formation marker alkaline phosphatase was slightly below normal range in both short-term and long-term SCI groups.

Neural lesions and hormonal changes may also be involved in this process (7). Some proposed mechanisms include: 1) increased renal elimination and reduced intestinal absorption of calcium leading to a negative calcium balance; 2) vitamin D deficiency; 3) disrupted gonadal function with inhibition of the osteoanabolic action of sex steroids; 4) hyperleptinemia, in which serum levels of leptin are elevated (leptin is a hormone that plays a central role in regulating energy intake and energy expenditure); 5) pituitary suppression of thyroid stimulating hormone (TSH); and 6) insulin resistance (7). Patients who have sustained a cerebrovascular accident may have further complications, including sensory and visual/perceptual deficits, which may increase their risk of falls and fractures.

PATIENT ASSESSMENT

History

Osteoporosis should be suspected in adults with neurologic disabilities who have an associated paraplegia, tetraplegia, or hemiplegia due to their underlying condition. Clinicians should inquire about prior workups for osteoporosis such as x-rays, bone density studies, and blood and urine tests. A review of those records is important to determine the extent of osteopenia and may minimize the need for duplication of tests. It is also important to get a history of any previous fractures and their impact on the patient's functionality. Inquiries about pain related to previous fractures should include location, duration, radiation, quality, intensity, and aggravating and alleviating factors. Treatments tried and reason for their success or failure should also be noted.

The patient should also be asked about any recent trauma to the paralyzed limb(s) that can range from mild to severe. Did they notice any subsequent swelling, hematoma, or deformity in that limb?

The assessment should also include questions that address the potential risk of falls in this high-risk population. A review of difficulties with transfers, dressing, bathing, and mobility can shed light on areas that could potentially be addressed with adaptive equipment and rehabilitation. A thorough medication review checking for possible drug–drug interactions or drug-related cognitive or balance side effects should be carried out. Key questions to ask are outlined in Table 16.1.

Physical Examination

Since the adult with a neurologic disability is at risk for a fall-related fracture, the physical examination should attempt to identify physical findings that are associated with an increased risk of falls. These include an assessment of vision, balance, proprioception, range of motion, strength, transfers, and gait if the patient is ambulatory.

Table 16.1

Medical History

Fracture History
1. What caused the fracture-(i.e fall, range of motion exercises...)
2. Which limb(s) were fractured?
3. How was the fracture treated? (i.e cast, soft splint...)
4. Any pain associated with the fracture? If yes:
   Location, Intensity, Quality, Duration, Radiation, Aggravating and Alleviating factors.

Trauma History
1. Any recent trauma to the paralyzed limbs? If yes:
2. Any associated swelling, hematomas or deformities, low grade fever following the trauma?

Functionality:
1. Any falls or near falls with transfers, dressing, bathing or ambulation (if applicable)?

Balance
1. Any balance difficulties with transfers or ambulation?

Vision:
1. Loss of vision
2. Loss of depth perception
3. Difficulties with visual adaptations going from light to dark

The paralyzed limbs should also be inspected for any swelling, hematomas, or deformities, as these may be signs of an underlying fracture. Tenderness on palpation or pain with range of motion should be noted in patients with sensation in the weakened limb(s). Table 16.2 outlines some of the pertinent areas of the physical examination.

Diagnostic Tests

Osteoporosis is diagnosed with a bone mineral density test utilizing dual energy x-ray absorptiometry (DEXA), the gold standard, or is presumed to exist following an insufficiency fracture. Screening with a BMD is recommended to establish a diagnosis as well as to help gauge response to therapeutic treatments.

In SCI patients, immobilization affects the bone density of the proximal femur. Bone density in turn may be used to quantify fracture risk in SCI patients. Decreases of bone density are related to increased fracture risk. Bone density is reported as a T-score, which is that value compared to controls. Osteopenia is defined as a T-score from –1 to –2.5, while osteoporosis is defined as a T-score of –2.5 or less. Bone density should be performed initially as a baseline prior to starting antiosteoporotic medications, and then either annually or biannually (8).

Table 16.2

Physical Examination

- Paralyzed or paretic limbs
  o Range of motion and presence of contractures
  o Swelling
  o Deformities
  o Hematomas
  o Pain with range of motion.
- Neurologic examination
  o Strength testing
  o Balance
    o Ask patient to stand on one leg (if applicable)
    o Perform Romberg (have patient close eyes while assessing balance)
  o Sensation: assess light touch, pinprick, and temperature in lower extremities
  o Vibration and position sense in lower extremities
- Vision: assess vision and in particular assess field of vision
- Functional examination
  o Transfers: wheelchair to exam table or mat.
  o Ambulation
    o Ask patient to perform tandem gait on a straight line in the office
    o Watch patient ambulate down a long hallway or corridor (if applicable)

In addition to BMD, blood and urine studies may be performed to rule out underlying causes of osteoporosis. Serum studies such as 25-hydroxyvitamin D, intact parathyroid hormone (PTH), and urinary NTX may be performed to rule out conditions such as rickets or vitamin D deficiency and hyperparathyroidism. It is recommended that 25-hydroxyvitamin D be greater than 30 nmol/liter for optimal bone health. The normal laboratory values of intact PTH are 10–65 ng/liter. Urinary NTX should typically be maintained in the range of 20–40 nmol BCE/liter for the adult.

TREATMENT

The treatment of osteoporosis can be broken down into pharmacologic and nonpharmacologic treatments.

Pharmacologic Treatment

Heightened awareness of osteoporosis and ongoing bone loss in the patient with neurologic disability is essential. Appropriate osteoporosis treatment is often forgotten, particularly in the setting of the medically fragile patient. In one trial evaluating the use of antiosteoporotic medication and calcium and vitamin D in the stroke patient, small percentages of patients were found to be taking these medications. Among inpatients with stroke, 7.1% were taking osteoporosis medications, 11.3% were taking calcium supplements, and 5.9% were taking vitamin D supplements, while among outpatients with stroke, 5.7% were taking osteoporosis medication, 5.8% were taking calcium supplements, 2.2% were taking vitamin D supplements, and 16.0% were taking multivitamin supplements (9).

Pharmacologic management of osteoporosis should include, at a minimum, calcium and vitamin D. Calcium citrate and calcium carbonate are both widely available, with the former preferred due to its ease of absorption. Calcium carbonate requires an acidic environment to be activated, and therefore any individual who is taking antacids or who lacks gastric acidity should take calcium citrate. Daily recommendations for intake are 1500 mg of calcium and 800 IU of vitamin D.

Bisphosphonate medications inhibit osteoclast function and bone resorption and therefore represent an excellent treatment option for the patient with neurologic disability. One study demonstrated that the use of the bisphosphonate etidronate had virtually no effect on cortical osteoclasts, but reduced the number of trabecular osteoclasts (10). Another study found that etidronate preserved bone density in SCI patients who became ambulatory compared to all other patients who showed a loss of bone density over time (11).

Alendronate has also been shown to be effective in SCI patients taking it for 6 months (12) and was shown to be effective in one patient taking it for 2 years (13). Overall, specific long-term, comprehensive studies in SCI patients are lacking, but existing literature docs appear to support their use.

Oral bisphosphonates such as alendronate and etidronate represent one option, but in patients in whom oral administration is not possible or recommended (14), the intravenous bisphosphonates represent alternative options. While there have been no comprehensive trials utilizing these agents in patients with neurologic disabilities, inferences may be made based on trials in postmenopausal women with osteoporosis. In one recent trial, zoledronic acid administered during a 3-year period was found to reduce risk of morphometric vertebral fracture by 70% and reduce the risk of hip fracture by 41% compared to controls (15). In this study, the only reported differences in the two groups was an increased incidence of atrial fibrillation in the group treated with the zoledronic acid.

Calcitonin and teriparatide may also represent treatment options for the patient with neurologic disability. Calcitonin appears to provide only vertebral fracture protection and therefore has limited use. Teriparatide is a daily injectable anabolic medication whose target is the osteoblasts. It is unclear what role teriparitide may have in the patient with neurologic disabilities, given the typical mechanism of bone loss (significantly increased osteoclastic activity). To the author's knowledge, there have been no reported trials involving teriparatide in patients with neurologic disabilities. Commonly used medications for the treatment of osteoporosis are briefly described in Table 16.3.

Special Considerations for Adults with Neurologic Disabilities

Existing trials in this population are lacking both in quantity and in their ability to comment on long-term consequences of treatment. Currently, there is a dearth of trials investigating chronic use of antiosteoporotic medications in this population. It appears that just as with the general population, further research is needed to clarify the optimal treatment regimen for these patients.

Currently, there is no clear-cut consensus on the exact duration of treatment for the osteoporotic patient. While it remains clear that bisphosphonate medications may be safely administered for many years, as multiple studies have demonstrated their use to be safe after 10 years' use (16,17), it is less clear what the ideal algorithm is and what the long-term sequelae are. Teriparatide is a newer medication whose long-term safety profile is unknown at present based on clinical trials.

Nonpharmacologic Management

Nonmedical management should complement the pharmacologic treatment of this patient population and includes physical therapy exercise and appropriate positioning. Exercises such as tilt table, standing, and electrical stimulation may be beneficial to this population (18), as is appropriate wheelchair positioning in wheelchair-bound patients. One review of 65 studies involving exercise in SCI patients demonstrated that reconditioning training programs after SCI have a direct impact on function and quality of life (19). These programs help facilitate participation in physical activities in addition to daily living activities.

Table 16.3

Pharmacologic Treatment

Name	Dosage	Side effects	Drug–drug interactions	Significant adverse events
Alendronate	70 mg PO Q wk or 10 mg PO QD	GI distress	Food, calcium and other minerals reduce the absorption of risedronate. It should be taken with water only.	Caution in severe renal impairment, maintain adequate calcium and vitamin D to avoid hypocalcemia
Risedronate	35 mg PO Q wk or 5 mg PO QD	GI distress	Food, calcium and other minerals reduce the absorption of risedronate. It should be taken with water only.	Caution in severe renal impairment, maintain adequate calcium and vitamin D to avoid hypocalcemia
Pamidronate (intravenous)	30 mg IV once Q 3–4 months	Fever, stomach pain, loss of appetite, nausea, constipation, or initial increase in bone pain may occur	None reported	Avascular necrosis of the jaw is a rare complication. Caution in severe renal impairment, maintain adequate calcium and vitamin D to avoid hypocalcemia.
Zoledronate (intravenous)	4 mg IV once annually	Fever, fatigue, anemia, muscle aches, swelling in the feet or legs, flu-like symptoms	None reported	Avascular necrosis of the jaw is a rare complication. Caution in severe renal impairment, maintain adequate calcium and vitamin D to avoid hypocalcemia.

Weight bearing clearly has positive benefits on BMD in the SCI patient. In a study by Saltzstein et al. (20), the authors demonstrated a strong correlation between mobility and bone density utilizing single photon absorptiometry. Furthermore, there may be a role for additional treatments, including functional electrical stimulation cycling. In one study, functional electrical stimulation cycling exercises after 6 months resulted in significant increases in BMD of the distal femur, and proximal tibia PT increased significantly (21). However, the effect was not found to be permanent. Instead, it diminished after cessation of the exercises.

Assistive devices and orthotics such as walkers, canes, and posterior leaf spring orthotics may all enable patients with neurologic disabilities to have optimal mobility despite their specific deficits. Hip protectors are external orthoses which are similar to bicycle pants with pads placed over the trochanters. The goal of the protectors is to absorb some of the forces sustained by a fall in order to miminize fractures. The literature has been both positive and negative on their efficacy, with participants consisting of elderly osteoporotic patients (22–24). Randomized controlled trials have shown that they can help to prevent hip fracture (19). However, they may be most beneficial to those in institutionalized settings, and perhaps less effective in home dwellers (22,23). Hip protectors can increase one's self-efficacy, or belief in one's own ability to prevent a fall (25). However, they have been shown not to be as efficacious in preventing falls in patients with more limited mental status (26), and drawbacks include complaints of discomfort and impracticality. Hip protectors may therefore be most appropriate in the higher-functioning patient and may have more limited use in patients with severe neurologic disabilities who need a great deal of assistance in activities of daily living since they are somewhat difficult to don and doff. There have been no specific studies in the patient with neurologic disabilities to the author's knowledge.

Patients and their caregivers should also be instructed in fall-prevention techniques and have their homes modified to minimize the risk of falls. Examples of home modifications include: 1) tub bench, 2) raised toilet seats, 3) hand-held showers, 4) grab bars, 5) nonskid rugs, and 6) night lights in commonly traveled corridors such as the bedroom to the bathroom. Patients with impaired transfers and ambulation would also benefit from a "refresher" rehab program addressing these deficits.

Osteoporosis-related fractures are often precipitated by a fall in which there is either a direct trauma to the paralyzed or paretic limb or engagement in a seemingly mild activity such as range of motion of an osteopenic limb. These fractures typically occur in the lower extremities (but can be seen in paralyzed upper extremities as well) and can be challenging to detect in the insensate patient.

Clinicians should have a high index of suspicion in a patient that presents with a history of trauma and has swelling, hematomas, and deformities in the paralyzed limb(s) on physical examination. Radiologic tests such as x-rays can help to detect a fracture. Treatment in a nonfunctioning limb typically involves soft tissue splinting to allow healing in good anatomic alignment. Caution should be used if rigid casts are utilized since these can irritate the underlying skin and cause pressure ulcers. It is important to maintain the patient's level of function as much as possible during the healing process and to provide adequate DVT prophylaxis (27).

Patient Safety

Patient safety can be promoted with the appropriate precautions in mind:
- Screening and treating osteoporosis is essential in adults with neurologic disabilities. This includes not only the initial treatment, but appropriate monitoring as well.
- Provide assistive devices and training to minimize the risk of falling.
- Avoid aggressive range of motion in the lower extremities of nonambulatory adults.
- Clinicians should be vigilant for the presence of a lower extremity fracture in a paralyzed and insensate limb.
- Caution should be used in prescribing biphosphonates (especially in patients with suspected renal disease). Intravenous Pamidronate and Zoledronate have been associated with avascular necrosis of the jaw.
- The main side effect of one of the most commonly prescribed class of anti-osteoroprotic medications, the oral bisphosphonates, is on the digestive tract. Patients who have serious gastrointestinal conditions such as ulcers or esophageal strictures should avoid oral bisphosphonates and instead may opt for parenteral bisphoshponates.

Patient Education

Physicians should educate their patients about the importance of osteoporosis and fractures. Some key points include the following:
- Fall prevention is an important part of preventing osteoporosis-related fractures. A home evaluation by a physical or occupational therapist can be very helpful in identifying high-risk areas and provide recommendations for adaptive equipment such as grab bars, tub benches, night lights, and non-skid rugs. It is also often very helpful for the patient to undergo a "refresher" training program in transfer training and ambulation (if applicable).
- It is essential that patients consume the recommended calcium and vitamin D. This is needed in addition to prescribed antiosteoporotic medication. Most patients with neurologic disabilities may be less likely to receive adequate sunlight exposure and therefore may be at higher risk for vitamin D deficiency.

- Oral bisphosphonates must be taken on an empty stomach first thing in the morning with only a glass of water. Other food, drink, or medication should be avoided for at least 30 minutes. Patients must remain upright during this time in order to minimize the potential for GI complications.
- Patients who have sensory deficits and paralyzed limbs should be alerted to the signs and symptoms of fractures, which include swelling, erythema, increased spasms, low-grade fever, and deformity of the affected limb.

REFERENCES

1. Jiang SD, Dai LY, Jiang LS. Osteoporosis after spinal cord injury. Osteoporos Int 2006; 17(2):180–192.
2. Garland DE, Stewart CA, Adkins RH, et al. Osteoporosis after spinal cord injury. J Orthop Res 1992; 10(3):371–378.
3. Maimoun L, Fattal C, Micallef JP, Peruchon E, Rabischong P. Bone loss in spinal cord-injured patients: from physiopathology to therapy. Spinal Cord 2006; 44(4):203–210.
4. Ikai T, Uematsu M, Eun SS, Kimura C, Hasegawa C, Miyano S. Prevention of secondary osteoporosis postmenopause in hemiplegia. Am J Phys Med Rehabil 2001; 80(3):169–174.
5. Beaupre GS, Lew HL. Bone-density changes after stroke. Am J Phys Med Rehabil 2006; 85(5):464–472.
6. Reiter AL, Volk A, Vollmar J, Fromm B, Gerner HJ. Changes of basic bone turnover parameters in short-term and long-term patients with spinal cord injury. Eur Spine J 2007; 16(6):771–776.
7. Jiang SD, Jiang LS, Dai LY. Mechanisms of osteoporosis in spinal cord injury. Clin Endocrinol (Oxf) 2006; 65(5):555–565.
8. Lazo MG, Shirazi P, Sam M, Giobbie-Hurder A, Blacconiere MJ, Muppidi M. Osteoporosis and risk of fracture in men with spinal cord injury. Spinal Cord 2001; 39(4):208–214.
9. Greenberg JA, Roth EJ, Wuermser LA, Almagor O, Schnitzer TJ. Osteoporosis treatment for patients with stroke. Top Stroke Rehabil 2007; 14(2):62–67.
10. Chappard D, Petitjean M, Alexandre C, Vico L, Minaire P, Riffat G. Cortical osteoclasts are less sensitive to etidronate than trabecular osteoclasts. J Bone Miner Res 1991; 6(7):673–680.
11. Pearson EG, Nance PW, Leslie WD, Ludwig S. Cyclical etidronate: its effect on bone density in patients with acute spinal cord injury. Arch Phys Med Rehabil 1997; 78(3):269–272.
12. Moran de Brito CM, Battistella LR, Saito ET, Sakamoto H. Effect of alendronate on bone mineral density in spinal cord injury patients: a pilot study. Spinal Cord 2005; 43(6):341–348.
13. Sniger W, Garshick E. Alendronate increases bone density in chronic spinal cord injury: a case report. Arch Phys Med Rehabil 2002; 83(1):139–140.
14. Poole KE, Reeve J, Warburton EA. Falls, fractures, and osteoporosis after stroke: time to think about protection? Stroke 2002; 33(5):1432–1436.
15. Black DM, Delmas PD, Eastell R, A et al. Once-yearly zoledronic acid for treatment of postmenopausal osteoporosis. N Engl J Med 2007; 356(18):1809–1822.
16. Bone HG, Hosking D, Devogelaer JP, et al. Ten years' experience with alendronate for osteoporosis in postmenopausal women. N Engl J Med 2004; 350(12):1189–1199.
17. Liberman UA. Long-term safety of bisphosphonate therapy for osteoporosis: a review of the evidence. Drugs Aging 2006; 23(4):289–298.
18. Frey-Rindova P, de Bruin ED, Stussi E, Dambacher MA, Dietz V. Bone mineral density in upper and lower extremities during 12 months after spinal cord injury measured by peripheral quantitative computed tomography. Spinal Cord 2000; 38(1):26–32.

19. Devillard X, Rimaud D, Roche F, Calmels P. Effects of training programs for spinal cord injury. Ann Readapt Med Phys 2007; 50(6):490–499.
20. Saltzstein RJ, Hardin S, Hastings J. Osteoporosis in spinal cord injury: using an index of mobility and its relationship to bone density. J Am Paraplegia Soc 1992; 15(4):232–234.
21. Chen SC, Lai CH, Chan WP, Huang MH, Tsai HW, Chen JJ. Increases in bone mineral density after functional electrical stimulation cycling exercises in spinal cord injured patients. Disabil Rehabil 2005; 27(22):1337–1341.
22. Parker MJ, Gillespie WJ, Gillespie LD. Hip protectors for preventing hip fractures in older people. Cochrane Database Syst Rev 2005; (3):CD001255.
23. Parker MJ, Gillespie WJ, Gillespie LD. Effectiveness of hip protectors for preventing hip fractures in elderly people: systematic review. BMJ 2006; 332(7541):571–574.
24. Sawka AM, Boulos P, Beattie K, et al. Do hip protectors decrease the risk of hip fracture in institutional and community-dwelling elderly? A systematic review and meta-analysis of randomized controlled trials. Osteoporos Int 2005; 16(12):1461–1474.
25. Cameron ID, Stafford B, Cumming RG, et al. Hip protectors improve falls self-efficacy. Age Ageing 2000; 29(1):57–62.
26. Jensen J, Nyberg L, Gustafson Y, Lundin-Olsson L. Fall and injury prevention in residential care—effects in residents with higher and lower levels of cognition. J Am Geriatr Soc 2003; 51(5):627–635.
27. Little JW, Burns SP. Neuromusculoskeletal complications of spinal cord injury. In: Kirschlum S, Campagnolo D, DeLisa J, eds. Spinal Cord Medicine. Philadelphia: Lippincott, 2002: 241–252.

17 | Musculoskeletal System

Amit Dholakia
Mohamed S. Ahmed
Adrian Cristian

Musculoskeletal pain is very common in adults with neurologic disability, and it can have a significant impact on the functionality and quality of life of those afflicted with it. This chapter will review some common musculoskeletal conditions that effect the lumbar spine, shoulders, hips, and knees in people living with impairments brought on by spinal cord injury (SCI), traumatic brain injury (TBI), multiple sclerosis (MS), and cerebrovascular accidents (CVA).

LOW BACK PAIN

Low back pain is very common in adults with neurologic disabilities. Causes include myofascial pain, spinal stenosis, degenerative changes of the spine, and radiculopathy. These conditions are also commonly seen in the general population, but can pose additional functional limitations when present in this population. They may also be aggravated by the neurologic disability itself. For example, poor seating in a wheelchair, ambulation with an altered gait, and ill-fitting orthoses can all precipitate or aggravate low back pain.

Anatomy

Degenerative changes have been observed in the lumbosacral spine. These can include loss of disc height, osteophytes, thickening and buckling of ligamentum flavum, as well as facet joint arthritis. All of these can lead to narrowing of the intervertebral and spinal canals, which in turn can place pressure on nerves. Inflammation and irritation of pain sensitive structures in the spine and surrounding structures (i.e., facet joints, ligaments, and paraspinal muscles) can also lead to pain. Presence of spasticity, spinal instrumentation, healing fractures, poor trunk control, muscle weakness, and poor posture can all contribute to low back pain in adults with neurologic disabilities.

217

Patient Assessment

Whereas the actual pain generator in low back pain is not often identified, there are often hints obtained in the medical history and physical examination that point to a possible diagnosis. Spinal stenosis pain has been described as a vice-like, squeezing, and achy sensation, often in the thighs and calves, that is aggravated by prolonged standing. Facet joint pain is localized to the low back, but can radiate to the buttocks and is worsened with extension. In thin adults there may be associated tenderness on palpation of the lumbosacral spine. Radiculopathy-related pain is described as electrical in nature and radiating into the lower extremities in a dermatomal pattern. Myofascial pain should be suspected when there is tenderness on palpation of a specific "trigger point" associated with a radiation to adjacent tissues.

It is worthwhile to mention that in a patient with absent or impaired sensation and motor weakness, the presentation of the pain may be altered from that commonly described in the general able bodied population (Table 17.1).

Diagnostic Tests

Commonly used diagnostic tests include x-rays, magnetic resonance imaging (MRI), computed tomography (CT) scans, and electrodiagnostics. It is important to review previous tests and to determine if the test ordered will add sig-

Table 17.1

Assessment of Low Back Pain in Adults with Neurologic Disabilities

Medical history	Physical examination
1. Inciting cause, location, quality, intensity, duration, radiation, aggravating and alleviating factors for the pain	1. Observation for presence of spinal deformity (i.e., kyphosis, scoliosis) and pressure ulcers (sacrum, ischial tuberosities, greater trochanters, and heels)
2. Impact of pain on functionality for everyday activities, sleep, work, and personal relationships	2. Palpation for tender points along the spine and lower extremities
3. Diagnostic tests performed and their results (x-rays, MRI, CT scans)	3. Range of motion of the spine in flexion, extension, lateral bending, and rotation as well as in the lower extremities (i.e., contractures at hips, knees, and ankles)
4. Treatments tried for the pain and their level of success (physical therapy, chiropractic care, massage therapy, acupuncture, injections, medications, surgery)	4. Motor strength, sensation, reflexes, presence of spasms in the lower extremities
5. Fever, chills, weight loss, weakness in the lower extremities (i.e., foot drop), loss of bowel/bladder function	5. Evaluation of peripheral pulses
6. Previous history of injuries to the low back.	6. Gait analysis
	7. Wheelchair seating assessment in wheelchair-bound patients with special emphasis on the cushion and back
	8. Ill-fitting lower extremity orthosis

nificant information that will help determine the treatment plan, since some of these tests can be uncomfortable.

Treatment

Prior to the initiation of treatment, it is always best to try to identify the cause of the pain. This may not always be possible, and the patient should be informed of this early on. Common treatment options include medications (i.e., nonsteroidal anti-inflammatory drugs [NSAIDs], opioids, antiepileptics), injections (i.e., trigger point, epidural, and facet joint injections), physical therapy, chiropractic, massage, braces, biofeedback, acupuncture, and lumbosacral orthoses.

The replacement of an ill-fitting lower extremity orthotic, an appropriately sized wheelchair with adequate cushion and back, adaptive equipment for everyday activities, or an appropriate cane or crutch can often be surprisingly effective in the treatment of low back pain in this population.

SHOULDER PAIN

Shoulder pain is very common in adults with neurologic disabilities. The prevalence of shoulder pain in CVA, TBI, and SCI has been reported to be 62, 69, and 40%, respectively (1,2). Shoulder pain has also been reported in 59% of tetraplegics and 42% of paraplegics (3). It may be directly due to the impact of the neurologic impairment on the joint (i.e., shoulder subluxation post stroke in a hemiplegic limb) or as a secondary problem brought on by repetitive stress to the joint (i.e., wheelchair propulsion).

Common causes of shoulder pain and loss of function in this population include 1) adhesive capsulitis, 2) subluxation, 3) impingement syndrome, 4) rotator cuff tear, and 5) bicipital tendonitis.

Anatomy

The humeral head articulates with the glenoid fossa and is stabilized by the rotator cuff and deltoid muscles, tendons, ligaments, and an articular capsule. The rotator cuff is composed of four muscles: the supraspinatus, infraspinatus, teres minor, and subscapularis. They stabilize the glenohumeral joint and prevent excessive upward movement of the humeral head (4). The subacromial bursa is located beneath the acromion, partially covering the supraspinatus and humeral head (5). The long head tendon of the biceps lies in the bicipital groove of the humerus between the greater and lesser tuberosities and inserts into the gleno-humeral joint structure. A synovial sheath covers the tendon lying in the bicipital groove. The long head of the biceps not only participates in flexion and supination of the forearm, but helps stabilize the humeral head during abduction and external rotation.

Adhesive capsulitis (commonly referred to as "frozen shoulder") is loss of both active and passive range of motion of the shoulder due to adhesions of the joint capsule and synovial membrane of the glenohumeral joint. Prolonged immobilization from shoulder paralysis, pain from shoulder impingement, upper extremity spasticity, and sling use can all contribute to the development of this condition (6).

Shoulder subluxation is partial slippage of the humeral head out of the glenohumeral socket. It can occur due to 1) an inability of a weakened supraspinatus muscle to maintain the humeral head within the glenoid fossa or 2) weak scapula-stabilizing muscles causing downward rotation of the scapula, changing glenoid fossa depth, ligament laxity, and functional scoliosis (7).

Inflammatory Conditions

Bicipital tendonitis is an inflammation of the bicipital tendon and synovial sheath that can be associated with repetitive overuse of the shoulder. Rotator cuff tendonitis is an inflammation of the rotator cuff muscle tendons. The supraspinatus is most commonly affected. Subacromial bursitis is inflammation of the subacromial bursa.

Impingement Syndrome

The rotator cuff muscles, primarily the supraspinatus, and subacromial bursa are compressed between the humeral head and coracoacromial arch upon shoulder elevation. Repetitive shoulder motions can lead to inflammation of these structures. Blood supply to the supraspinatus tendon is often insufficient, leaving the tendon prone to degeneration.

This condition is extremely common in adults with neurologic disabilities. It has been estimated that two thirds of shoulder pain in SCI is due to chronic impingement syndrome. This can strongly affect manual wheelchair propulsion, transfers, activities of daily living requiring overhead reaching, occupational duties, and sleep (8).

Repetitive use of the upper extremities is a major cause of impingement syndrome. Heavy reliance on upper limb functioning for transfers, ischial pressure reliefs, maintaining truncal stability, and wheelchair propulsion put mechanical pressure on the rotator cuff and bursa. Rotator cuff fatigue can also lead to superior migration of the humeral head by the stronger deltoid further squeezing these structures (6).

Repetitive trauma to the rotator cuff tendons causes bony changes to the acromion occur, making impingement syndrome likely. Neurologic impairment is also a contributing factor. Flail scapula stabilizers and muscle imbalances between shoulder adductors and abductors lead to increased stress on the rotator cuff muscles, resulting in microtrauma and inflammation. Spasticity of the deltoid, scapula stabilizers, and internal rotators of the humeral head can result in impingement of the subacromial bursa and supraspinatus. Increased thoracic kyphosis due to poor trunk control and poor posture may affect the scapula and glenohumeral relationship, predisposing to shoulder impingement (6). Other causes include contractures, heterotopic ossification, and the presence of a syrinx. Long-standing impingement syndrome can lead to partial or complete rotator cuff tears, osteoarthritis, and glenohumeral laxity.

Patient Assessment

In the assessment of shoulder pain in adults with neurologic disabilities, it is important to obtain a thorough medical history of the problem, which includes inciting cause, location, quality, intensity, duration, radiation, and aggravating and alleviating factors for the shoulder pain. It is equally important to determine the impact of this pain on functionality, quality of life, and sleep. Physical examination should target losses of range of motion, weakness, subluxation, spasticity, contractures, and painful structures (Table 17.2).

Diagnostic Tests

AP and lateral x-rays are helpful in ruling out the presence of fractures, subluxation, and heterotopic ossification but are not very helpful for conditions such

Table 17.2

Assessment of Shoulder Problems in Adults with Neurologic Disabilities

Medical history	Physical examination
1. Inciting cause, location, quality, intensity, duration, radiation, aggravating and alleviating factors for the shoulder pain	1. Inspection (i.e., deformities, contractures, subluxation, shoulder "shrugging," atrophy of the shoulder musculature)
2. Shoulder pain with overhead activities or reaching behind the back	2. Palpation (i.e., tenderness over the biceps tendon, shoulder musculature)
3. Shoulder pain with wheelchair propulsion or transfers	3. Shoulder range of motion (passive and active for flexion, abduction, adduction, extension, internal rotation, and external rotation) and range of motion for the rest of the upper extremities
4. Impact of shoulder pain on sleep, work and personal relationships	
5. Neck pain, electrical sensations in the arms and fingers	4. Scapular retraction, protraction and elevation
6. Fever, chills, weight loss, weakness	5. Neurologic examination: motor strength, sensation, and reflexes
7. Diagnostic tests performed and their results (x-rays, MRI, CT scans)	6. Special tests and maneuvers: Yergason's test, speed test, Neer sign, test for shoulder dislocation, drop arm sign, empty can sign, Hawkins sign
8. Treatments tried for the pain and their level of success (physical therapy, massage therapy, acupuncture, injections, medications, surgery)	7. Radial pulses
	8. Spasticity evaluation in the upper extremities (i.e., Ashworth scale)

as adhesive capsulitis, rotator cuff tears, and bicipital tendonitis. However, in impingement syndrome, x-rays may reveal a "hooked acromion," osteophytes along the inferior surface of the acromion, sclerosis, cysts, and joint space narrowing between the humeral head and the acromion, which can be associated with a rotator cuff tear. Arthrography, MRI, and arthroscopy can be used to substantiate an adhesive capsulitis. A subacromial injection of lidocaine can often localize the pain source to the shoulder if pain relief is noted after the injection. Similarly, injection of lidocaine near the bicipital groove that results in pain relief may help differentiate bicipital tendonitis from other causes of shoulder pain. MRI is the imaging study of choice for rotator cuff tears and inflammation.

Treatment

The main goals of the treatment of the painful shoulder in this population include: 1) reduction of pain, 2) restoration of range of motion and strength, and 3) maximizing function.

To achieve these goals, the following are some common treatment options:

- Medications (NSAIDs, acetaminophen, tramadol, opioids)
- Rehabilitation: range of motion exercises (especially in scapular mobility and external rotation for adhesive capsulitis), modalities (deep heat, ultrasound, ice, electrical stimulation), muscle strengthening program, and training in activities of daily living to minimize stress on shoulders
- Wheelchair modifications for proper posture and body mechanics during wheelchair propulsion in wheelchair-dependent patients (power wheelchairs may be indicated if the use of a manual chair is too difficult and painful for patient to use)
- Corticosteroid injections-(i.e., subacromial, bicipital tendon region)
- Acupuncture
- Proper limb positioning (especially in subluxed and hemiplegic limb) to minimize traction on the limb
- Neuromuscular stimulation and shoulder taping for shoulder subluxation (8)
- Manipulation under anesthesia for adhesive capsulitis (5) (however, avoid in osteopenia, fractures, and heterotopic ossification)
- Spasticity management (i.e., botulinum toxin injections)
- Avoid or minimize use of slings (8)
- Surgery for rotator cuff tears: surgical repair for rotator cuff tear, if found early, with aggressive postoperative therapy may be beneficial. However, longstanding rotator cuff tears with muscle atrophy, superior migration of humerus, and limited range of motion, may not be ideal surgical candidates. Orthopedic consultation is recommended.

HIP PAIN

Hip pain can have a significant impact on ambulation, functionality, and quality of life in ambulatory adults with neurologic disabilities. Common causes of hip pain include osteoarthritis and greater trochanteric bursitis.

Osteoarthritis

Anatomy

The hip joint is commonly referred to as a ball-and-socket joint. The articulation between the cartilaginous surfaces of the femoral head and acetabulum serve as the framework of this joint. Numerous factors such as muscle imbalance, increased tone, repetitive abnormal mechanical stresses, and impaired gait and proprioceptive feedback (5) in this population place increased mechanical stresses on the joint, accelerating the degenerative process.

The trochanteric bursa is a large bursa located on the greater trochanter of the femur and covered by the gluteus maximus muscle. The bursa helps facilitate movement of the muscle over the greater trochanter. Inflammation of the bursa can occur from imbalance of the hip girdle. This can occur from gait dysfunction and lower extremity spasticity.

Patient Assessment

Symptoms of osteoarthritic hip pain are usually described as achy or sharp and aggravated with walking. The pain may radiate to the groin, thigh, or knee. Activities of daily living such as putting on pants and tying shoelaces can be painful. Pain due to greater trochanteric bursitis is usually localized to the outer aspect of the greater trochanters and may radiate to the lateral aspect of the leg and knee. Sleeping on the affected side may exacerbate symptoms. Table 17.3 lists some key questions and physical examination findings.

Table 17.3

Assessment of Hip Problems

Medical history	Physical examination
1. Cause of the pain, location, quality, intensity, duration, radiation, aggravating and alleviating factors	1. Inspection: i.e., deformities, contractures, atrophy of the hip
2. Groin pain	2. Palpation: tenderness over the greater trochanters and hip musculature
3. Pain with walking, transfers, dressing (pants, shoes), and sleep	3. Range of motion: passive and active hip range of motion-flexion, extension, abduction and adduction
4. Pain with lying on the affected side	4. Neurologic examination: motor strength, sensation, reflexes
5. History of trauma to the hip or falls	5. Special tests: i.e., Patrick test
6. Low back pain	6. Gait
7. New-onset numbness, weakness in the toes	
8. Fever, chills, weight loss, or bowel/bladder problems (new onset)	
9. Diagnostic tests performed and their results (x-rays, MRI, CT scans)	
10. Treatments tried for the pain and their level of success (physical therapy, acupuncture, injections, medications, surgery)	

Diagnostic Tests

AP and lateral radiographs of the hip may reveal 1) fractures, 2) heterotopic ossification, and 3) degenerative changes (i.e., narrowing joint space, osteophyte formation, subchondral sclerosis, and/or subchondral cyst formation). Calcific deposits may also be seen above the trochanter. Injection with a local anesthetic (lidocaine) to the greater trochanter gives immediate relief and confirms the diagnosis. This can also be therapeutic if a corticosteroid is mixed with anesthetic.

Treatment

Treatment options include:
- Medications (acetaminophen, NSAIDs, tramadol, opioids)
- Injections (corticosteroid injections for greater trochanteric bursitis; hip joint injection)
- Gait devices (cane, crutches)
- Acupuncture
- Rehabilitation interventions (i.e., range-of-motion exercises, modalities such as ultrasound, strengthening of weak hip musclesm and gait training)
- Surgical interventions (i.e., hip replacement)

KNEE

Osteoarthritis of the Knee

Anatomy

Painful osteoarthritis of the knee can limit ambulation, transfers, and functionality in the ambulatory adult aging with a neurologic disability. It is believed to be due to degenerative changes in the joint and may be accelerated in ambulatory adults with neurologic disabilities due to altered gait biomechanics, contractures, and impact of spasticity in the lower extremities (i.e., excessive knee hyperextension).

Patient Assessment

Onset may be insidious, and symptoms may include achy pain, joint stiffness, pain with weight-bearing activities, and buckling. Table 17.4 lists some key questions and physical examination findings.

Diagnostic Tests

Weight-bearing AP radiographs should be obtained whenever possible. Radiographs may show 1) fractures, 2) heterotopic ossification, and 3) degenerative changes (narrowing of joint space, subchondral sclerosis and cyst formation, and osteophytes). It should be noted that radiographs may not correlate with the symptoms.

Table 17.4

Assessment of the Osteoarthritic Knee in Adults with Neurologic Disability

Medical history	Physical examination
1. Cause of the pain, location, quality, intensity, duration, radiation, aggravating and alleviating factors	1. Inspection: i.e., deformities, contractures, swelling, erythema
2. Pain or stiffness with walking, transfers, stairs, prolonged sitting	2. Palpation: tenderness over the joint line
3. "Buckling" and "locking " of the knee	3. Range of motion: passive and active flexion and extension
4. Swelling of the knee	4. Neurologic examination: motor strength, sensation, reflexes
5. History of trauma to the knee or falls	5. Special tests: tests for varus/valgus instability, McMurray test, Lachman test
6. New-onset numbness, weakness in the toes	6. Foot deformities
7. Diagnostic tests performed and their results (x rays, MRI)	7. Gait analysis
8. Treatments tried for the pain and their level of success (physical therapy, acupuncture, injections, medications, surgery)	

Treatment

Common treatment interventions for osteoarthritis of the knee include:

- Medications (NSAIDs, glucosamine and chondroitin sulfate, acetaminophen, tramadol, opioids)
- Injections (corticosteroid, visco-supplementation)
- Acupuncture
- Braces (neoprene sleeves, medial knee compartment unloading braces, heel wedges)
- Weight loss
- Cane
- Rehabilitation program (range of motion, strengthening exercises of knee extensors, stretching exercises to hamstrings, gait training)
- Surgery (i.e., knee replacement)

Table 17.5

Risks, Benefits, and Contraindications for Injections

Intervention	Risks	Benefits	Contraindications
Trigger point injection	Skin infection, bleeding, pneumothorax (if near intercostal space), allergic reaction to agent	Pain relief, improvement in function	Systemic infection, local infection, allergy to agent Relative—anticoagulation
Peripheral corticosteroid joint injection	Tendon rupture and ligament rupture, bleeding, hyperglycemia, infection, adrenal gland suppression	Pain relief, improvement in function, confirm diagnosis	Systemic infection, local infection, allergy to agent Relative—anticoagulation, diabetes mellitus
Visco-supplementation	Increased joint pain, swelling, erythema, itching	Pain relief, may slow progression of osteoarthritis, improvement in function	See trigger point
Fluoroscopic interventional spinal injection	Nerve root injury, spinal cord injury, bleeding, infection, dural puncture, spinal headache, vasovagal syncope, allergic reaction, cerebrovascular accident, epidural abscess, epidural hecatomb, adrenal gland suppression	Pain relief, confirm diagnosis, may improve function	Pregnancy, systemic infection, local infection, acute spinal cord compression, bleeding disorder, anti-coagulation Relative—diabetes mellitus (corticosteroids)

Patient Safety

1. Excessive use of acetaminophen may cause liver damage.
2. Chronic use of NSAIDS may cause gastric, renal, or hepatic complications.
3. Clinicians should be knowledgeable about the risks and contraindications of the various types of injections used to treat musculoskeletal pain (Table 17.5).
4. Medical causes of lower back pain (e.g., metastatic cancer, infections of the spine) and spinal fractures or unstable spine need to be excluded prior to initiation of conservative treatments. Traction and manipulation in patients with unstable spines, recent fractures, or spinal surgeries should be avoided.

Patient Education

1. Patients should be educated on strategies to minimize trauma to peripheral joints and spine from repetitive use.
2. Patients should be encouraged to have their orthotic devices and wheelchairs evaluated on a regular basis to ensure that they are functioning well and are still appropriate for the patient's condition.

REFERENCES

1. Leung J, Moseley A, Fereday S, Jones T, Fairbairn T, Wyndham S. Prevalence and characteristics of shoulder pain after traumatic brain injury. Clin Rehabil 2007; 21(2):171–181.
2. Alm M, Saraste H, Norrbrink C. Shoulder pain in persons with thoracic SCI: prevalence and characteristics. J Rehabil Med 2008; 40(4):277–283.
3. Curtis KA, Drysdale GA, Lanza RD, Kolber M, Vitolo RS, West R. Shoulder pain in WC users with tetraplegia and paraplegia. Arch Phys Med Rehabil 1999; 80(4):453–457.
4. Mehta AJ. Common Musculoskeletal Problems. Philadelphia: Hanley & Belfus Inc., 1997.
5. Waters RL, Ien HS, Adkins RH. The musculoskeletal system In: Whiteneck G, et al., eds. Aging with Spinal Cord Injury. New York: Demos Publications, 1993:53–71.
6. Braddom RL. Physical Medicine & Rehabilitation, 3rd ed. Philadelphia: Saunders Elseveir, 2007.
7. Dyson-Hudson TA, Kirshblum SC. Shoulder pain in chronic spinal cord injury, part I: epidemiology, etiology, and pathomechanics. J Spinal Cord Med 2004; 27(1):4–17.
8. Little JW, Burns SP. Neuromusculoskeletal Complications of Spinal Cord Injury In: Kirshblum S, et al., eds. Spinal Cord Medicine. Philadelphia: Lippincott Williams and Wilkins, 2002:241–252.

18 | Patient Safety

Adrian Cristian

Patient safety and medical errors have become very important topics in recent years, attracting the attention of patients, clinicians, and healthcare insurance providers. Thirty-four to 40% of Americans has either experienced or knows someone whom has experienced a medical error. Forty-eight percent of Americans are concerned about the safety of their medical care (1).

Types of medical errors include: 1) diagnostic (failure or delay to diagnose a problem or to monitor it once diagnosed), 2) treatment-related (technical error in performing a procedure or surgery or prescribing a medication), 3) preventive (failure to provide preventive measures before the problem arises) (2), and 4) communication-related, including poor communication or lack of communication between clinicians, especially at transition points in care; missing parts of the medical record; missing medical records; and mislabeled specimens (3).

Adults with neurologic disabilities are inherently at risk for medical errors for the following reasons: 1) impaired cognition, 2) impaired communication, 3) multiple medical problems, 4) polypharmacy, 5) narrow margin of good health due to the impact of neurologic disease on their body, and 6) limited support system and income.

The goal of this chapter is to provide clinicians with information on basic patient safety principles that can be used in everyday clinical practice in both an outpatient and an inpatient setting

PATIENT ASSESSMENT: THE HISTORY AND PHYSICAL EXAMINATION

Patient safety begins with a thorough medical history and physical examination of the adult with a neurologic disability.

Medical History

Some general principles include the following:

229

1. Allow ample time for patients to describe their symptoms and concerns. This is especially important when evaluating a patient with cognitive and/or communication impairments. Information provided should also be corroborated with caregiver.
2. Ask open-ended questions at an appropriate literacy level.
3. An interpreter should be used when evaluating non–English-speaking patients, unless the clinician is fluent in the patient's language.
4. Assess for the presence of "red flags" of a high-risk patient (low literacy level, different culture, limited social support system and income, cognitive/communication impairment).

A thorough review of all medications taken (including over-the-counter medications, herbs, nutrients) should be performed. This should include indications, effectiveness, how and when they are taking the medication, name of prescribing physician, and presence of any side effects. Nonadherence with medications is a very common occurrence. Types of nonadherence include: 1) not filling prescriptions, 2) missed doses of medications, 3) taking medications at irregular intervals, 4) discontinuing medications without telling the physician, and 5) use of someone else's medications. Adults with cognitive impairments; limited support systems; limited financial resources, and illiteracy are especially at high risk (1).

All allergies should be noted. These can include medication allergies as well as food allergies. A description of what actually happens when these substances are ingested is important to distinguish a true allergy from a side effect.

Inquiries should be made about alcohol intake, use of illicit substances (cocaine, marijuana, heroin, etc.), depression, and suicidal ideation.

It is important to ask patients about their current level of function for everyday activities, such as bathing, dressing, feeding, hygiene, bowel/bladder care transfers, and ambulation, as well as higher level activities such as shopping, cooking, cleaning, driving, work, and hobbies. How much assistance do they typically require, and how have their current symptoms impacted on these activities? The patient's level of family and community support should also be assessed.

Physical Examination

Key points of the physical examination with a special emphasis on safety are outlined in Table 18.1. It is important to document any cognitive, communication, or swallowing impairments as well as evidence of muscle weakness or insensate areas of the body. Skin check for pressure ulcers or incontinence as well as evidence of malnutrition should also be noted.

It is worthwhile to ask the patient as part of the evaluation to perform some basic tasks that are important for identifying potential patient safety concerns. These can include performing basic math calculations, which would be important in the administration of medications, reading a medication label, and opening a pill bottle (Table 18.1).

Table 18.1

Patient Assessment

Medical History

1. Don't hurry patient! Allow ample time for patients with cognitive and or communication impairments.
2. Corroborate medical history with caregiver/family member and patient's primary care physician.
3. Assess for "red flags" of a high-risk patient for safety (limited income/social support; impaired cognition/communication).
4. Level of function for basic and advanced activities of daily living and impact of current illness on those functions.
5. Medication history: names, indications, administration, effectiveness, and name of prescribing providers. It is helpful to ask the patient bring all medication bottles for review at the time of appointment.
6. Allergies.
7. Substance abuse: alcoholism, cocaine, marijuana, heroin, etc.
8. Support systems: extent of family and community support.

Physical Examination

1. General appearance: evidence of malnutrition/dehydration/cachexia, etc.
2. Vital signs: blood pressure, respiration, pulse, temperature.
3. Orientation, concentration, memory (immediate and delayed recall), and basic math skills (important for understanding how to take medications).
4. Speech, swallowing, and communication.
5. Vision (including ability to read a pill bottle).
6. Hearing.
7. Balance and coordination.
8. General strength and sensation in the upper and lower extremities.
9. Hand dexterity.
10. Skin check for pressure ulcers.
11. Evaluate for deep vein thrombosis.
12. Functional exam: transfers, ambulation.

COMMUNICATION

Communication Between Providers

Communication between providers is essential to ensure patient safety. This is especially important at points of transition in the patient's care. Some common points of transition include: 1) admission to a rehab unit from another medical institution; within the same medical center or from home, 2) transfer from rehab unit to an acute medical, surgical, or intensive care unit in the same medical center or an outside institution, and 3) discharge to home or a long-term facility. The information should be complete, clearly presented, and provided in a timely fashion to appropriate providers. At a minimum it should include a medical history, recent lab values, diagnostic test results, a comprehensive medication list, allergies, advanced directives, reason for transfer, and names of treating clinicians (physicians, nurses, therapists, etc.) in both settings.

Patient Communication

It is important to recognize that the patient and his or her caregiver are at the center of his or her medical care. As such, clinicians need to understand the patient's treatment beliefs and goals and actively involve the patient in their care. Much of patient care centers on good communication between the clinician and the patient so that the patient can make informed decisions. By involving the patient in the decision-making process and addressing any potential barriers to the implementation of the treatment plan, the clinician helps to ensure that the treatment plan will be carried out.

Table 18.2 outlines some key points of patient communication.

PATIENT SAFETY

Medications

According to the Institute of Medicine's landmark publication "To Err Is Human," 1 of 131 outpatient deaths and 1 of 854 inpatient deaths are related to medication errors (2). Hospitalized patients are subject to at least one medication error per day, and 25% of all medication errors are preventable. Thirty

Table 18.2

Communication with Patients

---

1. Take into account patient's treatment preferences, values, and financial limitations as much as possible.
2. Assess the self-management beliefs and patterns of the patient and his/her caregiver.
3. Treatment goals should be set taking into account the patient's wishes. These goals should be reevaluated on a regular basis.
4. Medical information should be provided taking into account the patient's level of literacy, age, language, and culture.
5. Treatment plan should be thoroughly discussed with patient and/or caregiver and his/her primary care physician.
6. Patient and caregiver should be given concrete instructions on the treatment plan. Clinician should check for understanding.
7. All treatment options should be discussed, including:
   a. Functional impact on activities of daily living, work, and hobbies
   b. Expected outcomes of treatment plan
   c. Risks and benefits and likelihood of their occurrence
   d. Potential barriers to adherence to treatment plan and ways to overcome them
8. Patient and caregiver should be educated on symptoms and side effects of potential treatment plan and what to do if they notice them.
9. Medical errors—if an error has occurred, it is important to tell the patient what has happened, what will be done about it, and how it can be prevented in the future.

percent of patients seen in emergency rooms for medication problems had no understanding of their medications (1). There are at least 1.5 million preventable adverse drug events per year with an estimated cost of $2 billion for inpatient admissions (1,2).

Medication errors can occur at any step in the medication use process: prescription, dispension, and administration (Table 18.3). For hospitalized patients the most common errors occur during the prescription and administration stages. Most common types of administration errors are due to dosing errors, incorrect drugs prescribed, incorrect routes of administration, miscommunication, miscalculation of doses, staffing shortages, and incomplete documentation. It has been estimated that there are between 11 and 30% prescribing errors per patient per day in hospitalized medical units (1).

Adults with neurologic disabilities often take many medications for various health-related ailments. Polypharmacy can increase the risk of medication-related adverse events. Thirty percent of adults take at least five medications and 11.8 prescriptions per person per year have been filled in the United States (1).

Special concern has been raised for patients receiving intravenous medications since this route of administration leads to a faster onset of action, the medications have a very high potency, and patients are often sicker (1).

Table 18.4 shows some key points to consider when prescribing medications.

Rehab Interventions

Whereas the vast majority of rehab interventions are tolerated well, one must not forget that adults with neurologic disabilities often have multiple comorbidities, which place them at increased risk of adverse effects while undergoing rehabilitation.

Safety in the rehab setting begins with a thorough medical history and physical examination, as described above. Once the assessment is completed, the rehab prescription serves as an excellent source of communication between the referring physician and treating therapists. In this prescription, specific precautions should be described to ensure safety while the patient is receiving treatments.

Some of these precautions are listed in Table 18.5.

Table 18.3

Common Medication-Related Errors

1. Wrong medication ordered
2. Wrong medication administered
3. Wrong dose ordered
4. Wrong abbreviation
5. Wrong unit of measurement used
6. Not asking about allergies
7. Failure to take into account kidney or liver disease in the dosing of the medication

Table 18.4

General Safety Considerations in the Prescribing and Administration of Medications

---

1. Avoid verbal orders—but if given, person on the receiving end should read it back, including spelling out the name of the medication and dose units.
2. Prescriptions should be written in print with units of measurement and decimal points double checked for accuracy.
3. Use only standardized abbreviations and dose designations.
4. Physician should avoid any distractions when writing out a prescription. High-traffic, high-noise areas such as nurse's station should be avoided and quiet areas sought out.
5. Keep the total number of daily admissions and discharges per physician to a rehab unit to a minimum to avoid prescribing errors.
6. Doublecheck prescription after it is written.
7. Don't multitask while writing out prescriptions.
8. Keep in mind renal and liver function and geriatric considerations in dosing of medications.
9. Be very specific in the language used on the prescription to instruct patients
10. Be careful with dose units and conversions (kilogram, milligram, microgram, etc.)
11. Clarify patient instructions on use of medication. All providers should be giving the patient the same instructions.
12. All medications should be reviewed at time of transition both within and outside a medical center or nursing home (e.g., rehab ward to medical ward to intensive care unit).
13. Medications should also be reviewed at all outpatient visits for effectiveness, side effects, and continued need.
14. Monitor blood level of medications whenever possible.
15. Ask about medication and food allergies.
16. Be knowledgeable about drug–food interactions whenever applicable.
17. Be wary of "sound-alike" and "look-alike" medications.
18. Be careful with dosing of intravenous and intrathecal medications.
19. List of medications should be compared at transition points in care. Names, dosages, and routes of administration should be clarified and verified and reassessed for continued need.

Table 18.5

Patient Safety Precautions in the Rehab Setting

---

1. Cardiac
2. Risk for orthostatic hypotension
3. Pulmonary
4. Wound-specific precautions
5. Weight-bearing status
6. Risk for hypoglycemia
7. Falls
8. Impaired communication
9. Sensory deficits/insensate areas of the body
10. Range-of-motion restrictions
11. Vital signs should be obtained before, during, and after exercising

Procedures

Interventional procedures are commonly used in the diagnosis and treatment of various conditions in adults with neurologic disabilities. Cognitive and communication impairments make this population more vulnerable to adverse events associated with procedures. Table 18.6 lists some key points for providers to consider when performing invasive procedures in this population.

Injection safety techniques are important to prevent the transmission of infectious diseases between clinician and patient as well as between patients in addition to preventing needle stick injuries. The Centers for Disease Control and Prevention (CDC) provides some very useful information on this topic: (www.cdc.gov/ncidod/dhqp/injectionSafetyFAQshtml#Q1).

Fall Prevention

Adults with neurologic disabilities are at risk for falls in both the home and medical and nursing home settings.

Preventing Falls in the Home

To minimize the risk of falls in the home, it is often important to perform a home safety assessment. This includes an evaluation of the rooms and corridors commonly used by the patient for the following: 1) adequate lighting, 2) clutter-free passageways, 3) presence of loose rugs, 4) safety equipment in the bathrooms (grab bars, tub bench, raised toilet seats, hand-held shower), and 5) chairs and tables with legs that stick out.

Since the cause of falls in the home is often multifactorial, caregivers for patients with cognitive impairments should be advised as to the following:

1. Safely administer medications and monitor for side effects such as dizziness and impaired balance.
2. Orient and reorient the patient to the environment.
3. Assist patient with toileting, especially prior to bedtime.
4. Place commonly used items such as glasses and telephone within the patient's reach.

Fall Prevention in Medical and Institutionalized Settings

Strategies to prevent falls in a healthcare setting are in many ways similar to the ones described above for the home setting. They include: 1) orienting and reorienting patients to their environment, 2) instructing high-risk patients to ask for assistance when getting in and out of bed, 3) checking on the patient often during all shifts, 4) keeping personal belongings within reach of patient, 5) assisting patient with bowel and bladder elimination, especially at bedtime and in the early morning, 6) using low beds and bed alarms whenever necessary, and 7) identifying high-fall-risk patients with visible markers (e.g., colorful wrist band).

It is important for caregivers to communicate about high-fall-risk patients between shifts and at transition points within the institution (e.g., rehab ward

Table 18.6

Patient Safety During Procedures

---

1. The clinician with the appropriate competency and the most experience available should perform the procedure.
2. Protocol to be used in performing procedure should be rehearsed by the team on a regular basis to establish and maintain competencies.
3. Patient's identification should be double-checked prior to the procedure. This can include verification by clinician of the patient's name, Social Security number, address, and body part that will undergo the procedure. If patient cannot provide this information, then appropriate surrogate should be contacted.
4. "Right vs. left" considerations should be double-checked prior to the procedure.
5. Proper body part should be marked or identified prior to the procedure.
6. "Time out" should be taken before the procedure by team members to check identity of patient, procedure to be performed, body part, and clinician whom will be performing the procedure
7. Clinician should discuss with patient:
   a. The type of procedure
   b. The risks and benefits
   c. Consequences of not undergoing procedure
   d. Who will be actually performing the procedure? Will residents or clinicians in training be involved?
   e. Alternatives to the procedure
   f. How long and what will the recovery process be like following the procedure?
8. Patient should be encouraged to have an advocate who can speak on his/her behalf if he/she cannot communicate his/her needs.
9. Patient should be given a copy of the test/procedure results for his/her records.

to medical ward) and to closely monitor for adverse medications or a worsening in their condition, as these can contribute to confusion, dizziness, and impaired balance (4).

Pressure Ulcers

Adults with neurologic disabilities who are wheelchair or bed bound are at high risk for the development of pressure ulcers. Pressure ulcers are a source of pain and infections and are associated with both increased costs and prolonged hospitalizations. It is important for clinicians to identify high-risk patients and then implement strategies to prevent them from developing.

High-risk patients present with any of the following problems: 1) limited mobility, 2) urinary or fecal incontinence, 3) poor nutrition, 4) dehydration, 5) multiple medical and surgical problems, and 6) impaired circulation. These patients should have their skin examined thoroughly at time of admission to a medical or nursing setting or at time of transition from one medical setting to another. In addition, daily skin checks should be performed and documented in the medical chart. Areas that especially prone to pressure ulcers include the buttocks, heels, and elbows.

Strategies to prevent pressure ulcers include: 1) maximizing nutrition and hydration, 2) appropriate padding over high-risk areas (e.g., heels), 3) reducing moisture (sweat, incontinence)—this can be accomplished with the use of mild skin cleaners, undergarments, and appropriate wound and fluid drainage (ideally these items should be kept at the patient's bedside for ready access by nursing staff), 4) turning and repositioning of immobilized patients every 2 hours, and 5) use of a pressure-relieving mattress. The use of an alarm clock to remind staff can be helpful (5).

Hospital-Acquired Infections

According to the CDC there are 1.7 million infections and 99,000 associated deaths each year in American hospitals due to healthcare-associated infections. The most common types of infections are urinary tract infections (32%), surgical site infections (22%), pneumonia (15%), and bloodstream infections (14%) (6). Table 18.7 lists some common strategies to prevent infections in the medical setting. In addition, the reader is referred to the CDC website for additional information www.cdc.gov.

Table 18.7

Prevention of Hospital-Acquired Infections

1. Hand washing:
   a. Wash hands in between patients; before eating; after touching garbage.
   b. Hands should be washed with antibacterial soap with vigorous rubbing for 15 seconds; they should be rinsed and dried well; a paper towel should be used to turn off the water (www.publichealth.va.gov/InfectionDon'tPass It On).
   c. Use of alcohol-based hand cleaners is encouraged.
   d. Hands should also be washed after gloves are taken off.
2. Nails must be kept short—less than ¼ inch. Fake nails should not be worn.
3. Urinary catheters (www.cdc.gov/ncidod/dhqp/gl_catheter_assoc.html):
   a. Personnel identified to insert indwelling catheters should receive adequate training and be deemed competent to perform this procedure. They should also receive periodic training as well.
   b. Indwelling urinary catheters should be removed as soon as possible.
   c. Hand washing should be done soon after the urinary catheter is inserted or handled.
   d. Urinary catheters should be inserted using aseptic technique.
   e. Indwelling catheters should be properly secured after insertion to prevent traction.
4. Advice for clinicians with a respiratory infection:
   a. Wash hands often.
   b. Cover mouth if coughing or sneezing.
   c. Don't share food or drink with anyone.
   d. Stay home.

Patient Education

Patient education is an important component of patient safety. It has been reported that 50% of all Americans have difficulty understanding and acting upon health information (1).

Patients and their caregivers should receive education about the patient's condition, prognosis, and treatment at an appropriate literacy level that takes into account the patient's age, language, culture, values, and beliefs.

Patients should be provided ample education time using appropriate educational material with staff deemed competent as patient educators. Special emphasis should be placed on preventive measures to reduce the risk of injuries (e.g., education about fall prevention).

Patients and their caregivers should be educated on the medications and procedures recommended for their medical condition. For medications, that education should include: 1) the name of the medication, 2) indications, 3) anticipated benefits, 4) common side effects and their likelihood of occurrence, 5) significant adverse effects, 6) drug–food and drug–drug interactions, and 7) impact on their level of function, and 8) alternatives.

For procedures, information should include: 1) the name of the procedure, 2) a description of the procedure, including the possibility of associated pain, 3) anticipated benefits of the procedure, 4) risks of the procedure and their likelihood of occurring, and 5) alternatives.

Patients and their caregivers should also receive a basic education on how to monitor their own health (taking blood pressure, finger sticks, and recording results). They should also be encouraged to be partners in their own care, advocate for their needs, and, when they cannot, identify someone who can advocate for them. The Agency for Healthcare Research and Quality (AHRQ) provides a useful patient brochure that patients can bring with them when they have an appointment with their physician (www.ahrq.gov/qual/beprepared.pdf]. Patients should be encouraged to carry a personal medical record with them that identifies, at a minimum: 1) the main medical diagnoses, 2) a complete medication list, 3) allergies, 4) name and contact information of their primary care physician, 5) advanced directives, and 6) emergency contact information (1).

REFERENCES

1. Preventing Medication Errors: Quality Chasm Series. National Academies Press, 2007.
2. To Err Is Human: Building a Safer Health System. National Academies Press, 2000.
3. Woolf SH, Kuzel AJ, Dovey SM, Phillips RL Jr. A string of mistakes: the importance of cascade analysis. Ann Family Med 2004; 2(4):317–326.
4. Lancaster AD, Ayers A, Belbot B, Goldner V, Kress A, Stanton D, Jones P, Sparkman L. Preventing falls and eliminating injury at ascension health. Joint Commission Journal on Quality and Patient Safety Clinical Excellence Series 2007; 33(7):367–375.
5. Duncan KD. Preventing pressure ulcers: the goal is zero. Joint Commission Journal on Quality and Patient Safety 2007; 33(10):605–610.
6. www.cdc.gov/ncidod/dhqp/hai.html.

19 | Clinical Pharmacology and Medication Safety in the Patient with Neurologic Disability

Shai Gavi

One of the most commonly employed tools of physicians is the writing of a prescription or an order for a medication. The use of medications in neurologically disabled patients is especially high. Most common types of medications are aimed at the treatment of the specific neurologic disorder (e.g., multiple sclerosis). However, many medications utilized for the treatment of individuals with neurologic diseases are aimed at alleviating the sequale of the neurologic disease (e.g., spasticity, pain, neurogenic bladder, neurogenic bowel). Many of these individuals suffer from chronic and acute medical illnesses and are commonly prescribed cardiovascular medications, analgesics, gastrointestinal agents, and antibiotics. The use of multiple medications predisposes such individuals to adverse drug events. As such, an understanding of key concepts of clinical pharmacology is essential for the successful use of medications in the patient with a neurologic disability.

PHARMACOLOGY

Pharmacokinetic Principles

The goal of administering a drug is to achieve a desired therapeutic effect with minimal adverse effects. The selection of a drug formulation, dose, frequency of dose administration, and adverse events are governed by the principles of pharmacokinetics. Pharmacokinetics is the study of the body's mechanism of delivering a medication to the site of action. This involves the processes of absorption, distribution, metabolism, and elimination (1–3).

Absorption

Absorption is the process of transfer of drug from site of administration to the blood. Routes of administration include oral, sublingual, transdermal, rectal, inhalation, subcutaneous, intramuscular, and intravenous. Each of these routes affects the quantity of drug and the time it takes to reach the drug site. Drug administration by nonintravenous routes often involves an absorption process with increasing plasma level to a maximum value after some time of administration and then declining as the rate of drug elimination exceeds the rate of absorption. The peak concentration is lower and occurs later than if the drug is given with the same dose by intravenous injection. Absorption of a medication commonly occurs by passive diffusion across a membrane barrier to the systemic circulation. The rate of drug absorption is determined by the free drug concentration or at times by the rate of delivery from a sustained-release preparation. The extent of drug absorption that reaches the systemic circulation is termed bioavailability (1,2).

Distribution

The distribution phase is the initial phase following drug administration and the subsequent phase of decline in drug concentration. The volume of distribution describes the amount of drug in the body as it relates to the plasma concentration. The volume of distribution is useful for calculating the loading dose and explains why certain body composition changes can affect a drug's half-life. The loading dose of a drug is calculated by multiplying the volume of distribution by the desired drug concentration. At the end of the distribution phase the drug leaves the circulation and enters the tissues. The drug is first delivered to well-perfused tissues and later to areas that are less perfused.

Metabolism

Drugs are predominantly eliminated by metabolism in the liver or by renal filtration or secretion. Following oral administration, many drugs are absorbed intact from the small intestine and transported via the portal circulation to the liver, where they are metabolized by phase I and II reactions. This process is called the "first-pass" effect and may greatly limit the bioavailability of orally administered drugs. Most drugs are hydrophobic and therefore are not readily excreted by the kidneys. Biotransformation within the liver of hydrophobic parent drug to hydrophilic metabolites enhances drug excretion by the kidneys. Phase I reactions via oxidations, reductions, and hydrolyses add a polar group to the parent compound to make it more polar. Cytochrome P450 of the phase I reaction is the most abundant enzyme, making it the rate-limiting step in hepatic drug oxidation. Certain drug substrates may induce or inhibit the cytochrome P450 system and affect the half-life of the drug. The metabolites produced by phase I reactions are usually not polar enough for rapid elimination. Phase II reactions involve adding an endogenous substance such as glucuronic acid, sulfuric acid, or acetic acid to form a highly polar conjugate. Such conjugation transforms the drug to a very polar compound, which is readily excreted by the kidneys. While most drugs are metabolized by the liver, some drugs are metabolized in the small intestine, lungs, skin, and kidneys (2,3).

Elimination

Most drugs are eliminated by renal filtration or secretion by "first-order" (linear) kinetics—the amount of drug being eliminated is directly proportional to the plasma concentration. However, certain drugs follow an elimination of "zero-order" kinetics; these drugs have dose-dependent, nonlinear, saturation kinetics. As the dose of the drug increases and the plasma concentration increases, the amount of drug being eliminated increases until the rate of the drug metabolism is at its maximum. At this point, the drug concentration starts to increase much more with each subsequent increase in dose. Phenytoin is eliminated by zero-order kinetics. Half-life is defined as the amount of time needed to decrease the concentration of a drug in half. A drug can be considered to be totally eliminated after three to five half-lives (1–3).

For most medications the therapeutic effects occur over a wide range of drug concentration, whereas with some medications, the therapeutic effects are within a narrow therapeutic concentration. Serious toxicity can develop outside of this narrow range of concentration (Table 19.1). Such medications require drug concentrations to be used as a guide. To adequately interpret such assays, the timing of blood collection is very important. If sampling is done too early, the drug level may still be in the distribution phase and very high and will not reflect drug concentration at the tissue level. The continuation of administration of a drug either as repeated doses or as a continuous infusion results in accumulation until a steady state occurs. Steady state is the point where the amount of drug being administered equals the amount being eliminated so that the plasma and tissue levels remain constant. Steady state is achieved in three to five half-lives. For many drugs administered intermittently, a trough level at steady state obtained before administration of the next dose is most useful for determining dosing adjustments. The trough level at steady state drug concentration provides the best correlation between drug concentration and toxic effect. Trough levels are generally sampled 30 minutes before the fourth dose. Peak drug levels measured 30 minutes to 1 hour after drug administration documents the maximum drug concentration to assess if it is within the therapeutic concentration. Drug levels can be misinterpreted in the presence of altered protein levels. Many drugs are bound to serum proteins to a large extent and are therefore inactive. However, serum assays usually measure the inactive protein bound as well as free active drug. Therefore, assessment

Table 19.1

Drugs with Low Therapeutic Index

- Antispasmodics: baclofen, tizanidine
- Anticoagulation: warfarin, heparin
- Antiepileptic: phenytoin, carbamazepine, valproic acid
- Psychiatric medications: tricyclic antidepressants, monoamine oxidase inhibitors
- Analgesics: opiode narcotics

of true free drug concentration is unknown, especially when protein levels are altered (2,3).

Pharmacodynamic Principles

Once a drug reaches it site of action, a cascade of cellular responses occur, which manifest as a desired effect of the drug. The molecular response of a drug is highly variable between individuals. This often explains different responses to therapies in different individuals (e.g., opioids, warfarin). Furthermore, the response of the target receptor may be altered by other factors, such as prior exposure to similar agonists or antagonists or receptor up- or downregulation due to disease state or genetic variability (1,2).

PATIENT ASSESSMENT

An appropriate history and physical examination is an important part of the safe prescription of medications. Clinicians should obtain from their patients a thorough medication history for all their medical problems as well as a history of allergies to foods and medications. Reasons for the discontinuation of medications can shed light on possible drug sensitivities. An important distinction is between drug allergy and side effect. Experiencing a drug side effect is not a true allergy to a medication and therefore does not preclude one from taking that medication again. Restrictive diets (e.g., vegan) and use of over-the-counter medications and herbs are also important to note. Clinicians should inquire about a history of renal and liver disease. Recent surgeries, infections, and hospitalizations can point to a frailer individual who would need adjustments made to medication dosing or frequency. Age-related changes of increasing adipose tissue, decreased lean body mass, decrease in plasma proteins, and a decrease in renal function may lead to higher drug concentration in the elderly.

Physical examination should include vital signs, cognitive assessment, and targeted systems such as the cardiopulmonary and gastrointestinal systems. The presence of malnutrition, cachexia, or fluid overload should also be noted.

PRINCIPLES OF DOSE SELECTION

The desired drug effect should be defined when drug treatment is initiated. However, the onset of efficacy for some drugs may be delayed for weeks to months. The nature of anticipated toxicity will determine the starting dose. If the side effects are minor, it may be acceptable to start at a dose highly likely to achieve efficacy and downtitrate if side effects occur. If a drug dose does not achieve its desired effect, a dosage increase is justified only if toxicity is absent and the likelihood of serious toxicity is small. Failure of drug effects may be due to drug interaction and noncompliance. Noncompliance occurs in over

25% of patients; this is exaggerated by use of multidrug regimen with multiple doses per day.

Alteration of drug effects is usually achieved by changing the drug dose but not the dosing interval. However, this is only done if an increase in the dose does not result in a peak concentration that is toxic and a decrease in the dose does not result in a trough value that falls below the minimum effective concentration. Alternatively, dosing may be changed by either decreasing or increasing the frequency of the dose but not the amount. Generally, doses are given at intervals equal to the drug's half-life. If the dosing interval is equal to the drug's half-life, fluctuation is approximately twofold. The dosing interval will usually reflect the magnitude of drug concentration above and below the steady state. Drugs with short half-lives have a smaller change above and below the steady-state level, whereas drugs with long half-lives have a greater change above and below the steady-state level. While for most drugs a change in drug effect can be achieved with changing the dose amount or dose frequency, in drugs with a narrow therapeutic range, a small increase in dose can cause toxicity, whereas a small decrease in concentration can lead to loss of efficacy. As such, changes in the dosage should not exceed 50% of the previous dose, and dose change should not occur more frequently than every three to four half-lives. With such drugs, the dose frequency would remain the same as their half-life to minimize fluctuations in drug concentration above and below steady state. The concept of *start low and go slow* is important when prescribing medications with a narrow therapeutic window (1–3).

ADVERSE DRUG REACTIONS

An adverse drug reaction is an untoward effect produced by a drug at standard doses. The incidence of adverse drug reactions varies from 10 to 20% depending on the population studied and setting. Adverse drug reactions are the fourth to sixth leading cause of death in hospitalized patients. The most common offenders include drugs with narrow therapeutic concentrations that are taken in combination with other drugs (Table 19.1). The mechanism of adverse effects can be an exaggerated but predictable drug response or a toxic/immunologic and unpredictable response. Exaggerated response may be due to altered pharmacokinetic or pharmacodynamic properties in the patient. Altered absorption, body composition, or renal function can alter the distribution and half-life of a drug. In addition, changes with aging or genetic variability can explain altered pharmacodynamic changes in response to a drug. A toxic effect of a drug may be the direct effect of a drug or its metabolite on an organ. Immunologic reactions usually involve the binding of a drug to a protein to form an antigenic drug–protein complex. Drugs in themselves are too small to elicit an immune response. Diagnosing an adverse drug reaction requires a high index of suspicion, especially in individuals with multiple illnesses and medications. Any new symptoms in such individuals should be considered as a potential adverse effect of a medication.

DRUG–DRUG INTERACTIONS

The co-administration of several drugs can produce an untoward effect. A drug effect can be exaggerated or diminished by the effect of another medication. This may be due to alteration in pharmacokinetics or pharmacodynamics. The challenge of remembering all drug interactions is daunting; therefore, a high index of suspicion is essential. Common risk factors for adverse drug–drug interactions include the use of medications with low therapeutic index, polypharmacy (risk increases proportionally to the number of medications with a range of 2.5–50.6%), and patients with multisystemic illness with poor homeostatic reserve. The administration of drugs can also interact with foods or herbal products. Drugs can affect the absorption, distribution, and metabolism of other drugs. Furthermore, drugs can affect the receptor sensitivity to other drugs. Methods to prevent drug interactions are initiated by a meticulous history of prescription medications, over-the-counter products, alternative health agents, and unusual diet patterns (e.g., vegetarian diet). Minimizing the number of medications prescribed is critical, as is maintaining a high index of suspicion for drug–drug interactions. Common drug interactions in patients with a neurologic disability involve the coadministration of medications that have an effect on the central nervous system (e.g., antispasticity agents, antiepileptic agents, opiods, antidepressants). Of the antiepileptic agents, gabapentin has minimal drug interactions without a significant clinical effect. The coadministration of these medications may lead to increase somnolence, disorientation, and falls. Other interactions have been described with these agents (Table 19.2). Interaction between tiaznidine and drugs that inhibit the cytochrome P450 CYP1A2 (e.g., fluroquinolones, antiarrythmics, cimetidine, acyclovir) should be avoided.

DRUG–DISEASE INTERACTIONS

Disease states may often contribute to alteration in pharmacokinetics and pharmacokinetics of drugs and need to be considered (Table 19.3). Diseases of the gastrointestinal tract can affect the rate and extent of medication absorption. Alteration of small bowel motility, surface area, and pH can affect absorption of various medications. Change in body composition from disease states (e.g., fluid overload, cachexia, and malnutrition) can affect drug distribution of hydrophilic drugs, hydrophobic drugs, and highly protein-bound drugs. Furthermore, disease states affecting the liver and kidneys can affect metabolism and elimination of medications. A medical history of such disease states would require dose adjustment or drug substitution.

PHARMACOGENETICS

Modern molecular tools have revealed the genetic makeup of the humans with appreciation of common polymorphism. As such, genetic makeup may have an important influence on a drug's pharmacokinetic and pharmacodynamic profile between different individuals. Variability in the cytochrome P450 leads

Table 19.2

Drug–Drug Interactions

Drug–Drug	Pharmacologic effect
• Baclofen + tricyclic antidepressant	Exacerbate depression, hypotension
• Baclofen + monoamine oxidase inhibitor	Exacerbate depression, hypotension
• Lamotrigine + phenytoin, phenobarbital, rifampin	Decrease lamotrigine serum levels by 40%
• Phenyotin + enteral nutrition	Decrease phenytoin levels
• Phenytoin + methyphenidate	Increase phenytoin levels
• Phenytoin + diazepam	Increase phenytoin levels
• Tizanidine + clonidine	Hypotension, syncope
• Tizanidine + ciprofloxacin	Increase tizanidine levels
• Tizanidine + vluvoxamine	Increase tizanidine levels
• Tizanidine + oral contraceptives	Increase tizanidine levels
• Dantrolene + calcium channel blockers	Hypotension, hyperkalemia
• Tramadol + carbamazepine	Reduce tramadol levels
• Tramadol + tricyclic antidepressant	Reduce seizure threshold
• Tramadol + selective serotonin reuptake inhibitors	Reduce seizure threshold, serotonin syndrome
• Tramadol + opioids	Reduce seizure threshold
• Tramadol + monoamine oxidase inhibitor	Reduce seizure threshold, serotonin syndrome
• Methylphenidate + guanethidine, clonidine	Hypotension
• Amantadine + anticholinergic agents	Dry mouth, urinary retention, constipation
• Amantadine + quinine or quinidine	Increase amantadine levels
• Amantadine + live attenuated influenza vaccine	May inhibit replication of live vaccine virus

Table 19.3

Drug–Disease Interactions

Drug–Disease	Physiologic effect
• Phenytoin–Diabetes	Increase glucose levels
• Phenytoin–Osteoporosis	Decrease vitamin D metabolism
• Phenytoin–Liver disease	Impaired phenytoin metabolism
• Baclofen–Chronic kidney disease	Impaired clearance
• Baclofen–Epilepsy	May reduce seizure threshold
• Tizanidine–Liver disease	Impaired clearance
• Tizanidine–Renal disease	Impaired clearance
• Tramadol–Seizure	May reduce seizure threshold
• Methylphenidate–Cardiomyopathy	Sudden cardiac death
• Methylphenidate–Hypertension	Increase blood pressure
• Methylphenidate–Epilepsy	Reduce seizure threshold
• Amantadine–Glaucoma	May precipitate attack of glaucoma
• Amantadine–Psychiatric disease	May exacerbate underlying psychiatric disorder, increase suicide risk
• Amantadine–Benign prostatic hyperplasia	Urinary retention
• Opioids–Constipation	Increase constipation
• NSAIDS–Chronic kidney disease	Worsen renal function, hyperkalemia

to altered rate of metabolism of certain drugs (e.g., acetaminophen, warfarin); however, this cannot be tested in the clinical setting at this time. Variability in amino acid sequence of drug receptors has elucidated different response to physiologic stimuli as well as pharmacologic agents (e.g., variability in β-adrenergic pharmacodynamic has effect on effectiveness of β-agonist inhalers or prevalence of heart failure in certain populations). This may also explain the variability of drug effects between different ethnicities.

MEDICATION SAFETY

The Institute of Medicine report noted that as many as 98,000 people die each year from medical errors—7000 from medication errors alone—and that 2–3% of hospital admissions are for illnesses attributed to drugs (4). The in-hospital cost attributed to medication-related errors has been estimated to be greater than $3.5 billion. A new Institute of Medicine report in 2006 highlighted the need for efforts to reduce medication errors (5). A medication error can be defined as an unintended act of omission or commission. More than half of all medication errors of near misses were due to lack of drug knowledge (6). These errors could have been prevented by checking the dose and identity of drugs and providing patients with information. Health professionals need to have drug information at the time of medication prescribing. Lack of information about the patient or a drug accounts for 40% of serious injury due to errors (6).

An adverse drug event is defined as an injury form a drug-related intervention. An adverse drug event may be due to errors in prescribing, dispensing, and administration. Adverse drug events have been categorized as preventable, nonpreventable, and potential. At least 1.5 million preventable adverse drug events occur each year in the United States (6). As such, adverse drug events are the most frequent single source of iatrogenic mishap. Aspirin, nonsteroidal anti-inflammatory drugs (NSAIDS), opioids, digoxin, anticoagulants, diuretics, antimicrobials, glucocorticoids, antineoplastics, hypoglycemics, and insulin account for most adverse drug events (6). Many adverse drug events are preventable. Adverse drug events may be prevented by standardizing and simplifying core medication processes, redesigning medication-delivery systems, and education (Table 19.4).

Table 19.4

Principles of Prescribing Medications Safely

- The benefit of drug therapy should always outweigh the risk.
- Start low and increase slow.
- Any new symptom may be an adverse drug event until proven otherwise.
- The smallest dosage necessary to produce the desired effect should be used.
- The number of medications and doses per day should be minimized.
- Computers and hand-held devices should be used to readily access drug information.
- Prescribers should use a limited number of drugs with which they are thoroughly familiar.

High-alert medications are medications that are most likely to cause harm to the patient, even when used as intended. The Institute for Safe Medication Practices reports that although errors may not occur more frequently with the high-alert medications, the consequence of the error is greater (6). These medications include anticoagulants, narcotics and opioids, insulin, and sedatives (Table 19.5).

Anticoagulants account for 4% of preventable adverse drug events and 10% of potential adverse drug events and are associated with more serious adverse drug events in both inpatient and outpatients. Warfarin is commonly involved in adverse drug events due to the complexity of dosing and monitoring, patient compliance, drug–drug interactions, and interaction with dietary intake. Guidelines such as "The Pharmacology and Management of the Vitamin K Antagonists" provide the tools necessary for the safe use of warfarin (7).

Narcotics and opioids are other medications associated with frequent adverse drug events, even with appropriate dosing. Adverse drug events include oversedation, respiratory depression, confusion, lethargy, nausea, vomiting, and constipation. Nausea and vomiting are estimated at 34.5 and 18.2%, respectively (8). In addition, bradypnea and oxygen desaturation occurred in 0.5 and 1.6%, respectively. The use of patient-controlled analgesia also poses potential harm but has a lower likelihood of adverse events than frequent administration of short-acting opioids. Inappropriate use of sedatives, in combination with opioids or alone, is associated with oversedation, hypotension, delirium, and lethargy and may contribute to falls. Importantly, opioid conversion tables are essential to prevent adverse drug events during change of opioids (1,2).

Optimizing glucose control is important in diabetic patients. The use of insulin to optimize glucose control is complex. The pharmacology of the drug, dosing and interval, administration, and variety of insulin forms make the use of insulin challenging and complex. Standardized protocols to manage hyperglycemia are valuable to promote the safe use of insulin. The Institute for Healthcare Improvement and the American Diabetes Association have information to help reduce harm from insulin.

Table 19.5

High-Alert Medications

- Anticoagulants
- Anticonvulsants
- Antiarrhythmics
- Digoxin
- Insulin
- Lithium carbonate
- Opioids
- Oral hypoglycemics
- Theophylline

Methods to improve the safety of medications include development of order sets, preprinted order forms, and the use of protocols and electronic medical records. Additional methods to prevent harm at the time of ordering or administration of medications include: 1) minimized variability by standardizing concentrations, dose strength, 2) clear labeling, 3) reminders and information for patients regarding appropriate monitoring parameters (8). Methods to help include ensuring that: 1) lab information necessary to write the medication is available, 2) protocols for delivering reversal agents are available, and 3) antidotes and reversal agents are readily available.

It is important to maintain an accurate medication list to avoid errors such as conflicts or unintentional omissions at times of transition of care (6). Therefore, accurate medication reconciliation must take place at all points of transition of care. Medication reconciliation is the process of comparing the medication the patient was taking prior to admission or entry to a new setting or level of care with what the organization is providing at the time of admission to the new setting.

Patient Safety

Patients should be assessed for renal and liver disease, history of drug allergies, malnutrition, cachexia, and fluid overload. A thorough review of current and prior medications is also strongly recommended.

Drug–drug interactions and drug–disease interactions should be strongly considered when prescribing medications to adults with neurologic disabilities. Key points are outlined in Tables 19.2 and 19.3. Principles of prescribing medications safely are shown in Table 19.4, and common sources of medication errors are outlined in Table 19.6. Caution should be used when prescribing high-risk medications such as anticoagulants, opioids, sedatives, and insulin (Table 19.5).

Table 19.6

Common Causes of Medication Errors

- Lack of information about the patient
- Lack of information about the drug
- Medication reconciliation at time of transition of care
- Look-alike and sound-alike drugs
- Unsafe drug standardization, storage, and distribution
- Inadequate patient education
- Lack of supportive culture of safety and error-reduction strategies

Patient Education

Patients and their caregivers should be educated on all aspects of the medications being prescribed for them. This education should include reason for use, dosage, frequency, route of administration and specific instructions (e.g., titration or complex schedule), potential side effects (including their likelihood of occurring), and potential drug–drug interactions.

Clinicians should check for comprehension of instructions by having the patient or caregiver recite back the instructions. Written material at an appropriate reading level and in a language commonly spoken by the patient are also important.

REFERENCES

1. Brunton L, Lazo J, Parke K. Goodman & Gilmans's The Pharmacological Basis of Therapeutics, 11th ed. New York: McGraw-Hill, 2005.
2. Katzung BG. Basic and Clinical Pharmacology, 9th ed. New York: McGraw-Hill, 2003.
3. Bateman DN, Eddleston M. Clinical pharmacology: the basics. Surgery 2006; 24;9:291–296.
4. Kohn LT, Corrigan JM, Donaldson MS. To Err Is Human; Building a Safer Health System. Washington, DC: National Academy Press, 2000.
5. Aspden P, Wolcott J, Bootman JL, Cronenwett LR. Preventing Medication Errors: Quality Chasm Series. Washington, DC: National Academy Press, 2006.
6. Cohen MR. Medication Errors, 2nd ed. Washington, DC: American Pharmacists Association, 2007.
7. Ansel J, Hirsh J, Poller L, Bussey H, Jacobson A, Hylek E. The pharmacology and management of the vitamin K antagonists: the seventh ACCP Conference on antithrombotic and thrombolytic therapy. Chest 2004; 126:204–233.
8. www.ihi.org. Protecting 5 Million Lives from Harm: Institute for Healthcare Improvement.

20 | Pharmacologic Management of Behavior and Cognitive Impairment in Adults with Brain Injury

John L. Rigg

The annual incidence of traumatic brain injury (TBI) in the United States is 1.5 million cases. It has been estimated that at least 5.3 million Americans are living with the effects of a TBI. Leading causes of TBI are motor vehicle accidents, falls, and gunshot wounds. The use of alcoholic beverages and recreational drugs is highly associated with TBI (1).

More than 4 million people in the United States have survived a stroke and are living with stroke-related impairments. Risk factors for stroke include hypertension, diabetes, tobacco use, elevated cholesterol, and obesity (2).

The goal of this chapter is to provide clinicians with information about the pathophysiology, assessment, and management of the cognitive impairments commonly associated with TBI and stroke. These include memory and attention deficits and mood disorders such as apathy and agitation.

ANATOMY, PHYSIOLOGY, AND PATHOPHYSIOLOGY

The actual damage to the brain resulting in a TBI can be divided into two processes. The first is the initial traumatic event leading to shearing, laceration, and/or contusion of brain tissue that occurs at the time of the trauma. The second process consists of a cascade of molecular events that develop in the minutes, hours, and days following the trauma. These physiologic changes occur on the cellular and molecular level and may include any one, or combination of, the following: ischemia, hemorrhage, alterations in ion and neuromodulator levels, oxidative stress caused by free radicals, increased permeability of the blood-brain barrier, and edema.

The primary injury typically is caused by both impact and inertial forces—the actual impact of the head with a solid object and the consequent sudden change in velocity that generates the inertial (acceleration/deceleration) forces. Brain parenchyma damage then occurs as the result of compressing, stretching, or shearing of brain tissue caused by the impact and inertial forces.

Impact forces are responsible for skull fractures, epidural and/or subdural hematomas, and coup contusions. Inertial forces have both a linear (or translational acceleration) component and a rotational acceleration component. The inertial forces created by translational acceleration contribute to both focal and diffuse injury. These inertial forces can be responsible for the development of contra coup contusions, intracerebral hematomas, and subdural hematomas (3).

Diffuse injury results in white matter damage and the loss of normal communication between different areas of the brain. As a result, neurocognitive pathways such as the reticular activating system, mesocortical and mesolimbic pathways, limbic system, and raphe nucleus may be damaged, giving rise to the multitudes of neurologic deficits found in the TBI population (4).

Diffuse axonal injury (DAI) is the most significant cause of morbidity in patients with traumatic brain injury. It is characterized by diffuse damage to the white matter, as a result of rotational trauma. DAI is typically accompanied by loss of consciousness. It cannot be seen on computed tomography (CT) or magnetic resonance imaging (MRI), although one may often see petechial hemorrhages at the gray–white matter junctions that suggest the presence of a DAI. Petechial hemorrhages occur due to the shearing forces generated as a result of the difference in density between the gray and white matter. If this force is strong enough to cause vascular injuries with resultant petechial hemorrhages, it is likely to also have caused shearing of axons resulting in a DAI. Two thirds of DAI lesions occur at the gray–white matter junction.

The significant difference between the damage that occurs to the brain during a TBI and a stroke is that the typical injury in a stroke is a focal injury. Whether the injury is the result of a hemorrhage or ischemia, a specific focal area of the brain is affected, leading to deficits that correspond to the location of the injury. However, these focal injuries can also cause disruption of neuropathways (white matter tracts), resulting in deficits unrelated to the anatomic area that has been damaged. On the cellular level, blood flow that is interrupted by an embolism, thrombus, or hemorrhage leads to the death of neurons. Around this area of developing necrosis are other neurons that are hypoperfused, which may not be receiving enough blood supply to keep them alive. This area is called the penumbra. Additional cell death can be expected in this area if reperfusion is not established soon after the stroke. One of the major goals of acute stroke care and of research focus is to reestablish adequate perfusion as expeditiously as possible to lessen the effects of a stroke (5).

Disabilities arising as a consequence of neurologic injury typically include problems with: a) motor abilities—strength, coordination, and balance; b) cognition-concentration, memory, and judgment; c) sensation—particularly special senses such as vision, smell, and tactile sensation; and d) mood-emotional instability/impulsivity.

In order for patients' recovery to proceed, they must be able to participate in their occupational, physical, and speech therapy programs. This necessitates attainment of a satisfactory level of baseline arousal and control of agitation and restlessness along with minimizing the use of medications that could make the patient lethargic and unable to participate and learn. A patient's mood will also have a large effect on his or her recovery and must be considered throughout treatment. Also, brain injury patients commonly present with sleep disorders that must be dealt with because sleep deprivation will interfere with a patient's ability to fully participate and benefit from the therapeutic program (6).

Knowledge of medications that may actually impair recovery is critical. Often in the acute/trauma setting, patients are placed on drugs to control restlessness and agitation, which may potentially impede their neurorecovery (Table 20.1). If any of these drugs are being used, they should be tapered appropriately and replaced by medications that do not have negative effects on brain function.

PATIENT ASSESSMENT

Patients who have sustained a brain injury should be assessed for problems with initiation (abulia), disinhibition, alertness, attention, memory, restlessness, agitation, mood, and sleep disturbance. These symptoms may be difficult to assess. In the inpatient setting, the nursing staff, physical, occupational, and speech therapists will be able to supply very valuable information regarding how the patient is performing in therapies and what issues may be interfering with recovery. In the outpatient setting, family members and friends can often provide information on these problems in the home and community settings (Table 20.2).

Table 20.1

Medications with Potential to Interfere with Neurorecovery

- Typical and atypical antipsychotics—dopamine receptor antagonists
- Benzodiazepines—potentiate GABA and negatively affect memory formation
- Metoclopramide—antagonizes central and peripheral dopamine receptors
- Anticholinergics—may interfere with formation of new memories
- α_1-Adrenergic antagonists (Prazosin) and α_2-agonists (clonidine)
- Phenobarbitol and phenytoin (carbamazepine and valproate are better choices for seizure prophylaxis)

Table 20.2

Assessment of the Patient with Cognitive Impairment

- Level of alertness
- Communication and speech—Intelligible? Fluent?
- Ability to follow instructions
- Orientation: name, date, time, place
- Memory: immediate and delayed recall—five items, four trials
- Concentration: serial 7s, reverse number sequences

In a focal injury, the deficits appear as a result of damage to specific anatomic areas of the brain and manifest as a malfunction of those areas. For example, injury to the orbito-frontal area may result in disinhibition, impulsive behavior, or poor judgment and insight. Damage to the frontal convexity manifests as unopposed restraint/inactivity/apathy, often accompanied by motor programming deficits. Damage to the medial frontal lobe can result in decreased spontaneous movement and verbal output, lower extremity weakness, and incontinence.

TREATMENT

The effective management of cognitive and behavioral problems in adults with TBI and stroke often include a combination of both pharmacologic and non-pharmacologic interventions (Table 20.3).

Pharmacologic treatment is aimed at correcting and improving damaged brain signals through the manipulation of neurotransmitter supplies in the brain. A typical course of treatment begins with neurostimulatory medications to improve arousal, attention, and initiation. The frontal lobes are rich in dopaminergic pathways, and destruction of or damage to these pathways can clinically manifest as frontal lobe syndrome, which may be characterized by disinhibition, impulsiveness, antisocial behavior, impairment of normal functioning and planning, hypomanic like behavior, apathy/abulia, negligence about personal appearance, perseveration, and depression. Treatment with dopaminergic psychostimulant drugs may improve communication between the areas of the frontal lobes and resolution of some of the previously mentioned symptoms (7).

Treatment for the symptoms mentioned above may be started at any time in a patient's recovery. If the above-mentioned symptoms are found during acute hospitalization or even years after injury, they may benefit from treatment. It is important to remember, however, that patient response to medications may vary greatly during their course of recovery. A medication that may have worked at one time may cease to work, or a medication that was not effective at one time in the recovery may prove to become efficacious at a later date. Medications are not likely to be needed long term. Typically, a 3- to 6-month

Table 20.3

Mangement of Cognitive and Behavioral Problems in Adults

- Memory aids: notebooks, "to-do" lists, digital recorders, pocket electronic organizers, GPS systems
- Minimizing agitation: consistent caregivers, 1:1 observation, minimal auditory and visual stimuli, similar surroundings, low light, one visitor at a time, frequent rest periods during day, reestablish sleep-wake cycle

treatment course will be enough to trigger a new course of recovery, and medications may be tapered and discontinued without consequent setback. There is no well-researched algorithm for length of treatment with these medications. When the desired effect is achieved and maintained for a period of time on a consistent basis, tapering and discontinuation of the medication should be attempted in order to minimize the number of medications that a patient is taking. If the patient experiences a setback, he or she may be restarted.

When treating a patient with a brain injury, it is imperative to remember that an injured brain can be more sensitive to medications and their side effects. A drug's idiosyncratic effects are difficult to predict in the brain injury population. An injured brain is likely to be more sensitive to the effects of medications, both positive and negative. Typically one would be able to treat a brain-injured patient with smaller doses than normal to attain the desired result (8).

It is often difficult for a physician to assess the effectiveness of neuropharmacologic treatments on a daily basis. It is therefore very important to obtain relevant information provided by nursing staff, therapists, and family members who spend more time with the patient.

Neurostimulatory Medications

The following medications are presented in a usual sequence of initiation. Multiple neurostimulatory medications may be used (Table 20.4). Constant vigilance and monitoring of side effects that may present suddenly or insidiously is imperative.

Amantidine/Symmetrel: The first medication typically used in the course of a patient's recovery from a brain injury. It is used to improve a patient's attention and initiation. It may improve arousal, processing time, psychomotor speed, mobility, vocalization, anxiety, motivation, and agitation. It functions

Table 20.4

Neurostimulatory Medications

	Drug	Dosing (mg)	Frequency
Arousal, initiation	Amantadine	100	q7am and q12pm
Attention, focus	Methylphenidate	10	q7am, q1pm
	Atomoxetine	18	q7am for 3 days then increase to 40 mg q7am, may titrate to maximum of 80 mg daily
	Bromocriptine	2.5	q7am and q12pm, may increase by 2.5 mg per dose
	Modafinil	100	every 3 days as tolerated to max of 60 mg daily
			q am, may titrate to maximum of 400 mg/day

by augmenting dopaminergic neurotransmission and as a weak N-methyl-D-aspartic acid (NMDA) receptor antagonist. Adverse affects may include dizziness, lowering of the seizure threshold, hallucinations, irritability, depression, psychosis, and ataxia. It should not be used in patients with a penetrating head injury, history of seizures, or risk for seizures. Dosing will typically start and be maintained at 100 mg in the morning and an additional 100 mg at 1 P.M. It is important to dose this medication no later than lunch time in order to prevent interference with a patient's sleep pattern.

Methylphenidate/Ritalin: Another dopaminergic stimulant used to increase alertness and activity level. It is dosed 10 mg in the morning and an additional 10 mg with lunch in order to avoid insomnia. Contraindications include a history of Tourette's sydrome, cardiovascular disease—particularly arrhythmias—bipolar disorder, psychosis, and hypertension.

Bromocriptine/Parlodel: A dopamine agonist that provides direct stimulation of dopaminergic receptors. Its use in brain-injured patients has been shown to help with improvements in mood, cognition, and behavior, particularly with abulia. Starting dose is 2.5 mg bid dosed in the morning and at lunch time. This dose may be increased every 3 days to a maximum of 60 mg daily. Common side effects include nausea, headaches, drowsiness, dizziness, and fatigue. The most common serious side effect is seizures.

Atomoxetine/Strattera: A selective norepinephrine reuptake inhibitor. Norepinephrine is considered important in regulating attention, impulsivity, and activity levels. Treatment of TBI patients with Strattera may improve their cognition, memory, understanding, impulsivity, and even sleep. Dosing of this medication would be 18 mg in the morning. If tolerated well, it may be increased after 3 days to 40 mg in the morning. Maximum recommended dose is 80 mg per day. Most common side effects include dry mouth, abdominal pain, dyspepsia, nausea, and insomnia.

Carbidopa-Levodopa/Sinemet: This particular combination of medications inhibits peripheral dopamine decarboxylation, allowing greater penetration of the blood-brain barrier by levodopa to serve as a dopamine precursor. Starting dose is 10/100 mg tid for 1 week. Dose may then be increased to 25/250 mg tid. Maximum recommended dose in Parkinson's patients is 200/2000 mg/day. Between 70 and 100 mg/day of carbidopa are necessary to saturate peripheral dopa decarboxylase and minimize adverse effects.

Modafinil/Provigil: A wake-promoting agent with apparent cognitive properties that was initially developed for narcolepsy. It is highly specific to sites distinct from the classic neurostimulants as it does not act via enhancement of neurotransmitter activity. It is active in the hypothalamus with less cortical activity than the typical stimulants and may be useful if arousal alone is desired without psychomotor activation. It can be useful in patients with cardiac histories who may not be able to tolerate a medication like Ritalin. Dosing begins at 200 mg daily or 100 mg daily in the elderly. Maximum recommended dose is 400 mg per day. Common side effects include headache, nausea/vomiting, rhinitis, diarrhea, nervousness, or pharyngitis.

Memory Improvement

The medications used for memory improvement (Table 20.5) in TBI patients are the acetyl cholinesterase inhibitors (as listed below) and memantine/namenda. These medications have been reported to not only improve memory but also to help in decreasing agitation. The neurostimulant medications would typically be used first to ensure attention, which is critical to memory formation. Once the patient is able to participate fully in therapy with respect to alertness and initiation, these medications may be started.

Donepezil/Aricept: 5 mg qhs for 4 weeks, increase to 10 mg daily if needed.

Rivastigmine/Exelon: 1.5 mg bid, increasing 1.5 mg per dose every 2 weeks as tolerated to a maximum of 12 mg/day.

Galantamine/Razadyne: 4 mg bid, increasing 4 mg bid every 4 weeks to 12 mg bid as tolerated to a maximum of 24 mg/day. Animal studies have suggested that galantamine has an acetylcholine agonist effect in addition to its acetylcholinesterase inhibition effect. Typical side effects of the acetyl cholinesterase inhibitors include nausea, vomiting, and diarrhea.

Memantine/Namenda: An NMDA antagonist that can be used to augment/enhance the effect of the acetylcholinesterase inhibitors as the maximum dose is approached. It can be dosed at 5 mg daily, increasing 5 mg per week to a maximum of 20 mg/day as tolerated. Adverse reactions may include dizziness, headache, confusion, and constipation.

Agitation

It is first necessary to clinically make the distinction between agitation and restlessness. Both of these behaviors can cause significant disruption of therapeutic

Table 20.5

Medications for the Improvement of Memory

	Drug	Dose (mg)	Frequency	
Memory issues—begin treatment with one of these acetylcholinesterase inhibitors	Galantamine	4	Bid	Increase 4 mg bid every 4 weeks to 12 mg bid as tolerated to a maximum of 24 mg/day
	Donepezil	5	Daily	5 mg qhs for 4 weeks, increase to 10 mg daily if needed
	Rivastigmine	1.5	Bid	Increase 1.5 mg per dose every 2 weeks as tolerated to a maximum of 12 mg/day
Use as an adjunct to the acetylcholinesterase inhibitors above	Memantine	5	Daily	5 mg daily increasing 5 mg per week to a maximum of 20 mg/day as tolerated

goals, but they are distinctly different forms of behavior requiring appropriate management. They are both accompanied by akathisia (inability to remain motionless), disinhibition, and emotional lability. Agitation is characterized by excesses of behavior often accompanied by aggressiveness, combativeness, and destructiveness, whereas restless behavior is characterized by constant activity that a patient may be able to briefly inhibit.

Post-TBI agitation restlessness may be caused by psychiatric disease (panic, premorbid personality, agitated depression, anxiety), pain, alcohol/drug withdrawal (licit and illicit), headaches, infection, seizures, postictal state, metabolic (endocrine, hepatic, renal, electrolyte), cardiac/pulmonary problems, or a central nervous system mass lesion. These causes should obviously be assessed and treated appropriately.

Restlessness in TBI patients can often be treated by allowing the patient to "burn off" their excess energy. In a patient who has no motor deficits, allowing them to walk the hallways of a low-stimulation environment Brain Injury unit with a 1:1 companion can result in decrease in their symptoms. Bedside therapies with active and passive range of motion exercises for non-ambulatory patients is also an option.

In agitated patients, it is important to reestablish the sleep/wake cycle. The first step is to provide a low-stimulus environment. The use of trazadone, which is effective for sleep maintenance, is an important treatment option. In the initial treatment phase, short one-to-one treatment sessions should be considered. Initiating therapy too soon may be excitotoxic.

The goal is behavioral control using modalities, a low-stimulation environment, and medications (Table 20.6). The typical and atypical antipsychotics and benzodiazepines are known to interfere with cognitive processing and memory and should be limited in use.

For a patient who is truly agitated, of propranolol, 20 mg bid, should be initiated. The dose may be increased as tolerated, dependent upon heart rate and blood pressure. If behavioral control is not achieved after initiation of the above suggestions, the use of an anticonvulsant/membrane stabilizer such as valproic acid or carbamazepine should be considered. Treatment may begin as outlined in Table 20.6. Valproic acid will usually be very effective in controlling even the most agitated patients once it has been titrated up to an effective dose. Blood levels should be checked to insure that toxic levels are not reached. It is not important to maintain the patient in therapeutic range unless they are also being treated for seizures. To summarize, effective control of agitation can usually be achieved by: 1) creating and maintaining a low-slim environment, 2) ruling out other causes of agitation as listed above, 3) re-establishing sleep-wake cycle, 4) treating with propranolol as tolerated by blood pressure and heart rate, 5) treatment with valproic acid, titrated up to effective levels. There will be occasions when a situation will call for the use of an antipsychotic medication or a benzodiazepine to prevent harm to the patient or staff but these situations can be greatly limited by applying the above algorithm.

Pharmacologic treatments for anxiety are outlined in Table 20.7.

Table 20.6

Medications for Agitation

Drug	Dose	Common side effects	Significant adverse events	Drug–drug interactions	Comments
Propranolol	Starting dose: 20 mg bid Can be increased as tolerated by blood pressure and heart rate	Fatigue, dizziness, bradycardia, hypotension, depression, insomnia, constipation	CHF, severe bradycardia, heart block, Raynaud's	Thioridazine	May reduce agitation significantly with no cognitive side effects
Valproic Acid	Starting dose: 250 mg bid Can be titrated up to 15mg/kg divided tid	Headache, nausea, vomiting, loss of energy and strength, somnolence, thrombocytopenia, and dizziness	Hepatotoxicity	Clonazepam, ginkgo biloba, rifampin	Liver function tests and valproic acid levels should be evaluated weekly
Carbamazepine	Starting dose: 200 mg bid Can be titrated up to 1200 mg/day divided tid	Dizziness, drowsiness, and loss of coordination, nausea, vomiting, and blurry vision	Hypersensitivity reaction, Stevens-Johnson syndrome	All MAOIs, azole, antifungals, nefazodone, protease inhibitors	Liver function tests and carbamazepine levels should be evaluated weekly

Table 20.7

Medications for Anxiety

Drug	Dose	Common side effects	Significant adverse events	Drug–drug interactions	Comments
Escitolopram	10 mg daily for a week, then increase to 20 mg daily	Nausea, delayed ejaculation, insomnia, diarrhea, somnolence, sweating	Suicidality, worsening depression, serotonin syndrome, withdrawal syndrome, hyponatremia, SIADH	All MAOIs, phenothiazines, pimozide	
Propranolol	Beginning dose 20 mg bid	Fatigue, dizziness, constipation, bradycardia, hypotension	Severe bradycardia, CHF, heart block	Thioridazine	Titrate up as tolerated by blood pressure and heart rate
Buspirone	Beginning dose is 7.5 mg bid, may increase to 20–30 mg divided bid or tid to max dose of 60 mg/day	Drowsiness, dizziness, headache, nausea	Serotonin syndrome, akathisia	Nonselective MAOIs	Has very slow onset of action
Mirtazapine	Beginning dose is 15 mg qhs, may increase dose to 30 or 45 mg qhs if starting dose not effective	Dry mouth, somnolence, appetite stimulation, constipation	Neutropenia, agranulocytosis	All MAOIs	Side effect is appetite stimulation —may be valuable in patients who are not eating
Venlafaxin	Starting at 37.5 mg bid increasing to 45 mg daily if necessary	Headaches, somnolence, nausea, dry mouth	Seizures, worsening depression, suicidality	All MAOIs, phenothiazines, cisapride, ranolazine	

Nutritional Supplementation

There is interest in maximizing patients' nutritional intake in order to optimize the body's ability to heal itself after a brain injury. Although research is being done in this field, no specific nutritional protocol has been recommended to accelerate or allow increased levels of recovery. There are data, mainly from animal model studies, that show improved cognitive and motor recovery after treatment with the nutritional supplements listed here. Fortunately, the side effect profile for these supplements is very low except for the precautions mentioned here. These medications can be used together without fear of interaction and with minimal precautions. There are no known interactions with any of the pharmacological treatments reported above, and consequently these supplements may be used with any of the pharmacologic agents listed.

The following doses and scheduling were determined after evaluating a number of studies and may not represent optimal dosing or the effectiveness of the supplements themselves, as this has not yet been established. Although it is generally considered that early initiation of treatment will result in the best outcome, it may be possible that improvements can occur at any time postinjury. These supplements may be initiated in the following order.

CiticolineI (cytidine-5-diphosphate choline) is an essential intermediate in the biosynthetic pathway of structural phospholipids, which are important constituents of all biologic membranes, including neuronal membranes. Research has shown positive results with respect to neurologic recovery after TBI and cerebral vascular accident (CVA). It has also been shown to decrease memory loss in aging. Dosing is generally recommended at 1000 mg bid-tid.

Methylcobalamin is the form of vitamin B_{12} that is active in the brain. It is thought to promote regeneration of nerve tissue and protect against glutamate-induced neurotoxicity. Dosing is generally recommended at 4000 μg daily sublingually as methylcobalamin can be broken down by stomach acids.

Hydergine is an an ergoloid mesylate. It has been used extensively to treat dementia, and, although once thought to improve cognitive function by improving oxygen flow to the brain, it is now believed that it works by affecting synaptic transmission via stimulation of the dopaminergic and serotonergic receptors and blocking α-adrenoreceptors. Usual dose is 2.25–9 mg daily built up gradually. Side effects have been reported to be nausea and headaches, which can be avoided by titrating the dose up slowly.

Branched-chain amino acids (leucine, isoleucine, and valine) were found to positively affect cognitive recovery in severe TBI cases. It can be taken in dosages of 5–20 g per day as tolerated. Care should be taken in administering any amino acids to patients with liver or kidney disease.

Antioxidants are being investigated for their ability to control the cascade of molecular events in secondary injury that are triggered by the production of reactive oxygen species and free radicals. Typical antioxidants used may include vitamin C dosed at 1000 mg bid-tid, vitamin E (α-tocopherol) 400 units daily, and CoQ-10 80–120 mg daily.

Acetyl-L-carnitine is reported to increase the density of neurotransmitter receptors and the levels of acetylcholine and dopamine, both of which are linked to recall and memory retention. Typical daily dose is 100–400 mg once a day in the morning. Overstimulation and nausea may occur as side effects at dosages greater than 500 mg.

Ginkgo biloba has been used for thousands of year in traditional Chinese medicine as a neurocognitive enhancer and is generally well tolerated. However, there have been multiple case reports recently of bleeding, and current recommendation is to not use this herb in patients with history of a brain bleed. Dosing is 40–60 mg early morning and lunchtime. Additional side effects may include stomach or intestinal problems, headache, and allergic skin reactions. A rare but significant side effect is seizures, particularly in very old patients taking ginkgo biloba extract. Also, high doses of ginkgo biloba extract may aggravate seizures in patients with a previous history of seizures (9).

Vinpocetine has been found to inhibit the cascade of molecular events caused by the rise of intracellular calcium, dilate blood vessels, and enhance blood flow in the brain. It also has antioxidant properties and functions as platelet inhibitor. Dosing is 5 mg daily.

Piracetam is considered a cognitive enhancer, also known as a nootropic. It has been reported to improve memory, attention, and intelligence. It reportedly improves the function of the brain's corpus callosum, allowing greater brain potential. A common dosing is three 800 mg tablets bid to start, decreasing to one or two tablets twice a day after a month. Common side effects include nausea and headaches (9).

Centrophenoxine is thought to improve general brain function by reducing lipofuscin levels. Studies in both humans and animals have shown that high lipofuscin levels predict poor cellular health and low lipofuscin levels correlate

Patient Safety

- If evidence of hydrocephalus, gait disturbance, incontinence, or change in mental status occurs, an immediate MRI and referral to neurosurgery should be made.
- As previously stated, it is imperative to remember that an injured brain can be more sensitive to medications and their side effects. The effects of medications are often difficult to predict in the brain injury population. However, secondary drug effects can sometimes be used advantageously.
- It is important to remember that responses to any given medication are often unpredictable. The same drug given at different stages of recovery will likely have different activity—it is important to remember that brain injury is a moving target! Medications that may have been helpful when initiated can lose their effectiveness and become more significant for their side effects rather than the desired outcome.
- Avoid medications that can interfere with neurologic recovery.

Patient Education

- Patients and their families should be made aware of the course of recovery following brain injury and stroke.
- It is very important for the patient and his or her family to realize that recovery does not take place in a linear fashion. Brain injury recovery is better described as consisting of stages of advancements, stagnancy, and setbacks of variable duration.
- Emergence of new symptoms is common even months or years postinjury. These may include seizures, mood issues, memory, behavioral problems, and more.
- It is important to keep in mind that a TBI may magnify the premorbid personality.

with healthy cellular function. Centrophenoxine has been reported to improve glucose and oxygen uptake as well as increasing levels of neuronal RNA, allowing the synthesis of proteins that assist in encoding memory as well as repairing cell damage. Dosing in patients with significant injury would start at 750–1250 mg per day with breakfast and lunch to avoid insomnia. Side effects include insomnia, hyperexcitability, irritability, agitation, and restlessness. Shoulder muscle tension and headaches along with neck and jaw pain have been reported. Acetylcholine excess can be avoided by taking occasional breaks from the regular dose, usually recommended once per week.

REFERENCES

1. Centers for Disease Control and Prevention (CDC), National Center for Injury Prevention and Control. Annual Data Submission Standards: Guidelines for Surveillance of Central Nervous System Injury. Atlanta (GA): CDC, 1995. Revised 2000.
2. American Heart Association. 1999 Heart and Stroke Statistical Update. Dallas, Texas: American Heart Association. 1998.
3. Thurman D. The Epidemiology and Economics of Head Trauma. In: Miller L, Hayes R, editors. Head Trauma: Basic, Preclinical, and Clinical Directions. New York (NY): Wiley and Sons, 2001.
4. Halliday AL. Pathophysiology. In: Marion DW, ed. Traumatic Brain Injury. NY: Thieme Medical Publishers, 1999:29–38.
5. Williams GH, Brauwald E. In: Braunwald E, et al. Harrison's Principles of Internal Medicine. New York: McGraw-Hill, 1987:1024.
6. Woo BH, Nesathurai S. Overview. The Rehabilitation of People with Traumatic Brain Injury, Vol 1. Blackwell Science, Malden, MA, 2000:5–12.
7. Trimble MH, Psychopathology of Frontal Lobe Syndromes Seminars in Neurology, Volume 10, No. 3, September 1990:287–295.
8. Silver JM, McAllister TW, Yudofsky SC. Textbook of Traumatic Brain Injury. Arlington, VA: American Psychiatric Publishing Inc, 2005.
9. Zasler ND, Katz DI, Zafonte RD. Brain Injury Medicine, Principles and Practice. New York: Demos Medical Publishing, 2007.

21 | Pneumonia and Urinary Tract Infections

Michelle Stern
Alan Anschel
Kevin Sperber

Infectious diseases can be a significant cause of morbidity and mortality in patients with neurologic dysfunction. This chapter will focus on pneumonia and urinary tract infection (UTI) since these infections are very commonly seen in patients with spinal cord injury (SCI), cerebral vascular accident (CVA), multiple sclerosis (MS), and traumatic brain injury (TBI). These infections will be discussed in the context of each of these neurologic diagnoses since there are both similarities and differences in their presentations. Whereas all attempts were made to minimize overlap, the reader is also referred to the respiratory and genitourinary chapters in this book for additional discussion on the manifestation and treatment of conditions affecting these systems.

The antibiotic treatments for pneumonia and UTI are the same for all neurologic diagnoses, unless otherwise specified in the text. Consultation with an infectious disease specialist is recommended for complicated patients.

CEREBRAL VASCULAR ACCIDENT

Urinary Tract Infection

Epidemiology
The frequency of UTI has been reported as 11–24% in the postacute phase and 22–23% during a 6- to 30-month follow-up. It is only a serious complication in 1% of patients. Although UTIs are common in this patient population, literature on the subject is scant.

Risk factors for a UTI poststroke include older age, female, indwelling catheter, neurogenic bladder, immobility, and diabetes. Most of the urologic symptoms can be expected to resolve, except for those with severe neurologic deficits (1).

Pathophysiology
Under normal conditions the urinary tract is sterile. An uncomplicated UTI involves the bladder only and is termed cystitis. Involvement of the upper

tract of the kidney is termed pyelonephritis. Sterile conditions are maintained by urine acidity, emptying of the bladder at micturition, ureterovesical and urethral sphincters, and various immunologic and mucosal barriers. During the acute phase of stroke, incontinence is often present due to uninhibited bladder contractions secondary to depressed sacral reflexes. Urinary retention may also develop due to immobility.

A neurogenic bladder with incomplete bladder emptying can lead to an increase frequency of UTIs. A UTI is also more common in females due to short urethra and higher frequency of incontinence that makes entrance of uropathogens to the urinary system easier. Males can develop urinary retention due to the effects of an enlarged prostate combined with immobility and anticholinergic medication. Older patients are also at increased risk due to decreased immune function, decreased bladder capacity and compliance, and age-related decrease in kidney function. The lack of estrogen in older females also puts them at risk for UTI.

The most common causative organism for a UTI in patients with a stroke is *Escherichia coli.*

Patient Assessment

Cystitis in this population can present with urinary retention, urinary incontinence, frequency, burning, straining, hematuria, urgency, foul-smelling urine, suprapubic tenderness, and pain with voiding. Pyelonephritis would also include flank pain, chills, and fever. Patients with altered cognitive function or aphasia after a stroke may not be able to accurately report symptoms. A UTI can also lead to confusion as well as increased neurologic symptoms, especially in those patients who develop urosepsis.

Diagnostic testing that is suggestive of a urinary tract infection includes dipstick test positive for leukocyte esterase and/or nitrate, pyuria (either ≥10 white blood cells [WBC] per milliliter or ≥3 WBC per high-powered field of unspun urine), and organisms seen on Gram stain of unspun urine. Urine cultures positive for UTI have ≥100,000 colonies per milliliter, with no more than two species of organisms.

The presence of casts on a urinalysis should increase the suspicion of upper tract infection. A mid-catch urine culture is preferred for those patients who are able to void. A mid-catch specimen may be difficult to obtain in patients with a dense hemiplegia, visual-spatial difficulties, memory deficits, and incontinence; therefore, a catherized specimen may be most appropriate. In a patient with an indwelling catheter, it is suggested to change the catheter before obtaining the urine culture to obtain a more sensitive sample for the offending organism.

Baseline lab values such as complete blood count (CBC), hepatic profile, and basic metabolic panel should be ordered as antibiotic dosing may be affected by these values. Because patients with strokes commonly have hypertension and diabetes, these factors may also cause renal insufficiency, which will need adjustment of antibiotic dosing. Fever over 101°F or significant elevation of WBC count should prompt for blood cultures to rule out urosepsis.

Supportive measures include hydration, analgesia with phenzaopyridine (pyridium), and ensuring adequate emptying of the bladder with postvoid residuals (PVR) less than 50–100 cc after voiding. This can be difficult to measure in an incontinent patient. The use of a bladder scan in an inpatient setting can give the results of postvoid residual noninvasively. If a patient is retaining urine (>400 cc in bladder) or has a high postvoid residual, catheterization every 4–6 hours should be started or, if deemed necessary, the use of an indwelling catheter. Males may benefit from the addition of α-adrenergic blocking agents to help against urinary retention, but these can cause orthostatic hypotension and are best given before bedtime.

Pneumonia

Epidemiology

Pneumonia is the most common cause of fever within the first 48 hours after an acute stroke, and it is the most common medical complication 2–4 weeks following onset. It is also a leading cause of nonvascular death after stroke in both the acute and chronic care settings. Fourteen percent of patients develop pneumonia during the first 3 months. It occurs in 6.7–22% of hospitalized patients with stroke and confers a threefold increased risk of mortality. Pneumonia is also associated with a greater likelihood of discharge to a nursing home and increased length of hospital stay. Many cases of pneumonia occurring after stroke are preventable by appropriate evaluation of swallowing function and modification of oral intake (2,3).

Pathophysiology

Aspiration is the cause of about two thirds of poststroke pneumonias and is usually due to stroke-related dysphagia or to decreased level of consciousness. Stroke can also alter normal gastrointestinal function, which puts patients at risk for the development of aspiration pneumonia. Increased upper esophageal sphincter tone, decreased lower esophageal sphincter tone, delayed gastric emptying, intestinal tract distention, and impaired peristalsis have been shown to occur with stroke. Types of stroke most likely to have dysphagia include main stem middle cerebral artery (MCA), upper division MCA, and lateral medullary stroke (4).

Risk Factors

Risk factors for dysphagia are covered in greater detail in the dysphagia chapter in this book, but some risk factors include male gender, age greater than 70, disabling stroke, cognitive impairment, impaired pharyngeal response, incomplete oral clearance, and palatal weakness or asymmetry. A history of chronic obstructive pulmonary disease and smoking can also predispose to developing pneumonia. Dysphagia improves in most patients with unilateral stroke within 1 month. Patients with brain stem or bilateral hemisphere lesions require more time and may require a gastrostomy. Neglect can also lead to the development of aspiration pneumonia due to spillage of food contents from the oral cavity that the patient is unaware of (5).

Patient Assessment

In patients with pneumonia, the following physical findings may be present: 1) fever, 2) tachypnea, 3) tachycardia, 4) decreased breath sounds, 5) hypoxemia, 6) hypotension, 7) decreased oxygen saturation, 8) sputum production, 9) dullness to percussion over areas of consolidation cough, 10) rhonchi, and 11) increased confusion and change in mental status. In aspiration pneumonia, the right middle lobe is more likely to be affected.

Diagnostic tests include CBC, basic metabolic panel, sputum cultures, chest radiograph, and arterial blood gas. In unclear cases, high-resolution computed tomography (CT) scanning of the lungs may aid in the diagnosis. An increase in WBC count can be seen with pneumonia. Electrolytes are important to determine the fluid status of the patient as well as to determine if adjustment is needed in antibiotic dosing. Sputum culture should have fewer than 10 oral squamous epithelial cells per low-power field, and WBC count should be more than 25 per low-power field. A patient with a stroke may not be able to give an adequate specimen. Respiratory infections can also be caused by the influenza and parainfluenza virus and should be tested for, especially in those patients who are in the chronic stages of the disease. Blood cultures have poor sensitivity in pneumonia. Patients with a stroke may also be at risk for a pulmonary embolus, which can also produce fevers and low oxygen saturation. In these cases a ventilation-perfusion scan or spiral CT scan may be required to differentiate.

Treatment

Adequate hydration, oxygen, antibiotics, chest physical therapy, and the use of nebulizer treatment are all beneficial, as is early mobilization. For aspiration pneumonia, a swallowing evaluation is also warranted to help answer whether the patient can tolerate oral feedings and to determine an appropriate diet. In high-risk patients, aspiration precautions should be observed. These include: 1) head maneuvers for the patient to perform while eating (see Chapter 7), 2) having the patient upright at a 90-degree angle while eating and for at least an hour after eating, and 3) ensuring that patient is alert while eating. Patients with neglect may also need to have the oral cavity examined to ensure pocketing of the food is not occurring.

Interventions are available to prevent pneumonia among older patients, including influenza vaccination, pneumovax, and improved oral hygiene. Emphasizing the prevention of respiratory illness may substantially improve the long-term outcomes of patients with stroke. Vaccinations with influenza and pneumococcal vaccines are encouraged in this population (6).

Complications of pneumonia include effusion, empyema, abscess formation, and adult respiratory distress syndrome. Significant pleural effusions might require a thoracentesis to exclude an empyema. Patients with a prolonged hospital course or multiple medical comorbidities, critically ill patients, or residents of a long-term care facility may be more prone to developing pneumonia with a resistant organism. For critically ill patients or those at risk for resistant organisms, consultation with an infectious disease specialist for appropriate antibiotic coverage is recommended. A consultation with a pulmonologist may also be required for bronchoscopy or thoracentesis, especially in patients with severe respiratory distress.

SPINAL CORD INJURY

Urinary Tract Infection

After a complete spinal cord injury, the cerebral micturition centers are neurologically disconnected from the bladder. This disconnection radically impairs the genitourinary (GU) system, leading to devastating reproductive and urine-voiding impairments. As a result, UTIs are a common lifelong problem with significant morbidity in the SCI population. UTIs were once a major cause of mortality in the SCI, but with improved screening and treatment protocols, the associated mortality rate has been reduced significantly.

Pathophysiology

A UTI is defined as bacteriuria with tissue invasion and resultant tissue response with signs and/or symptoms. Typically the urinary tract becomes colonized by an ascending infection that travels from the distal urethra, often during sexual intercourse or catheterization. The high incidence of urinary tract infection after a spinal cord injury is due to abnormal emptying of the bladder. A complete spinal cord injury isolates the urinary apparatus from voluntary control and from the brain centers that coordinate contraction of the bladder with relaxation of the sphincter. Patients with upper-motor-neuron lesions may have a local reflex of bladder contraction (reflex voiding), but it often occurs against high sphincter pressure (bladder-sphincter dyssynergia), which in turn results in high intravesical pressure, thus contributing to the risk of infection and deterioration of the upper urinary tract. In patients with a flaccid bladder—for example, those with an injury of the conus medullaris—voiding can occur by overflow, with a large volume of residual urine and a high risk of infection. If the patient is voiding, postvoid residuals should be checked and ideally be less than 250 cc to confirm adequate emptying.

Patient Assessment

The classic triad of dysuria, urgency, and frequency can not be relied upon in the SCI patient. One should look for fever/chills or increasing fatigue. A patient might also note increasing urinary incontinence, cloudy and foul-smelling urine, an increase in spasticity, or autonomic dysreflexia.

Catheterization is an important risk factor in the SCI population. Indwelling catheterization (including suprapubic) and urinary diversion are the drainage methods most likely to lead to persistent bacteriuria. The risk of infection can be reduced through intermittent catheterization, particularly self-catheterization. In self-catheterization, one should note that clean technique (catheters can be reused if cleansed by soaking in an antiseptic solution or boiling water) is much cheaper than sterile technique and does not pose a greater risk of infection if reusable catheters are cleaned properly. More severely disabled people who require catheterization by others are at greater risk for UTIs. Surgical options include urinary diversion to increase bladder capacity and sacral anterior root stimulation (10).

Diagnostic Workup

Both a urine analysis (U/A) and urine culture must be sent if a UTI is suspected. Pyuria warrants treatment. The meaning of pyuria is unclear, as is the number of WBC that indicates pyuria. In our practice, more than 10 WBC per high-power field (either a clean catch or intermittent catherization specimen) constitutes pyuria. In patients with indwelling catheters, it is important to remove the current catheter and place a new one prior to collecting a urine sample when UTI is suspected (Table 21.1).

When the urine culture results come back, it is important to consider the etiology of the infection: reinfection, relapse, antibiotic resistance, or a new infection with a different organism. Antibiotic resistance is more likely when the infection involves the upper urinary tract and in complicated UTIs (e.g., neurogenic bladders, prostatitis, benign prostatic hypertrophy, nephrolithiasis, and polycystic kidney disease). This consideration will help direct antibiotic therapy toward the organisms most likely responsible for the infection.

In patients who appear acutely ill, further blood work is warranted: CBC, basic metabolic panel (BMP), and blood cultures. These labs will help determine the presence of leukocytosis or frank sepsis, as well as the level of current renal function (11).

In UTI, the goal of treatment is to avoid bacteremia, septic shock, and pyelonephritis—not to sterilize the urine. SCI patients frequently have asymptomatic bacteruria (especially if they have an indwelling catheter or suprapubic tube), which should not be treated in the absence of other findings. Multiple studies

Table 21. 1

Quantitative Urine Culture Criteria for Diagnosis of Bacteriuria	
Specimen type	cfu/ml
Catheter specimens from individuals on intermittent catheterization	$\geq 10^2$
Clean-void specimens from catheter-free males using condom collection devices	$\geq 10^4$
Specimens from indwelling catheters	Any detectable concentration

have revealed that there is no benefit in the routine use of antibiotic prophylaxis. Repeated antibiotic therapy increases the risk of selecting multiresistant bacteria without reducing either the incidence or the severity of symptomatic UTIs.

Pneumonia

Epidemiology

Respiratory diseases—particularly pneumonia—are the leading cause of death in the first year post-SCI. Of patients with complete tetraplegia, 21.6% develop atelectasis or pneumonia while receiving inpatient rehabilitation after acute care. Respiratory complications are the leading cause of readmission during the first 6 years postinjury. The age and affected neurologic level at the time of injury predict pneumonia related mortality, which is 37 times more likely in SCI patients than in the general population. The risk of death in a high-level motor-complete tetraplegic patient is even higher: 150 times greater than the risk of death in a neurologically intact individual due to respiratory complications (7).

Pathophysiology

Patients frequently develop respiratory disease secondary to difficulty clearing pulmonary secretions. Patients with a cervical or high thoracic SCI often have impaired innervation of the diaphragm, intercostal muscles, and abdominal muscles. Impaired innervation in turn leads to weak inspiratory and expiratory muscle function, impaired cough, and difficulty clearing pulmonary secretions.

In complete SCI, atelectasis and pneumonia are most likely to develop during the first 3 weeks after injury. The majority of pneumonias that develop soon after injury are left-sided due to difficulty with clearing secretions from the more acute takeoff angle of the left main stem bronchus. Bronchial mucus hypersecretion can also occur in some acute cervical level SCI.

Patient Assessment

Diagnosing pneumonia in SCI patients can be difficult. Symptoms and signs can range from nonspecific (malaise, fatigue) to specific, as noted above for CVA-related pneumonia. Additional findings of respiratory impairments are also discussed in Chapter 26.

Since fever is often the presenting complaint and the source of infection is often unclear, a fever workup is usually warranted. These workups should include a CBC with a differential, BMP, two peripheral blood cultures drawn from two different sites, urine analysis (UA), and urine culture. Chest imaging should also be obtained, and clinicians should have a low threshold for ordering a CT scan of the chest. Obtaining standard posterior-anterior and lateral x-ray views in a high paraplegic or tetraplegic patient is impractical and inadequate secondary to their compromised ability to take full inspirations.

Since patients may deteriorate rapidly, attempts to establish a bacteriologic diagnosis with sputum Gram stain, culture, and/or invasive sampling techniques such as bronchoscopy are generally warranted. Patients with tracheostomies will frequently have bacterial colonization, which can decrease the utility of sputum cultures.

Treatment

To date there have been no large-scale studies assessing trends in antimicrobial use in acute respiratory infections in SCI patients. It should be noted that the risk of developing multidrug-resistant bacteria can be high in those hospitalized for a prolonged period of time.

Clinicians should strongly consider inpatient management if the diagnosis is unclear; patients managed as outpatients require close follow-up. In SCI patients, pneumonia may present suddenly and rapidly progress to respiratory failure. Antibiotic treatment guidelines for pneumonia are comparable to those offered to nonneurologically impaired patients (Table 21.2).

Clearance of secretions is very important and can be assisted in a variety of ways. In patients with cervical or thoracic SCI, chest physical therapy (PT) is of the utmost importance. Chest PT includes encouragement of deep breathing through incentive spirometry, frequent changes of position, postural drainage of secretions, nasotracheal suctioning, and manually assisted coughing using forceful upper abdominal thrusts in a posterior and cephalad direction. β-Agonist bronchodilator therapy is also thought to enhance mucociliary clearance, but no studies have demonstrated this hypothesis. Insufflation-exsufflation devices may improve the clearance of secretions for those patients with a poor cough, but intermittent positive pressure breathing does not appear to be beneficial.

Acute respiratory decompensation requires intubation and positive pressure ventilation. Intubated SCI patients should be oriented with the head upright at a 45° angle in order to diminish the risk of aspiration of gastric contents. Patients who require chronic ventilation have a decreased survival rate because they have less residual respiratory muscle strength and are also exposed to the complications of chronic positive pressure ventilation, such as ventilator-associated pneumonia.

Prevention

It is highly recommended that SCI patients (especially for injuries that are T8 or higher) be given the flu vaccine annually and the pneumococcal pneumonia vaccine as early as possible when medically stable from their injury. The pneumococcal vaccine should be repeated every 10 years. It should be noted that prophylaxis in SCI has not been studied (8).

MULTIPLE SCLEROSIS

There is strong and consistent evidence that any infection, even a simple cold, can be associated with an increased risk of a MS exacerbation. Therefore, a

Table 21.2

Respiratory Tract Empiric Antibiotic Therapy Guidelines

Common infections	Definitions and common organisms	Primary recommended antibiotic therapy		Alternate antibiotic therapy
Bronchitis	S. pneumoniae, H. influenzae, M. catarrhalis, M. pneumoniae, C. pneumoniae		Azithromycin PO/IV or doxycycline PO/IV	
Community-acquired pneumonia	S. pneumoniae, H. influenzae, M. pneumoniae, M. catarrhalis, Legionella Suspected organisms altered by comorbidities (e.g., aspiration, alcoholism, structural lung disease, postviral)	Non-ICU	Ceftriaxone IV[a] + Azithromycin PO/IV OR If suspect aspiration: Ampicillin/sulbactam IV OR Piperacillin/tazobactam IV[a,b] ± Azithromycin PO/IV	If PCN-allergic: Levofloxacin IV (add Clindamycin IV if suspect aspiration)[a]
		ICU	Ceftriaxone IV[a] + Azithromycin IV OR If suspect aspiration: Piperacillin/tazobactam IV[a] ± Azithromycin IV	If PCN-allergic: Levofloxacin IV (add Clindamycin IV if suspect aspiration)[a]
Hospital-acquired ventilator-associated pneumonia	Presence of pneumonia defined by a new or progressive infiltrate plus at least two of the following three clinical features: • fever greater than 38°C • leukocytosis or leukopenia • purulent secretions Common organisms: P. aeruginosa, S. aureus, aerobic gram-negative rods Hospitalized and/or ventilated patients often colonized. Organisms isolated from respiratory cultures should only be treated if accompanied by the clinical signs/symptoms of pneumonia.	Non-ICU	Piperacillin/tazobactam IV ± Tobramycin IV	Levofloxacin IV + Tobramycin IV
		ICU	Piperacillin/tazobactam IV + Tobramycin IV ± Vancomycin IV	Levofloxacin IV + Tobramycin IV ± Vancomycin IV

[a] Consider the addition of vancomycin IV in patients with severe necrotizing and/or cavitating pneumonia (concern for community-acquired MRSA).

[b] If frequent contact with healthcare system or chronic care facility, the use of piperacillin/tazobactam over ampicillin/sulbactam may be warranted.

presenting symptom of an infection in this population may be a worsening of neurologic symptoms. Patients with MS may also be at risk for serious infections due to the side effects of the medications used in its treatment. Patients can present with change in neurologic function, fever, increased weakness, and unstable vital signs. Steroids may increase the risk for serious infection, and interferons can cause leukopenia. Natalizumab has been associated with serious infections and was investigated due to the association with progressive multifocal leukoencephalopathy, but was rereleased for treatment in 2006. The use of immunosuppressant agents such as mitoxantrone, cyclophosphamide, azathioprine, and methotrexate can also increase the risk of infection in the MS population. It is important to note the cognitive status of the MS patient as this can impair the ability to give a proper history and description of symptoms.

Urinary Tract Infection

Urinary tract dysfunction affects up to 90% of the MS population, and urinary tract infections are encountered in up to 74% of the tested population. A urinary tract infection also commonly precedes relapse and, when recurrent, is associated with neurologic progression.

Pathophysiology

Please refer to previous sections on stroke and SCI as the cause in MS is similar and depends on where the lesions are located. Since the MS patient could have lesions in either the brain or spinal cord, their voiding pattern is best evaluated by an urodynamic study (UDS). Patients with MS may demonstrate dyssynergia of the detrusor and the sphincter that can lead to upper tract damage.

Patient Assessment

Findings can include: 1) a change in neurologic status, 2) fever, 3) a change in voiding pattern, and 4) increased confusion. The bladder program for the patient should also be noted (intermittent catheterization, spontaneous voiding, and indwelling catheter placement). It is also important to note if the patient is in the relapsing remitting phase or progressive stage of the disease. In patients performing an intermittent catheterization program, the clinician should evaluate change in cognitive status or hand function that might interfere with the ability to perform the procedure cleanly.

Diagnostic Testing

The white blood cell count might be elevated in a UTI; however, a confounding factor might be the concurrent use of steroids to treat the MS exacerbation, which can also be associated with an increase in the white blood cell count. It should also be noted that the medications used to treat MS can also cause a leukopenia, so an increase in white cell count may not be seen.

Imaging studies
MS patients should undergo urologic evaluation with urodynamic studies and renal ultrasound (13).

Treatment

See Table 21.3 for antibiotic therapy guidelines. If a patient develops two urinary tract infections in less than a year and is voiding using a clean catch technique, consideration should be given to changing to a sterile catheter kit as this has been shown to reduce urinary tract infections.

Supportive measures for minimizing fever is important as heat can worsen the symptoms of MS. Consultation with an infectious disease specialist might be needed in the patient with frequent UTIs with resistant organisms, signs of serious infection with unstable vital signs, on immunosuppressant regimen or placement in a long-term care facility (which can lead to colonization with resistant organisms).

Pneumonia

Epidemiology
Swallowing disorders can occur in 3–20% of patients with MS, and this can potentially lead to aspiration pneumonia. Lesions in the brain can also affect cognition as well as oral-pharyngeal musculature. MS lesions in the spinal cord may lead to abdominal/respiratory muscle weakness with an impaired cough.

Pulmonary symptoms can be minimized with vaccines, but the use of immunizations in MS is a topic that requires further investigation. There is a possibility that patients with MS could be at an increased risk of exacerbation after immunization. Vaccination should be delayed during clinically significant relapses until patients have stabilized or have begun to improve from the relapse, typically 4–6 weeks after the start of the relapse. There is, however, no evidence regarding this practice. Influenza vaccine is currently recommended for yearly injections for every individual aged 50 or older. Current evidence has demonstrated that the influenza vaccine is safe and is not associated with a significantly increased risk of MS exacerbation. The use of the influenza vaccine in patients under 50 with MS is still under debate. The pneumococcal vaccine should be considered for patients with compromised pulmonary function (wheelchair-dependent or bed-bound) (12).

Immunosupressed patients warrant an infectious disease consult for appropriate antibiotic coverage. A neurology consult may also be needed to discuss changes in medication to treat MS.

TRAUMATIC BRAIN INJURY

In the acute phase after a moderate to severe TBI, patients are more vulnerable to infection due to a decreased immune response. The most common causes

Table 21.3

Genitourinary Empiric Antibiotic Therapy Guidelines

Common infections	Definitions and common organisms	Primary recommended antibiotic therapy	Alternate antibiotic therapy
UTI, uncomplicated	Uncomplicated UTI[a,b]: infection in a structurally and neurologically normal urinary tract (significant bacteriuria with pyuria or symptomatic) Most common organism: *E. coli*	Cephalexin PO	If PCN-allergic: TMP/SMX PO OR Levofloxacin PO
UTI, complicated, pyelonephritis	Complicated UTI[a]: infection in a urinary tract with abnormalities (e.g., UTI in men, pregnant women) Pyelonephritis: clinical syndrome characterized by flank pain or tenderness, or both, and fever, often associated with dysuria, urgency, and frequency (upper tract infection) Common organisms: Enterobacteriaceae (usually *E. coli*), enterococci	Ampicillin IV[b] + Gentamicin IV	If PCN-allergic: Levofloxacin IV + Gentamicin IV
UTI, catheter-associated	Catheter-associated UTI[a,c]: Significant bacteriuria with pyuria or symptoms Common organisms: *E. coli, K. pneumoniae, P. aeruginosa, Proteus mirabilis,* enterococci	Piperacillin/tazobactam IV ± Gentamicin IV[d]	If PCN-allergic: TMP/SMX IV/PO +Gentamicin IV[d]

[a] Diagnostic criteria for UTI: pyuria (>10 WBC/mm^3 of urine), significant bacteriuria: ≥10^5 bacteria/ml urine (≥10^4 for suspected pyelonephritis), symptoms of frequency, urgency, or dysuria. In certain settings, a CFU count < 10^5 may be indicative of a true infection.
Treatment of asymptomatic bacteriuria (defined as ≥10^5 bacteria found in two consecutive voided urine specimens in women or a single clean-catch specimen in men and ≥10^2 bacteria found in a single catheterized urine specimen in both men and women) is not recommended, EXCEPT in either pregnant women, or urinary tract structural abnormalities, or on immunosuppressive therapy, or about to undergo urinary tract instrumentation or manipulation.

[b] For urosepsis in patients with frequent healthcare system contact, who resides in a chronic care facility, or who are immunocompromised, the use of piperacillin/tazobactam over ampicillin may be warranted.

[c] Removal or changing of the urinary catheter is recommended. Treatment of asymptomatic bacteriuria without pyuria does not appear to be useful in decreasing complications and is not recommended (possible exceptions: neutropenic patients, solid organ transplant patients, pregnant women, and patients undergoing urologic surgery).

[d] History of significant antibiotic exposure or more systemic symptoms may warrant the use of tobramycin rather than gentamicin.

of infections in this population are pneumonia and urinary tract infections, whose diagnosis and management have been described earlier in the chapter. Pneumonia has been associated with increased mortality in both the acute phase and long term. Common causes of pneumonia include: 1) inability to manage secretions secondary to impaired cognition, 2) swallowing difficulties, and 3) the use of a ventilator or tracheostomy.

Aspiration of gastric contents is common in TBI. The risk of aspiration pneumonia can be minimized by: 1) keeping the bed upright while eating and for an hour afterwards, 2) ensuring the patient is alert while eating, and 3) regular chest physiotherapy in TBI patients with impaired cough. While reflux can contribute to aspiration, the use of metoclopramide should be avoided in this patient population as it may impair cognitive recovery.

Other common intracranial complications following an acute head injury include meningitis, which is usually associated with a basilar skull fracture or open-depressed skull fracture. Sinusitis is common in patients with nasotracheal or nasogastric tubes in place for several days and often subsides spontaneously with removal of the tubes.

Fever in patients with traumatic brain injury can result in increased length of stays and mortality rates and decreased functional outcomes. Interestingly, in up to 37% of patients, a cause for fever cannot be found and may relate to the degree of brain injury. Central fever can occur in patients with TBI, especially with lesions of the anterior hypothalamus. However, before a diagnosis of central fever can be given, a thorough fever workup should be performed to evaluate for a possible infection.

Heterotopic ossification is another source of fever in severely impaired TBI patients. Heterotopic ossification may occur around joints of the upper and/or lower extremities and should be differentiated from deep vein thrombosis (DVT) or cellulitis. This can be done by checking alkaline phosphatase levels and performing a triple-phase bone scan (14,15).

Patient Safety

1. Cognitive and communication impairments in adults with neurologic disabilities can often make it challenging to diagnose an underlying infection. Nevertheless, clinicians should have a high index of suspicion for pneumonia and UTI in this population and institute treatment early in the course of the infection.
2. Since aspiration is a common cause of pneumonia, clinicians should identify early high-risk patients for aspiration pneumonia and institute appropriate interventions to minimize the risk.
3. In dosing of antibiotics, clinicians should use renal and geriatric dosing whenever indicated.

Patient Education

1. Patients and their caregivers should be educated about the symptoms, signs, diagnostic tests, and treatment of pneumonia and UTI.
2. Patients and their caregivers should be educated on strategies to minimize the occurrence of pneumonia (e.g., aspiration precautions) and UTI (e.g., intermittent catherization).

REFERENCES

1. Ersoz M, Ulusoy H, Oktar MA, Akyuz M. Urinary tract infection and bacteriuria in stroke patients: frequencies, pathogen microorganisms, and risk factors. Am J Phys Med Rehabil 2007; 86(9):734–741.
2. Katzan IL, Dawson NV, Thomas CL, Votruba ME, Cebul RD. The cost of pneumonia after acute stroke. Neurology 2007; 68(22):1938–1943.
3. Sellars C, Bowie L, Bagg J, et al. Risk factors for chest infection in acute stroke: a prospective cohort study. Stroke 2007; 38(8):2284–2291.
4. Shigemitsu H, Afshar K. Aspiration pneumonias: under-diagnosed and under-treated. Curr Opin Pulm Med 2007; 13(3):192–198.
5. Singh S, Hamdy S. Dysphagia in stroke patients. Postgrad Med J 2006; 82(968):383–391.
6. Bravata DM, Ho SY, Meehan TP, Brass LM, Concato J. Readmission and death after hospitalization for acute ischemic stroke: 5-year follow-up in the Medicare population. Stroke 2007; 38(6):1899–1904.
7. Burns SP. Acute respiratory infections in persons with spinal cord injury. Phys Med Rehabil Clin N Am 2007; 18(2):203–16, v–vi.
8. Lammertse D. Maintaining Health Long-Term with Spinal Cord Injury. Topics in Spinal Cord Injury Rehabilitation: Aging with Spinal Cord Injury. Kemp B., Iss. Ed., David Apple, Ed., 2001; 6(5):15–17.
9. Salomon J, Gory A, Bernard L, Ruffion A, Denys P, Chartier-Kastler E. Urinary tract infection and neurogenic bladder. Progres Urol 2007; 17(3):448–453.
10. The prevention and management of urinary tract infections among people with spinal cord injuries. National Institute on Disability and Rehabilitation Research Consensus Statement, January 27–29, 1992. J Am Paraplegia Soc 1992; 15(3):194–204.
11. Haisma JAW, Stam LH, Bergen HJ, et al. Complications following spinal cord injury: occurrence and risk factors in a longitudinal study during and after inpatient rehabilitation. J Rehabil Med 2007; 39(5):393–398.
12. Rutschmann OT, McCrory DC, Matchar DB; Immunization Panel of the Multiple Sclerosis Council for Clinical Practice Guidelines. Immunization and MS: a summary of published evidence and recommendations. Neurology 2002; 59(12):1837–1843.
13. Stern M. Aging with multiple sclerosis. Phys Med Rehabil Clin N Am 2005; 16(1):219–234.
14. Hibbard MR, Uysal S, Sliwinski M, Gordon WA. Undiagnosed health issues in individuals with traumatic brain injury living in the community. J Head Trauma Rehabil 1998; 13(4):47–57.
15. Marion DW. Complications of head injury and their therapy. Neurosurg Clin N Am 1991; 2(2):411–424.

22 | Pressure Ulcers

Adrian Cristian
George A. Deitrick

The National Pressure Ulcer Advisory Panel (NPUAP) has defined a pressure ulcer (PU) as a localized injury to the skin and or underlying tissue usually over a bony prominence as a result of pressure or pressure in combination with shear and/or friction" (1). Pressure ulcers can have a profound impact on those who have them. They can cause pain or infections, prolong hospitalizations, limit mobility, restrict ability to perform activities of daily living, and have a negative impact on quality of life (2).

Pressure ulcers are very common in both acute and nursing home settings. The incidence and prevalence of pressure ulcers in both settings ranges from 2.7 to 29.5% (3). High-risk groups have a higher incidence of pressure ulcers. For example, elderly adults with femoral fractures have an incidence rate of 66%, whereas patients in critical care settings have a 33% incidence rate (3).

Among individuals living with a spinal cord injury (SCI), 30–40% develop pressure ulcers during their acute hospitalization and rehabilitation. Risk factors for pressure ulcers in this population include complete injuries, limited functional mobility, and longstanding injury. It has been reported that 29% of adults with SCI have a pressure ulcer even 20 years after their original injury (2). There is also a 35% recurrence rate of pressure ulcers—especially in smokers, diabetics, and those with cardiovascular disease.

It has also been reported that 1.3–3 million Americans have pressure ulcers (4) at a total cost of $1.335 billion per year (2,3). The goal of this chapter is to provide an overview of the assessment, prevention, and treatment of pressure ulcers in adults with neurologic disabilities such as SCI, traumatic brain injury (TBI), multiple sclerosis (MS), and cerebrovascular accident (CVA).

ANATOMY AND PHYSIOLOGY

The skin has been described as the largest organ in the body. Its function is to protect the body from the environment and maintain core body

279

temperature (2). The skin is made up of two layers: the epidermis and the dermis. The epidermis is the outermost layer and the dermis is the thick layer under it. Sweat glands, hair cells, nerve receptors, and capillaries are located in the dermis. Collagen is also located in the dermis and not in the epidermis. Pressure ulcers usually start in the dermis (2).

In the neurologically impaired skin, there is an increased breakdown of the existing collagen and less production of new collagen, making the skin less elastic and therefore more fragile. The new collagen being formed is less resilient (type 3 as opposed to type 1). There is also reduced subcutaneous fat and diminished blood flow with subsequent lowered tissue oxygenation and decreased nutrition (2,4). Muscle atrophy over bony prominences following a neurologic injury such as in SCI also leads to less padding over bony prominences (2).

Pressure ulcers are typically due to pressure between skin, bony prominences, and muscles, which compress blood vessels in the muscles, leading to ischemia of both muscles and skin (2). The pressures can be due to either direct continuously applied forces or shearing forces. Pressure ulcers usually begin deep inside tissues and extend to the surface since muscle is less sensitive to ischemia than skin (2).

There are four stages of pressure ulcers:

Stage 1: The skin is intact, but there is a persistent nonblanchable erythema in the dermis. The area may be tender, swollen, or warmer in comparison to nearby tissues (2,5). These patients need to be watched since they are at high risk for developing actual ulceration (4).

Stage 2: A superficial partial skin loss involves the dermis, epidermis and subcutaneous fat. It may look like a crater, blister, or skin abrasion (2,5). However a tiny blister or ulcer may be the "tip of the iceberg" (4).

Stage 3: These pressure ulcers involve the epidermis, dermis, and subcutaneous fat down to the fascia, but do not extend through it. The underlying bone and tendons are not visible or palpable (2,5).

Stage 4: These are full-thickness pressure ulcers that extend past the fascia and muscle and can include the underlying bone, tendon, and joint. Stage 4 pressure ulcers can also have sinus tracts (2,5). It is important to note that the true depth or staging of a pressure ulcer that is covered by a blackened eschar or "slough of different colors" cannot be determined until these are removed.

PATIENT ASSESSMENT

It is important to perform a thorough risk assessment for the development of pressure ulcers in all adults with neurologic disabilities. This includes obtaining a pertinent medical history as well as performing an appropriate physical examination targeting high-risk areas.

The medical history should include an evaluation of the patient's current medical status (e.g., acute illness), significant past medical history (e.g., previous pressure ulcers and their treatment, dementia, diabetes, peripheral vascular disease, collagen vascular disease), medication review, and psychosocial assessment (e.g., substance abuse, alcoholism, social support system, financial constraints). If the patient is predominantly wheelchair-bound or bed-bound, then a review of the pressure-relieving features of the current wheelchair and mattress is also necessary. Table 22.1 outlines key components of the medical history.

The physical examination begins with an evaluation of the patient's general appearance (e.g., acutely ill, overly sedated, malnourished, obese, poor personal hygiene) and then focuses on key systems such as the musculoskeletal and neurologic systems as well as the skin. Areas overlying bony prominences should be evaluated for presence of pressure ulcers. These include the sacrum, greater trochanters, ischii, knees, heels, elbows, scapulae, and occiput. It is important to note that pressure ulcers may be hard to detect in adults with dark skin pigmentation (2,5). Staging of a pressure ulcer may also be hard to determine if there is an overlying eschar, in which case the eschar would need to be removed to correctly determine the extent of the ulcer. Pressure ulcers may also be difficult to detect under casts and braces (3).

In wheelchair-bound and bed-bound patients it is also important to assess the wheelchair and mattress, respectively, to ensure that they are adequately relieving pressure over the bony prominences. Table 22.2 outlines key components of the physical examination of the patient at risk for pressure ulcers. Table 22.3 outlines some useful biochemical markers in the assessment of pressure ulcers.

Table 22.1

Medical History

1. History of present illness in hospitalized or acutely ill patient (4)
2. Pressure ulcer history: previous pressure ulcers and their treatment (2)
3. Past medical history: neurologic disease (duration, progression, and treatment), dementia, diabetes, peripheral vascular disease, collagen vascular disease, malignancy, depression, psychosis, SCI (autonomic dysreflexia, complete injury, tetraplegia)
4. Review of systems: incontinence (urinary and/or fecal), poor nutrition, poor appetite, weight loss or weight gain, pain with pressure ulcers (2,3).
5. Medications with significant cognitive side effects
6. Wheelchair-bound patients: no. of hours spent in a wheelchair per day; type of cushion; when the cushion was last evaluated (2)
7. Bed-bound patients: no. of hours spent in bed per day; type of bed (2)
8. Use of upper and/or lower extremity orthotics
9. Psycho-social history: 1) smoking (interferes with pressure ulcer healing), 2) alcoholism, drug abuse (may indicate self-neglect), 3) social support system, 4) amount of caregiver support, 5) financial limitations, 6) level of daily functional activity, 7) highest level of education achieved, 8) current employment status (2)

Table 22.2

Physical Examination

1. General appearance: e.g., poor hygiene, acutely ill appearance
2. Cognitive evaluation: a) orientation to name, place, date; b) immediate and delayed recall; c) concentration; d) presence of excessive sedation
3. Nutritional and fluid status: Is patient obese, cachectic, fluid overloaded?
4. Musculoskeletal: contractures in upper and lower limbs, kyphosis/scoliosis
5. Neurologic examination: motor strength, sensation, reflexes, trunk control
6. Skin evaluation: a) dry, flaky skin; b) excessive moisture (i.e., sweat, fecal and/or urinary incontinence)
7. High-risk areas for the development of pressure ulcers (greater trochanters, ischii, sacrum, knees, heels, elbows, scapulae, and occiput) should be checked daily
8. Pressure ulcer assessment (2,3): a) location, size, severity, length, width, and depth of pressure ulcer, evaluation for sinus tracts; b) ulcer base—is it clean of necrotic tissue and does it show evidence of granulation tissue (beefy red color, pearly shiny) or epithelialization (regrowth of epidermis across the surface of the pressure ulcer); is there presence of an eschar (black, dry, necrotic tissue) or "fibrin slough" (yellow); c) wound exudates (amount, odor, consistency, and color); d) longstanding pressure ulcers—irregular borders or evidence of nonhealing
9. Pressure ulcer infection: elevated temperature, erythema, warmth, induration, purulent drainage swelling may indicate cellulitis, osteomyelitis
10. Wheelchair evaluation: a) Does patient look as if he/she fits into the wheelchair? (Is the wheelchair too small or too big); b) Does the back of the wheelchair provide adequate support?; c) Poor posture control? Kyphosis? Scoliosis? Can patient do a pressure relief movement (perform a pushup, turn to each side, lean forward?; d) Does the current wheelchair cushion allow adequate pressure relief?
11. Mattress evaluation in bed-bound patients: Does the mattress and supportive padding provide adequate pressure relief over high-risk areas?
12. Check for ill-fitting braces

Table 22.3

Useful Biochemical Markers in the Assessment of Patients with Pressure Ulcers

1. Total protein
2. Albumin, prealbumin
3. Hemoglobin, hematocrit, transferrin
4. Total lymphocyte count
5. Hemoglobin A1C in diabetic patients

TREATMENT

Prevention

The saying that an ounce of prevention is worth a pound of cure is very appropriate when it comes to pressure ulcers. Clinicians should be vigilant about risk factors for pressure ulcers in adults with neurologic disabilities and be proactive in reducing them.

Assessment of the risk for pressure ulcers should be done in medical settings (e.g., medical, surgical, and rehab wards), long-term care settings, and in the home. In hospitalized or institutionalized patients, this risk assessment should be performed at time of admission. Reassessment should be performed in medical and rehab settings on a daily basis. In a long-term care facility it has been recommended that reassessment in stable patients should be performed weekly for 4 weeks following admission and then quarterly, but the frequency should be increased whenever there is a change in the patient's medical status (e.g., acute illness) (1,2).

The Braden and Norton scales have been used to identify patients at high risk for the development of pressure ulcers (1,2), but it is important to note that all patients who spend a majority of the day in a wheelchair or bed are at risk for developing them. The Braden scale consists of six subscales that measure the intensity and duration of pressure as well as the tolerance of tissues to pressure. These include activity, mobility, sensory perception, nutrition, moisture, friction, and shear. The Norton scale assesses risk by using five variables: mental condition, incontinence, mobility, activity, and physical condition (2).

Appropriate nutritional and fluid intake is very important in the prevention and treatment of pressure ulcers since increased energy expenditures and low-protein diets have been reported in adults with SCI and pressure ulcers (3). The reader is referred to Chapter 14 for additional information on this topic.

Table 22.4 lists some common measures to reduce the risk of the development of a pressure ulcer.

Pressure Relief

Pressure relief is an important part in both the prevention and the treatment of pressure ulcers. The goals of a support surface are: 1) increase the support surface area, 2) decrease pressure over high-risk areas, 3) reduce moisture retention, and 4) decrease shearing forces in a cost-effective manner (3). There are two broad types of pressure relief surfaces for bed-bound patients: static and dynamic.

Static support surfaces are indicated for high-risk patients who either don't have a skin breakdown or have a stage 1 pressure ulcer. They can be made out of foam, gel, or water and can be used as a mattress overlay. They don't require electricity (4). It is important to check the static support surface on a regular basis for adequate pressure relief. This can be done by placing the palm of the clinician's hand under the mattress overlay while the patient is lying on it. Inadequate support is present if there is less than one inch of support between the palm of the clinician and the patient.

Dynamic support surfaces are indicated for patients with stage 1 pressure ulcers developed while on static surfaces and for patients with existing stage3 and 4 ulcers (4). Examples of dynamic support surfaces include electrically driven alternating pressure surfaces, low-air-loss surface mattresses and air-fluidized beds (high air loss).

Table 22.4

Prevention of Pressure Ulcers

---

1. Daily visual and tactile skin inspections of high-risk areas (e.g., ischii, sacrum, coccyx, trochanters, knees, elbows, scapulae, and heels). This inspection should evaluate for moistness, blisters, warmth, and erythema. Clinicians should conduct a careful inspection, especially in adults with dark pigmentation (1,2).
2. Bed-bound patients should be turned every 2 hours (1,2,4).
3. Shearing motions in positioning and repositioning bed-bound patients should be avoided (e.g., dragging bed-bound patients on a bed surface). Hoyer lifts, trapeze, and sheets should be used to reposition patient (1,2).
4. Skin lubricants and protective dressings and padding should be used to reduce the risk of shearing (6).
5. Bed-bound patients should not be positioned on their greater trochanters, but rather on a 30° angle to the bed surface (2).
6. Pressure-relieving mattresses and overlays should be used in high-risk patients. It is important to regularly check these pressure-relieving devices to ensure that they are providing adequate pressure relief.
7. Pillows should be placed between the knees and other bony body parts that touch each other (2,4) in bed-bound patients.
8. In bed-bound patients, the head of the bed should be at the lowest level of elevation and for short periods of time (3,4).
9. Minimize moisture and heat over highrisk areas such as bony prominences (2).
10. Donut-type pressure-relieving devices should be avoided since they can decrease blood flow and cause localized swelling (2,6).
11. Skin should be cleaned on a regular basis and especially after soiling has occurred. Mild soap and lukewarm water should be used. Aggressive rubbing should be avoided. Skin should be patted dry to avoid trauma (1,2,7).
12. Dry skin should be treated with moisturebarrier moisturizing creams (2,4,6).
13. Minimize risk of skin burns (e.g., heating pads over bony and insensate areas) (2).
14. Avoid massage over bony areas (1).
15. Bedding sheets and clothing should be soft so that the skin is not irritated. They should be changed frequently (4).
16. Avoid the use of strong adhesive tape on skin because it can potentially lead to skin tears (4).
17. Bowel and bladder program should be instituted for incontinent patients. Appropriate undergarments and even an external collection device to collect stool should be considered (1).
18. Wheelchair-bound patients should be educated on performing weight shifts every 15–30 minutes. These include pushups, leaning forward and to each side (1,2,6).
19. Nutrition and fluid status should be maximized.
20. Range-of-motion and strengthening exercises should be performed on a daily basis (2,6).
21. In patients with plaster casts, consider cutting out pressure-relieving windows at pressure sites (4).

Alternating pressure surfaces relieve pressure intermittently, but have a reduced ability to reduce moisture and dissipate heat. Low-air-loss mattresses are better at managing moisture and heat than alternating pressure surfaces and are smaller and easier for positioning patients and patient transfers compared to air-fluidized beds (2).

Air-fluidized beds are indicated for patients with nonhealing stage 3 and 4 pressure ulcers and multiple pressure ulcers (3,4). They can be useful in the reduction of moisture but run the risk of dehydrating the patient and drying of moist dressings. They are also noisy, large, expensive, difficult during patient transfers, and require a significant amount of electricity (2).

Wheelchair cushions are important in the prevention of pressure ulcers in wheelchair-bound adults with neurologic disabilities. There are several different types of cushions, with foam, gel, and air cushions being the most common. Pressure mapping is often beneficial in identifying areas of pressure and in the selection of appropriate cushions.

Foam cushions are light and relatively inexpensive, but they retain heat and can lose their pressure-relieving properties quickly (2). Gel-filled cushions are effective in reducing shearing forces, distribute pressures well, have better skin temperature control, and are easy to clean, but they don't always provide the lowest pressure-reducing forces (2). Air cushions can provide good pressure relief and reduction of shearing forces and are light and easy to clean, but can be punctured and lose their pressure-relieving abilities if not adequately inflated. In addition, they require good posture control (2).

Clinicians should check the wheelchair cushions for adequate pressure relief in wheelchair-bound patients. This can be accomplished by placing the clinician's hand under the cushion with the patient on the cushion and estimating the distance between the patient and the clinician's palm. Inadequate support is present if there is less than one inch of support between the palm of the clinician and the patient (2).

The wheelchair back should also be examined for adequate support, since inadequate support of the patient's back can lead to increased pressures on the buttocks as well as increased shearing forces. The patient's ability to perform pressure relief should also be evaluated, and, if impaired, consideration for an alternate type of wheelchair should be given (e.g., tilt in space).

Nonsurgical Treatment

In order for a pressure ulcer to heal, the ulcer itself must be clean, free of necrotic tissue, and have granulation tissue present. Granulation tissue is beefy red, moist, and shiny and does not bleed easily (2).

Ulcers should be cleansed before each dressing change without traumatizing the ulcer itself. Normal saline is a good irrigating agent (2,3). Antiseptic solutions containing iodine should be avoided due to their cytoxic effects as well as the possibility of systemic absorption (2). Caution should be used in using gauze sponges to clean ulcers, since these may traumatize the wound itself. The ulcer should be cleansed centrally to peripherally to avoid contamination of wound.

Debridement of a pressure ulcer serves two general purposes: 1) removal of necrotic and/or infected tissues that can negatively impact on the healing process and 2) determining the size and stage of the pressure ulcer itself. Debridement can be performed at the bedside or in the operating room and should be performed by clinicians with the appropriate competency and experience.

There are different types of debridement: 1) autolytic, 2) enzymatic, 3) mechanical, and 4) sharp debridement. In autolytic debridement, a synthetic dressing (e.g., duoderm) is applied over the pressure ulcer and the eschar. The enzymes located inside the pressure ulcer digest the eschar. This type of debridement can be slow and is indicated for small noninfected pressure ulcers (3,4).

In enzymatic debridement, proteolytic enzymes (e.g., collagenase, papain) are applied to necrotic tissues, which are covered by a moist dressing, in order to digest the eschar. This type of treatment is recommended for patients with noninfected ulcers who are not surgical candidates (3,4).

Mechanical debridement can be accomplished by the application of wet/moist dressings, hydrotherapy, wound irrigation, or use of dextranomers. Dextranomers are beads that are placed in the wound and absorb debris and bacteria. Dressings can be applied wet to the pressure ulcer and removed along with necrotic tissues, once dried, 4–6 hours later. This process can be painful, so premedication with appropriate pain medications can be helpful. Mechanical debridement is not recommended for clean wounds with granulation tissue (2,3).

The advantage of sharp debridement or surgical debridement is the quick removal of necrotic and infected tissue; however, disadvantages are their invasive nature, bleeding, and possible trauma to healthy tissue (2–4). It has been recommended to avoid removing a dry, nontender, nonerythematous, nonpurulent heel eschar since it can act as a natural protective cover to the pressure ulcer (3).

Dressings have several roles, including: 1) keeping the ulcer base moist and the surrounding skin dry, 2) serving as a barrier to infection, and 3) facilitating debridement. There are different types of dressings, including transparent films, hydrogels, foams, hydrocolloids, alginates, and moist saline dressings.

Transparent films (e.g., tegaderm) are indicated for ulcers with little exudates. Hydrogels are cross-linked polymer dressings indicated for shallow wounds with little exudates. Foams form a moist environment for the healing of wounds and are also good for exudates. Hydrocolloids (duoderm, restore) are combinations of gelatin, pectin, and carboxymethylcellulose and are good for light to moderate exudates. Alginates (sorbsan) are indicated for copious exudate and bleeding after surgery (4).

Pressure ulcers should be loosely packed. Tight packing may cause tissue damage (2). The decision to change dressing types is usually influenced by increased pain, drainage, erythema, and a strong odor.

Complications of Pressure Ulcers

Complications of pressure ulcers include: 1) infections (cellulitis, osteomyelitis, sepsis, and abscess), 2) squamous cell carcinoma in a longstanding ulcer, 3) systemic effects of topical treatments of the ulcer (e.g., iodine toxicity), and 4) cutaneous fistulas (3,4).

Pressure ulcers should show signs of healing within 2–4 weeks (3). Poor risk factors for healing include: 1) incontinence, 2) immobilization, 3) dependency on others for activities of daily living, and 4) infection—especially if the bacterial count exceeds 10^5 organisms per gram of tissue (2). Stage 3 and 4 pressure ulcers are colonized with bacteria; therefore, swab cultures are never helpful. Bone biopsy or fluid needle aspirations are often needed to determine presence of a significant source of infection (3). In a clean nonhealing ulcer of 2–4 weeks duration, topical antibiotics such as silver sulfadiazine or a triple antibiotic have been recommended (3), but in the presence of sepsis or osteomyelitis, systemic antibiotics may be necessary. Signs of osteomyelitis include elevated temperature, erythema, swelling, foul odor, purulent discharge, and elevated white blood cell count. Consultation with an infectious disease specialist is helpful.

Patient Safety

Some patient safety concerns have been addressed earlier in this chapter, and the reader is referred to Table 22.4 for an overview.

The treatment of pressure ulcers is also an important area in which harm can be done to the patient. The following principles can help clinicians reduce the potential for harm in the treatment of patients with pressure ulcers:

- Avoid the use of strong tape adhesives, especially on fragile skin. The term "epidermal stripping" refers to the removal of the epidermis by pulling off the skin when strong adhesive tape is used (2).
- Avoid the use of antiseptic povidone-iodine solutions in the cleaning of pressure ulcers due to their cytoxic effects on the ulcerated tissues as well as the potential for systemic absorption of iodine (2).
- Caution is recommended in the use of gauze sponges to clean a pressure ulcer, since these may traumatize the ulcer bed itself.
- Surgical debridement should be performed by clinicians with competency and expertise in this type of debridement.
- Avoid removing dry and adherent eschar over heels with no evidence of infection, erythema, or drainage. They cover and protect the underlying healing ulcer. Their removal may also compromise distal circulation.

Patient Education

It is important for clinicians to educate patients and caregivers on the etiology, prevention, complications, and treatments of pressure ulcers. This education should be carried out at an appropriate level and in the patient's native language to ensure understanding. Table 22.5 outlines some key principles, and additional resources can be found in the reference section (1,2,6–8).

Table 22.5

Patient Education

- Daily skin inspections: Patients and caregivers should be educated on how to perform daily skin inspections of high-risk areas such as the heels, sacrum, ischii, coccyx, and trochanters in wheelchair-bound patients as well as scapulae, elbows, and knees in bed-bound patients. Skin inspection should evaluate for areas of erythema, blisters, warmth, drainage, and moisture (2).
- Pressure-relief techniques: Weight shifts should be performed for 30 seconds every 30 minutes or 60 seconds every 60 minutes for wheelchair-bound patients. Weight shift techniques include pushup on chair, leaning to each side and forward. Bed-bound patients should be turned every 2 hours.
- Skin should be kept dry, but if too dry, then moisturizers should be used (2).
- Clothing should be made of lightweight cotton. It should not be too tight, have a rough texture, or have metal fasteners. Tight socks, tight shoes, ill-fitting braces, and splints with poor padding should be avoided.
- Urinary leg bags with straps should be avoided since they can constrict blood flow.
- Maintain weight—an increase in weight may make it difficult to fit into a wheelchair and also may result in inadequate pressure relief.
- Minimize risk of skin burns (e.g., avoid using heating pads over insensate skin) (2).
- Exercise, stay active, and keep muscles as strong as possible (2).

REFERENCES

1. www.npuap.org—National Pressure Ulcer Advisory Panel, 2007. Pressure Ulcer Prevention Points.
2. Pressure Ulcer Prevention and Treatment Following Spinal Cord Injury: A Clinical Practice Guideline for Health Care Professionals.
3. www.ncbi.nlm.nih.gov/books—AHCPR Supported Clinical Practice Guidelines #15: Treatment of Pressure Ulcers.
4. www.merck.com—Pressure Ulcers, revised 11/05.
5. www.npuap.org—National Pressure Ulcer Advisory Panel, 2007.Updated Staging Systems.
6. www.ncbi.nlm.nih.gov/books—AHCPR Supported Clinical Practice Guidelines #3: Pressure Ulcers in Adults: Prediction and Prevention.
7. www.familydoctor.org—Pressure Sores; reviewed and updated 12/06.
8. www.nlm.nih.gov/medlineplus—Pressure Ulcer, updated 7/18/07.

23 | Preventive Screening

Gene Tekmyster
Avniel Shetreat-Klein

In years past, severe neurologic impairments were associated with dramatically shortened life spans. With progress in neurologic and rehabilitative treatment, survival rates have increased significantly, to the point where these conditions can now be considered chronic disabilities, with life spans in many cases nearing thos of the unimpaired. As a result, the usual prevention guidelines that apply to all adults must also be applied to adults with neurologic disability. It would not be unusual these days for an individual to survive a catastrophic stroke or traumatic brain injury (TBI) or spinal cord injury (SCI), only to end up further disabled by heart disease, diabetes, or other preventable illnesses.

This chapter is intended as an overview of basic preventative care as it applies to adults with neurologic disabilities such as stroke, SCI, TBI, and multiple sclerosis (MS). The goals of the chapter are to provide key points of preventive care. A list of general screening test by age is shown in Table 23.1. The main areas covered in this chapter are: 1) cardiovascular and metabolic health, 2) pulmonary health, 3) cancer screening, 4) musculoskeletal health, 5) mental health, and 6) pressure ulcer prevention. These topics are covered in greater detail in other sections of the book.

CARDIOVASCULAR AND METABOLIC HEALTH

Adults with neurologic disabilities are at risk for the development of hypertension, hyperlipidemia, diabetes mellitus, and obesity due to a variety of factors, such as inappropriate nutrition and sedentary lifestyle. These conditions are in turn associated with an increased risk of morbidity and mortality, such as myocardial infarction and stroke. It is important that clinicians screen for the presence of these conditions, initiate appropriate treatment, and provide regular monitoring for the effectiveness of the treatments.

Table 23.1

Most Common Screenings by Age for Adults with Neurologic Disabilities

Health activity	Ages 18–39	Ages 40–49	Ages 50–64	Age 65+
Physical exam	Annually	Annually	Annually	Annually
Blood pressure/ Pulse	Every office visit	Every office visit	Every office visit	Every office visit
Eye & ear exam	Baseline by 39	Every 2–4 years	Every 2–4 years; 60+ yearly	Yearly
Dental exam	Twice a year	Twice a year	Twice a year	Twice a year
Skin exam	Every office visit	Every office visit	Every office visit	Every office visit
Cholesterol/ Triglycerides	At age 20	Every 5 years	Every 5 years	Every 5 years
Blood sugar evaluation (diabetes)	Usually not needed	Every 3 years at 45	Every 3 years	Every 3 years
Bone density for osteoporosis	Annually	Annually	Annually	Annually

Hypertension

Hypertension is defined as a systolic blood pressure (BP) of >140 and diastolic BP >90, with prehypertension being systolic BP of 120–139 and diastolic BP of 80–89. Each office visit should include measurements of vital signs such as blood pressure and heart rate, with three separate measurements taken while the patient is sitting down. The careful monitoring of blood pressure is especially important for adults with spinal cord injuries above the T6 level, since they are at risk for the development of autonomic dysreflexia (AD). AD is characterized by a rapid rise in blood pressure as a result of a noxious stimulus below the level of the neurologic injury.

Lipid Disorders

The United States Preventive Services Task Force and the American Heart Association both recommend routine screenings of men (age > 35) and women (age > 45) for lipid disorders, as well as treatment of abnormal lipids in people who are at increased risk for coronary heart disease. Other recommendations are routine screening of younger adults (men ages 20–35, women ages 20–45) for lipid disorders if they have other risk factors for coronary heart disease (diabetes, family history of cardiovascular disease, family history of familial hyperlipidemia, tobacco use, hypertension). Screening for lipid disorders should include measurement of total cholesterol and low- and high-density lipoproteins (HDL) (normal values: total cholesterol < 200 mg/dl; LDL < 130 mg/dl; HDL: males > 29, females > 35 mg/dl; triglycerides: males 40–160, females 35–136 mg/dl). The lipid screening interval should not exceed 5 years and may be shorter in those with multiple risk factors. Nutritional and intensive behavioral dietary counseling are effective tools in the prevention and treatment of dislipidemia disorders.

Diabetes Mellitus

Adults with hypertension or hyperlipidemia should also be screened for diabetes mellitus. Effective screening should include a fasting blood sugar, 2-hour postload plasma glucose, and hemoglobin A1c (HbA1c). The American Diabetes Association recommends obtaining fasting plasma glucose level. persons with values > 126 mg/dl should be further evaluated by HbA1c and 2-hour postload plasma glucose to confirm the diagnosis of diabetes. The usual reference range for HbA1c is 4–5.9%. Values above 6% represent poor control of blood sugar levels over the past 3 months and warrant treatment. Testing should be performed every 3 years or more frequently if person is at higher risk for developing type 2 diabetes.

Obesity

Adults with neurologic disabilities are at risk for the development of obesity due to a sedentary lifestyle, increased caloric intake and decreased physical activity. Obesity screening using the Body Mass Index (BMI) should be concurrent with screenings for DM. The BMI is a helpful tool in categorizing patient risk and establishing an effective treatment protocol. The following are considered the standard values for BMI values for the general population:
- BMI of 25–29.9 is overweight
- BMI of 30 or more is obesity
  - Class I = BMI of 30–34.9
  - Class II = BMI of 35–39.9
  - Class III = BMI of 40 and above

Exercise along with a healthy and balanced diet is an important part of an effective weight-reduction program. Given their physical limitations, adults with neurologic disabilities are often at a disadvantage in participating in exercise and sports. This is often due to multiple factors including physical limitations, lack of access to gyms or sporting events, and inappropriate exercise equipment. Clinicians should screen high-risk patients for cardiovascular disease prior to inception of an exercise program. Patients should be encouraged to participate in an exercise program that combines both aerobic and strengthening components most days of the week. Exercise programs should incorporate the participant's physical limitations with appropriate precautions built in and should be supervised by a physical therapist or exercise physiologist, at least initially. This topic is discussed in greater detail elsewhere in the book.

Peripheral Arterial Disease

Although the U.S. Preventive Services Task Force recommends against routine screening for peripheral arterial disease (PAD), they do report that an ankle brachial index of >0.9 is "strongly associated with limitations in lower extremity functioning and physical activity tolerance." Once PAD is diagnosed, smoking cessation, physical activity, and lipid-lowering interventions can increase ambulation distance in men with early disease.

PULMONARY HEALTH

Patients with progressive neurologic decline should have measurement of pulmonary function to assess respiratory sufficiency at least once per year. This can be performed in the private office setting using incentive spirometry. If further evaluation is required, formal pulmonary function testing is generally performed by specialists, but the routine office visits should screen for any change in respiratory status such as increased frequency of respiratory infections, worsened vocal quality, increased difficulty clearing secretions, shortness of breath, or worsened dyspnea on exertion. Patients with respiratory muscle compromise should be vaccinated against pneumonia and influenza (Tables 23.2 and 23.3).

Smoking Cessation

Tobacco use is the single largest preventable cause of disease and premature death in the United States. Tobacco use has been linked with an increased incidence of stroke, heart attacks, peripheral vascular disease, and lung cancer.

Adults with neurologic disabilities should be asked if they smoke (including pregnant women) Strategy for assessment and treatment of tobacco use include: 1) asking about tobacco use, 2) advising to quit through clear personalized messages, 3) assessing willingness to quit, 4) assisting to quit, and 5) arranging follow-up and support.

Patients should be educated on the benefits of smoking cessation. These include decreased respiratory infections, improved endurance, better wound healing, and lower risk of cardiac and cerebrovascular events.

FDA-approved pharmacotherapy that has been identified as safe and effective for treating tobacco dependence includes nicotine replacement therapy and bupropion. Clonidine and nortriptyline have been found to be efficacious and may be considered. Counseling and support group environment have been shown to improve rates of smoking cessation.

CANCER SCREENING

According to the U.S. Preventative Task Force, there is insufficient evidence to recommend for or against screening of asymptomatic people for lung cancer using chest x-rays or low-dose computed tomography. Concerns raised

Table 23.2

Recommended Adult Immunization Schedule

Vaccine	Ages 19–49	Ages 50–64	Ages >65
Human papillomavirus (HPV)	Females up to the age of 26 (3 doses)	Not indicated	Not indicated
Influenza	Recommended if other risk factors present*	1 dose annually	1 dose annually
Pneumococcal	Recommended if other risk factors present*	Recommended if other risk factors present*	1 dose
Zoster			1 dose
Tetanus, diphtheria, pertussis (Td/Tdap)	1 dose Td booster every 10 years	1 dose Td booster every 10 years	1 dose Td booster every 10 years
Measles, mumps, rubella (MMR) (1 dose)	All persons who lack evidence of immunity	Recommended if other risk factors present*	Recommended if other risk factors present*
Varicella (2 doses at 0 and 4–8 weeks)	All persons who lack evidence of immunity	All persons who lack evidence of immunity	All persons who lack evidence of immunity
Hepatitis A (2 doses at 0 and 6–18 months)	Recommended if other risk factors present*		
Hepatitis B (3 doses at 0, 2, and 4–6 months)			
Meningococcal (1 or more doses)			

*Risk factors for determination of vaccinations include indications such as certain medical conditions, lifestyle, occupational or environmental hazards.
Source: Department of Health and Human Services Centers for Disease Control and Prevention. The recommendations in this schedule were approved by the CDC Advisory Committee on Immunization Practices, The American Academy of Family Physician, The American College of Physicians.

included the high rate of false positives and exposure to radiation and the significant morbidity and mortality rates associated with further diagnostic interventions. Nevertheless, symptomatic patients with a history of smoking should undergo a through and timely workup.

Colorectal cancer screening should begin at the age of 50 for both men and women. Screening for colorectal cancer and adenomatous polyps reduces both the mortality and incidence of this disease. Screening can be performed by fecal occult blood testing, flexible sigmoidoscopy, colonoscopy, or double-contrast barium enema. Colonoscopy is the most effective, sensitive, and specific test for detecting gastrointestinal abnormalities. The testing interval should not exceed 10 years. For those at high risk (positive family history of colorectal cancer),

Table 23.3

Vaccine Indication/Contraindications Based on Medical Conditions

Vaccine	Immuno-compromising conditions (excluding HIV)	HIV CD4 Count: >200 → >200 →	DM, CAD, COPD, Alcoholism	Asplenia	Chronic liver disease	ESRD	Health care personnel
Human papillomavirus (HPV)		3 doses for females through age 26 years at 0, 2, and 6 months					
Influenza		1 dose annually					
Pneumococcal		1–2 doses	1 dose				Recommended if other risk factors present*
Zoster		Contraindicated	1 dose				
Tetanus, diphtheria, pertussis (Td/Tdap)		1 dose Td booster every 10 years					
Measles, mumps, rubella (MMR) (1 dose)		Contraindicated	1 or 2 doses				
Varicella (2 doses at 0 and 4–8 weeks)		Contraindicated	2 doses at 0 and 4–8 weeks				
Hepatitis A (2 doses at 0 and 6–18 months)		Recommended if other risk factors present*	Recommended if other risk factors present*		All persons who lack evidence of immunity	Recommended if other risk factors present*	Recommended if other risk factors present*
Hepatitis B (3 doses at 0, 2, and 4–6 months)		Recommended if other risk factors present*	All persons who lack evidence of immunity		All persons who lack evidence of immunity	All persons who lack evidence of immunity	Recommended if other risk factors present
Meningococcal (1 or more doses)		Recommended if other risk factors present*	Recommended if other risk factors present*	1 dose	Recommended if other risk factors present*	Recommended if other risk factors present*	Recommended if other risk factors present*

*Risk factors for determination of vaccinations include indications such as certain medical conditions, lifestyle, occupational or environmental hazards.

Source: Department of Health and Human Services Centers for Disease Control and Prevention. The recommendations in this schedule were approved by the CDC Advisory Committee on Immunization Practices, The American Academy of Family Physician, The American College of Physicians.

the interval may be as low as 5 years. In spinal cord injury patients at risk for autonomic dysreflexia, blood pressure should be closely monitored. Some studies suggest that lidocaine anal block can decrease the incidence of AD during colonoscopy (11).

Breast cancer screening should be instated early, beginning with teaching breast exams as early as the age of 18 when risk factors are present (family history of breast cancer in a mother, sister, or daughter, history of atypical hyperplasia on breast biopsy, early age at menarche, null parity). Screening mammography, with or without clinical breast examination, should be done every 1–2 years for women aged 40 or older. Patients with a strong family history of breast cancer may be recommended for genetic screening and counseling (Table 23.4).

Cervical cancer screening with cytology testing should be done for women who have been sexually active beginning at the age of 18–21 and in all those under 65. Testing intervals should not be more than 3 years, with the recommended interval of one year. Human papillomavirus (HPV) testing is also appropriate, combined with cytology for cervical cancer screening of women over the age of 35 who are sexually active. HPV screening should be performed every 3 years. Discontinuation of testing after the age of 65 is appropriate.

Bladder cancer screening is recommended annually in those persons with a history of chronic indwelling catheter as well as in those with a history of smoking. Screening tests such as microscopic urinalysis and urine cytology have been used. Adults with urinary retention due to neurogenic bladder are at risk for increased urinary tract infection (UTI) and renal disease due to obstructive uropathy or due to high bladder pressures in the case of bladder dysenergia. In these patients annual assessment of the urinary tract includes a cystogram and kidney ultrasound. Cystogram is used for screening of bladder changes, vesicoureteral reflux, and urinary tract calculus. Kidney ultrasound is performed to evaluate the function of each kidney and screen for hydronephrosis.

The American Cancer Society recommends that prostate-specific antigen (PSA) testing along with a digital rectal exam should be performed annually in male patients over the age of 50. Those individuals with increased risk for prostate cancer (African descent, family history/first-degree relative) should begin screening at the age of 45.

Skin cancers, such as melanomas and squamous and basal cell carcinomas, are potentially lethal, but often curable when found in the early stages. The U.S. Preventative Services Task Force did not find sufficient evidence to recommend for or against a skin cancer screening program. However; it seems clear that appropriate awareness of suspicious lesions and proper patient education can be lifesaving. Referral to a dermatologist is indicated for further evaluation and management of suspicious lesions. The following are signs to look for:

- Basal Cell Carcinoma
  - Usually sun-exposed areas
  - Raised, smooth, pearly lesion
  - Crusting and bleeding of lesion is common
  - May be mistaken for nonhealing wound

Table 23.4

Breast and Cervical Cancer Screening by Age

	Ages 18–39	Ages 40–49	Ages 50–64	Age 65+	Comments
Pelvic exam by physician included Pap smear	Annually	Annually	Annually	Annually	Some doctors feel that after three or more consecutive normal results, Pap smears may be performed every 2–3 years on certain low-risk women
Human papillomavirus (HPV testing)	Every 3 years	Every 3 years	Every 3 years	Every 3 years	HPV vaccine is recommended for all women up to the age of 26
Breast self-exam (BSE)	Teach BSE by age 20	Monthly	Monthly	Monthly	Always call physician with concerns
Mammography	Usually not needed	Every 1–2 years	Every 1–2 years	Every 1–2 years	Risk level may require higher frequency
Breast exam by physician	Every 3 years	Annually	Annually	Annually	Risk level may require higher frequency

- Squamous Cell Carcinoma
  - Usually sun-exposed areas
  - Red, scaly, thickened patch
  - Ulceration and bleeding is common
- Melanoma
  - New or newly enlarged pigmented lesion
  - Irregular borders or coloration
  - Bleeding

MUSCULOSKELETAL HEALTH

Osteoporosis

Persons with spinal cord injuries are at a very high risk of osteoporosis—especially during the first year following the injury—and as such are at a high risk of developing osteoporosis-related fractures, commonly in the lower extremities. Clinicians should screen adults with spinal cord injuries for osteoporosis with bone density studies and initiate appropriate treatment. Patients should also be counseled about their increased risk of developing fractures in the extremities, including precautions to minimize that risk (e.g., avoid aggressive range of motion in osteoporotic limbs), and, in insensate patients, the signs and symptoms of a lower extremity fracture. This topic is covered in greater detail elsewhere in the book.

Overuse Injuries

Active manual wheelchair users are at high risk of developing overuse injuries to the upper extremities such as rotator cuff tears and carpal tunnel syndrome. These adults should be asked about upper extremity musculoskeletal symptoms at each office visit and undergo a focused physical examination of the upper extremities. Attention should be paid to the wheelchair itself during the patient visit. Cushions, brakes, tires, rims, footrests, and armrests should be checked for signs of excessive wear and tear.

Contractures

Contractures are fixed or nonfixed limitations in the range of motion of one or more joints that can significantly impact on the passive and active range of motion of the involved joint(s). These in turn can produce profound limitations on the functionality of the individual. Contractures often arise from positions of comfort in the bed or wheelchair. They typically occur in the shoulders, elbows, and wrists in the upper extremities and hip, knees, and ankles in the lower extremities. A recent decrease in range of motion in a particular joint should raise the possibility of heterotopic ossification (commonly at the knee and hip, less commonly at the shoulder).

Contracture prevention is truly a case where an ounce of prevention is worth a pound of cure, as contractures can often be prevented by vigilant range-of-motion exercises of joints that are at high risk. On the other hand, once a contracture is formed, reversing can be painful, time-consuming, and may require surgical intervention.

Pressure Ulcers

A decubitus or pressure ulcer is a common preventable condition with high morbidity in the adult with neurologic disability. During every follow-up clinic visit, patients that are at risk must be evaluated for decubitus ulcers by visual assessment and palpation of areas that are at high risk for skin breakdown. High-risk areas while supine are the sacrum, heel, and occiput. High-risk areas while seated are ischial tuberosities and trochanters. Immobility combined with sensory loss over the affected areas increases the risk of forming pressure ulcers. The key to preventing pressure ulcers is pressure relief. This topic is discussed in greater detail elsewhere in the text.

MENTAL HEALTH AND SUBSTANCE ABUSE

Mental illness and substance abuse are common in adults with neurologic disabilities. They may have been present prior or at the time of the injury (e.g., SCI and TBI) and worsened after the injury or may have developed after the injury. These subjects are discussed in greater detail elsewhere in this book. However, screenings for depression, suicidal ideation, and substance abuse are important preventive measures in the care of adults with neurologic disabilities.

Depression

There are many tools available to a clinician for the purpose of screening for depression. These include the Zung Self-Assessment Depression Scale, Beck Depression Inventory, General Health Questionnaire, and Center for Epidemiologic Study Depression Scale. Each physician can make his or her own clinical judgment as to which scale is best suited, but an effective method is to ask the following two questions:

Over the past 2 weeks, have you felt down, depressed, or hopeless?

Over the past 2 weeks, have you felt little interest or pleasure in doing things?

There is some evidence to show that these questions are just as effective a screening tool as using longer screening methods (7).

Suicidal Ideation

According to the U.S. Preventive Services Task Force, the strongest risk factors for attempted suicide include a history of suicide attempts, a history of mental illness, and a history of substance abuse. Clinicians should inquire about the presence of suicidal ideation—passive or active—at office visits, especially in those with risk factors.

Alcoholism

The definitions of alcohol abuse are as follows: 1) heavy drinking: women, 7 or more drinks per week or 3 in one sitting; men, 14 drinks per week or 4 drinks per occasion, 2) moderate drinking: 2 standard drinks or less per day for men and one drink per day for women and persons over the age of 65. Light alcohol consumption in adults has been found to have certain health benefits, such as reduced risk of coronary artery disease.

Several questionnaires are available to the clinician to screen for alcohol abuse. One of the more common and effective is the CAGE questionnaire:
- C = feeling the need to cut down
- A = annoyed by criticism
- G = guilty about drinking
- E = eye-opener in the morning

Any of the above questions that elicit a "yes" response should be further evaluated. Effective interventions for alcohol abuse cessation include counseling, feedback, and goal setting.

Opioid Medications

Pain is a common feature among patients with neurologic disability, and opioid medications are commonly prescribed for the management of pain. Patients receiving these medications for chronic conditions should be assessed for the possibility of abuse. Potential "red flags" include aberrant use of medications, evidence of "stockpiling "or "running out early" of medications, lost prescriptions, insistence on a particular medication, visits to multiple providers for medication, and a history of substance abuse.

REFERENCES

1. McDonnell GV, McCann JP. Issues of medical management in adults with spina bifida. Child's Nerv Syst 2000; 16:222–227.
2. Khan Y, Seddon PC. Respiratory problems in children with neurologic impairment. Arch Dis Child 2003; 88:75–78.
3. Klingbeil H, Baer HR, Wilson PE. Aging with a disability. Arch Phys Med Rehabil 2004; 85:68–73.
4. Meyers J, Lee M, Keratli J. Cardiovascular disease in spinal cord injury: an overview of prevalence, risk, evaluation, and management. Am J Phys Med 2007; 86:142–152.
5. Ditunno J, Formal CS. Chronic spinal cord injury. N Engl J Med 1994; 330:550–556.
6. Thompson AJ. Neurologic rehabilitation: from mechanisms to management. J Neurol Neurosurg Psychiatry 2000; 69:718–722.
7. U.S. Department of Health and Human Services, Agency of Healthcare Research and Quality. The Guide to Clinical Preventive Services, Recommendations of the U.S. Preventive Services Task Force, 2007.

8. Hopkins SC, Lenz ER, Pontes NM, Lin SX, Mundinger MO. Context of care or provider training: the impact on preventive screening practices. Prev Med 2005; 40:718–724.

9. Urdaneta F, Layon AJ. Respiratory complications in patients with traumatic cervical spine injuries: case report and review of the literature. J Clin Anesthesia 2003; 15:398–405.

10. Eyre H, Kahn R, Robertson RM. Preventing cancer, cardiovascular disease and diabetes, a common agenda for the American Cancer Society, the American Diabetes Association and the American Heart Association. Circulation 2004; 109:3244–3255.

11. Cosman B, Vu T. Lidocaine anal block limits autonomic dysreflexia during anorectal procedures in spinal cord injury: a randomized, double-blind, placebo-controlled trial. Dis Colon Rectum 2005; 48(8):1556–1561.

24 | Psychiatric Sequelae of the Spinal Cord–Injured Adult

Loran C. Vocaturo

Disability resulting from spinal cord injury (SCI) suddenly and unexpectedly changes the manner in which a person is able to relate to the environment. The psychological sequelae that often follow can be attributed to a combination of premorbid factors along with permanent physical and, sometimes, cognitive impairment. The role of the rehabilitation psychologist and neuropsychologist is to assess cognitive and psychological functioning, provide psychological interventions aimed to maximize the patient's rehabilitation, and improve the patient's adjustment to disability. Simply, the goal is to promote a sense of control out of a situation characterized by dependence. Rehabilitation physicians should be knowledgeable of the risks, symptoms, and subtle signs of psychological and cognitive sequelae that impact rehabilitation and long-term outcomes. Ordering psychological consults and interventions early in rehabilitation may help prevent the disabling effects of neuropsychiatric syndromes For many patients, feeling dependent upon others can result in a number of emotional and behavioral reactions. The prevention of psychological syndromes through education and early intervention is a significant part of rehabilitation and critical to rehabilitation success (1).

While the spinal cord–injured population is a fairly heterogeneous group, they do share a common consequence of a disability that penalizes them by reducing their freedom. The physical changes resulting from SCI are devastating, often producing both physical and sensory deficits, potential loss of control over internal organ functions, or in severe cases, the inability to breathe independently. Although normal cognitive function and intellectual faculties may remain intact, the psychological, emotional, and social implications can significantly affect the patient's adaptation to the resultant disability. Approximately 13% of patient with SCI will become clinically depressed, usually months or even years after the initial injury (2).

The goal of this chapter is to provide information about the prevalence, assessment, and treatment of different types of psychiatric sequelae following spinal cord injury.

PSYCHOLOGICAL ISSUES FOLLOWING SCI

Increased psychosocial stress associated with spinal cord injury puts patients at greater risk for the development of psychological symptoms. Early difficulties in adjustment and the long-term implications and consequences of SCI can eventually lead to the onset of clinical syndromes and psychiatric diagnoses. Common psychiatric diagnoses found among the SCI population include mood disorders (e.g., depression), anxiety disorders (e.g., panic disorder and post-traumatic stress disorder [PTSD]), and substance-related disorders.

It is important to note that like psychiatric disorders, SCI patients might also be at greater risk for suicide. Suicide rates for patients with SCI have been found to be two to six times greater than that of the able-bodied population (3). SCI patients who have a higher risk of suicide include those with comorbid psychiatric diagnoses (e.g., depression, schizophrenia), previous suicide attempt(s), substance abuse, poor coping skills, and limited social support (Table 24.1).

Although adjustment to SCI was previously thought to be largely dependent on certain physical variables, including level of injury, age of injury, and time since injury, new efforts have examined the role of individual variables in psychological adjustment, including premorbid coping and personality styles along with psychosocial resources and support (4). While a patient's reaction and adjustment to SCI are predictable by both physical and psychological variables, it is important to note that adjustment and adaptation to SCI are unique to each patient. Because the goal of acute hospitalization is survival and medical stabilization, often patients do not fully appreciate the long-term implications that SCI will have on daily life. Psychological symptoms may not be present in the early stages of recovery despite the existence of many acute stressors. Although the acute rehabilitation hospital represents an environment where the patient will be able to optimize his or her physical abilities, it is also place where he or she will come face to face with his physical challenges. Subsequently, this may also be a time when psychological symptoms and adjustment issues manifest, making psychological intervention critical.

Early emotional reactions vary among individuals after SCI, but denial, anger, helplessness, and anxiety are common clinical themes.

Denial (disavowal of the injury and resultant disability) differs from a lack of awareness of one's impairment, which results from organic brain damage (see Chapter 25). Denial is a normal response and coping mechanism in reaction to a life-altering, tragic event that represents the patient's attempt to maintain his or her premorbid identity and hope for recovery. Because it is often misunderstood, rehabilitation professionals may perceive denial as problematic. Denial, however, does not necessarily affect rehabilitation in a negative manner since it may not be a behavioral disavowal, but a cognitive or emotional one. Behavioral denial is present when patients refuse to try out adaptive equipment or perform activities of daily living because they believe that full recovery is pending and change unnecessary. It may represent a rigid and desperate

Table 24.1

Risk Factors and Warning Signs for Suicide

Risk factors	Assessment factors	Warning signs
Multiple previous suicide attempts	Personal characteristics; membership in at-risk groups (e.g., gender, age, ethnicity)	Sudden changes in behavior (e.g., withdrawal, depressed mood, irritability, agitation)
Resolved plans and preparations; suicide desire	Dispositional factors (e.g., threshold for pain, self-control, problem-solving skills)	Changes in eating or sleeping habits
Isolation; limited or loss of family or social support; limited or loss of daily activities	Situational factors (e.g., support system, stressors, possible triggers)	Increased drug or alcohol use
Comorbid psychiatric diagnosis (e.g., depression, schizophrenia)	Current symptoms (e.g., increased pain, increased suicidal intent, desire and ideation, level of agitation and anxiety, problem-solving deficits, dysfunctional assumptions, capacity for reality testing, increased self-loathing)	Sudden changes in appearance (e.g., neglect)
Family history of child abuse; maltreatment		Hypersensitivity to criticism; overly self-critical
Poor coping skills; impulsive or aggressive tendencies		Inability to recover from loss; continuous and overwhelming feelings of grief, hopelessness
Barriers to mental health services		Increased isolation and withdrawal from activities
Physical illness		Drastic personality or behavioral changes; feelings of rage, revenge
Access to means of committing suicide		Increased impulsivity, recklessness, or risk-taking behaviors
Unwillingness to seek help (e.g., stigma, substance abuse)		Threatening to commit suicide, openly talking about death
Cultural and religious beliefs		Giving away personal belongings, making final arrangements
Local epidemics of suicide		Sudden and inexplicable improvements in behavior or appearance

Source: Data from Centers for Disease Control and Prevention, National Center for Injury Prevention and Control: Suicide: fact sheet risk factors: www.cdc.gov/ncipc/factsheets/suifacts.htm, accessed October 2007.

attempt to maintain identity and refuse defeat. Denial becomes problematic when it leads to self-neglect and the development of secondary conditions (5).

When addressing denial, clinicians need to be careful not to destroy a patient's hope. It is often effective to suggest to patients that rehabilitation and recovery occurs in stages. The equipment needed to improve independence today may or may not be needed in the future; however, the current goal is to make the patient as independent as possible given the present circumstances.

Anger is understood among mental health clinicians as the outward expression of frustration with oneself or one's situation and represents how the person is internally experiencing his or her disability. While the etiology of anger may be different for patients with spinal cord injury than those with traumatic brain injury, it functions as an attempt on the patient's part to control his or her situation or destiny. It usually develops as the patient becomes aware of and acknowledges the physical magnitude and implications of the injury (5). Anger is a normal response to a devastating situation and may be motivating for some patients. If untreated, the patient may continue to have difficulty relating to others and eventually become alienated from a larger social network.

Failed attempts to maintain a sense of control, motivation, and hope for the future can lead to helplessness. A prolonged period of imposed helplessness along with limited return of independent activities puts patients at risk for developing depressive symptoms. As patients begins to grieve the associated losses of SCI, they may feel defeated by its consequences and implications. Reported feelings of guilt for the effects injuries have on loved ones and the fear of becoming a burden to family members contribute to the development of depression. It is important to note that depressive symptoms are commonly seen throughout the adjustment process and are manifested by affective, cognitive, and behavioral symptoms; however major depressive disorder is not usually seen in early rehabilitation.

Anxiety is also a common reaction that is precipitated by the patient's perception of fear and vulnerability. This fear might be in response to internal or external dangers that are real or imagined. For SCI patients, fear may be the result of a perceived loss of control of physical function, medical complications, or weaning from the ventilator. Anxiety reactions can result from anticipated limitations of functioning in an inaccessible world and rejection by the able-bodied community. Consequences of anxiety symptoms range from reduced social participation and isolation to the possible disabling effects of panic disorder or PTSD. The prevalence of PTSD following spinal cord injury is questionable with most studies, suggesting an incidence of approximately 15%.

RISK FACTORS FOR PSYCHIATRIC SEQUELAE FOLLOWING SCI

Level of SCI

Recent studies have shown that level of injury is not a significant predictor of long-term adjustment (4). Overall, patients with high-level injuries, including patients who are ventilator-dependent, report similar life satisfaction as paraplegic patients. Patients with incomplete injuries (partial preservation of sensory or motor function below the level of injury) generally have better functional outcomes; however, many experience problems and complications similar to complete injuries. To a larger social community, these patients may not appear to be spinal cord injured because they might ambulate, sometimes without the use of adaptive equipment. These patients continue to be faced with the challenges of disability and often are faced with adjustment difficulties as a result of attempts to function "as if" the disability did not exist. The Patient's identity is hindered by a body that does not function as it had prior to injury, nor "as well as" those of able-bodied people. While there is no evidence to suggest that the level of spinal cord injury or greater functional limitations affects the extent of emotional adjustment, the secondary medical complications that accompany SCI (e.g., pain and spasticity, pressure sores, bowel and bladder dysfunction, urinary tract infections) do play a role in long-term adjustment and contribute to overall life satisfaction and quality of life.

Pain Syndromes

Pain management in the SCI population is a complex clinical issue, which is often linked to psychological symptoms. While the initial pain associated with SCI usually resolves within weeks, some patients are left with various forms of chronic pain and muscle spasticity, which can by themselves be disabling. Somatic complaints may be a real consequence of SCI; however, pain is not strictly a physical phenomenon. The perception of and response to pain involves a psychological component. The psychological and social consequences of SCI make management of somatic complaints more difficult for patients. Studies have shown that psychosocial stress is directly related to the reported severity of already existing pain symptoms.

Rehabilitation psychologists must consider the psychological, social, and biological aspects of pain when treating patients with SCI since chronic pain puts patients at risk for developing psychological symptoms (e.g., depression) and may lead to decreased independent behavior, less participation in daily activities, and social withdrawal.

Bowel/Bladder Care

The inability of an individual to control his or her bladder and bowel function is one of the most difficult consequences of SCI. Managing bowel programs, learning catheterization techniques, and fear of incontinence or finding an accessible bathroom can result in withdrawal from social activities and isolation. While urinary tract infections (UTIs) are a common occurrence after SCI and most patients are able to identify the presence of a UTI over time, the somatic symptoms that are associated with these infections, especially in patients with chronic UTIs, may leave patients feeling discouraged and interfere with daily functioning.

Pressure Ulcers

The development of pressure ulcers is another potential, unfortunate consequence of SCI. Because the treatment for pressure ulcers requires decreased sitting time and, at times, hospitalization, employment activities and opportunities for social interaction can be limited. These imposed restrictions can lead to poorer adjustment and depression. Psychological factors such as depression and substance abuse can lead to self-neglect and the increased risk of developing pressure sores, ultimately having a significant negative effect on the quality of life (6).

Premorbid Psychiatric Disorders

Individuals with premorbid psychiatric disorders pose a challenging task to rehabilitation professionals. Psychiatric disorders including schizophrenia, bipolar disorder, and substance-related disorders are considered risks factors for SCI and can complicate the course of rehabilitation and long-term adjustment (7). Prior to their injuries, individuals with these types of disorders often have a history of struggling to maintain independence, sustain motivation, and utilize adaptive coping skills. Maintaining therapeutic levels of psychopharmacologic treatment in these patients can be complicated after SCI and can limit discharge placement options.

Substance Abuse

Patients with a premorbid history of chemical addiction may be at greater risk of having difficulty adjusting to their disabilities given that individuals with substance abuse problems have been found to spend less time in recovery and rehabilitation activities. The risk of developing chemical addictions after SCI is of particular concern because of the medical and psychosocial implications associated with long-term adjustment. These individuals tend to show a greater incidence of depression, anger, hopelessness, and anxiety soon and during the first year after injury (see Chapter 30).

Personality Disorders

These encompass a spectrum of mental health disorders characterized by a maladaptive and pervasive pattern in the way in which an individual perceives, interprets, and responds to the world. Individuals with personality disorders share a common disruption in identity formation, which makes them prone to affect instability, impulsivity, and difficulty managing interpersonal and situational stressors. They are more at risk for the development of other psychiatric disorders (e.g., mood disorders, substance-related disorders), which have been found to be a risk for SCI and can complicate rehabilitation. While SCI patients face common interpersonal and affective issues, there is no evidence to suggest the existence of a SCI personality syndrome.

Coping styles have been defined as cognitive and behavioral responses to overwhelming emotions and thoughts that result from a traumatic experience and have been found to be a strong predictor of adjustment to disability. The development and maintenance of coping styles has been linked to internal locus of control and social support. Individuals who cope with a traumatic experience by actively and extensively processing their emotions and thoughts through support seeking, problem solving, or venting utilize problem-focused coping. Emotion-focused coping style is a more avoidant approach, which includes mental distancing and suppression of distressing emotions (e.g., blocking, ignoring, distracting). Studies indicate that both problem-focused and emotion-focused coping are useful in successful rehabilitation and adjustment since both promote mental control, allowing patients to experience greater internal locus of control and predictability over the emotional implications of SCI. Consistent use of emotion-focused coping, however, has been associated with prolonged distress, psychological symptoms (e.g., depression, anxiety), and poorer adjustment (8).

Social and Family Support

Both researchers and clinicians agree that social and family support is one of the most significant predictors of positive adjustment after SCI. Premorbid family functioning plays an important role in successful adjustment, just as family adjustment plays a significant role in a patient's adjustment and quality of life. Patients with strong family and social support tend to report fewer feelings of helplessness and demonstrate greater participation in activities. Research consistently shows that families with cohesiveness, good communication, and low levels of conflict before the injury demonstrate better adjustment after SCI. On the basis of these findings, it is important to include family members as part of the patient's treatment team and provide psychological support to the family during the progressive stages of rehabilitation.

Personality Factors

These have consistently been linked to adjustment to SCI. It has been suggested that preinjury personality traits determine a patient's cognitive and behavioral responses to SCI and contribute to his adaptation to the limitations imposed by the injury. For example, patients who are more extroverted and assertive tend to endorse more problem-focused coping and health-focused lifestyles. These individuals tend to demonstrate more positive adjustment and fewer medical complications (e.g., pressure sores). Individuals with more introverted personality styles defined by catastrophizing or excitement-seeking behaviors may be less conscientious than those characterized as assertive. These patients tend to display less energy, less determination, less social participation adjustment ,and the development of psychiatric symptoms (e.g., depression) (9).

Cognitive Impairment

It has been estimated that approximately 50% of spinal cord–injured patients will also experience some level of traumatic brain injury (10). This may be manifested by cognitive impairment, personality, and/or behavioral changes. It is important to note that these symptoms may also represent certain psychological states and clinical mental disorders. For example, delirium is manifested by a change in mental status, cognitive function, and at times behavior (e.g., agitation), but if medically treated, the symptoms often subside. Similarly, mood disorders (e.g., depression, bipolar disorder) have cognitive, affective, and behavioral symptoms that could be misdiagnosed as a traumatic brain injury. Rehabilitation professionals must be cognizant of both organic and psychiatric conditions when developing and applying treatment plans to address these symptoms.

PATIENT ASSESSMENT

During the clinical interview, physicians should inquire about events that led up to the injury (e.g., was alcohol involved), type of spinal cord injury, treatment rendered at the time of the injury, and the presence of concurrent traumatic brain injury. The clinician should also inquire about the level of injury and complete versus incomplete, medical problems since the injury (e.g., pressure ulcers, bowel/bladder care management, pain syndromes, kidney or liver disease), medications, allergies, and current psychosocial factors.

It is important to note the patient's preinjury psychiatric history, level of education, level of independence and occupation, extent of family and community support, as well as any history of substance abuse or pain syndromes. The clinical interview should also include an assessment for depression and anxiety and substance abuse.

Physical examination should include a cognitive assessment (e.g., orientation, memory recall—immediate/delayed, and concentration) and thorough neuro-musculoskeletal, dermatologic, and functional evaluation.

Rehabilitation psychologists and neuropsychologists are able to identify the patient's symptoms and coping strategies by conducting a thorough assessment of the patient's psychological, social, and cognitive functioning. The clinical interview provides the initial opportunity to develop therapeutic rapport and assist the patient through rehabilitation. Standardized measures (e.g., neuropsychological batteries, personality scales, depression/anxiety scales) can be used to confirm and quantify the presence of symptoms. Standardized measures should be used to complement the clinical interview or treatment with the goal of capturing a comprehensive view of the patient's presentation and functioning. Given the physical limitations of individuals with SCI, certain measures will be restricted, and the validity of their results should be interpreted with caution.

Depression

Signs of depression may be manifested by traditional symptoms (e.g., apathy, worthlessness, and sleep/appetite disturbance), behavioral symptoms (e.g., refusal to participate in treatment or perform activities independently), or cognitive symptoms (e.g., decreased attention/concentration, preoccupation with somatic complaints). Although there may be medical explanations for some of the physical and cognitive symptoms, it is often a sign to the clinician that the patient feels psychologically defeated by his limitations. The refusal to participate in treatment, however, reinforces dependency and victimization and ultimately contributes to the depression.

Early identification of depressive symptoms can prevent the onset of full clinical syndromes and help sustain motivation for rehabilitation (Table 24.2). The Beck Depressive Inventory (BDI-II, BDI Fast Screen for Medical Patients) provides an easy and effective way to screen for signs of depression. SCI patients respond well to and benefit from supportive counseling and participation in peer support groups.

For some patients, more significant symptoms of depression will begin to manifest after discharge from the hospital. Depressive symptoms may result from failed attempts at community reintegration, chronic pain, and secondary medical conditions associated with SCI. Rehabilitation professionals should be aware of the clinical signs of depression and provide referrals for outpatient psychological counseling as needed.

A suicide risk assessment should be routinely conducted upon every patient's initial evaluation and repeated as necessary. Elevated suicide risk can be assessed through measures, including the Beck Depression Inventory, Beck Hopelessness Inventory, and Beck Scale for Suicidal Ideation, all of which demonstrate a significant correlation with suicide risk (Figure 24.1) (2).

Table 24.2

Signs and Symptoms of Depression

Affective	Cognitive	Behavioral
Depressed mood	Negative view of self	Tearfulness
Sadness or emptiness	Negative view of future	Changes in sleep habits
Irritability	Decreased concentration	(insomnia or hypersomnia)
Apathy	Decreased ability to make	Psychomotor agitation or
Markedly diminished interest	decisions	retardation
or pleasure in activities	Decreased ability to solve	Fatigue
Feelings of worthlessness	problems	Loss of energy
Inappropriate guilt	Short-term memory loss	Change in appetite with
Helplessness	Suicide ideation	associated weight loss or
Hopelessness		gain

Source: Data from American Psychiatric Association: Diagnostic and Statistical Manual of Mental Disorders, Washington, DC, 1994, American Psychiatric Association.

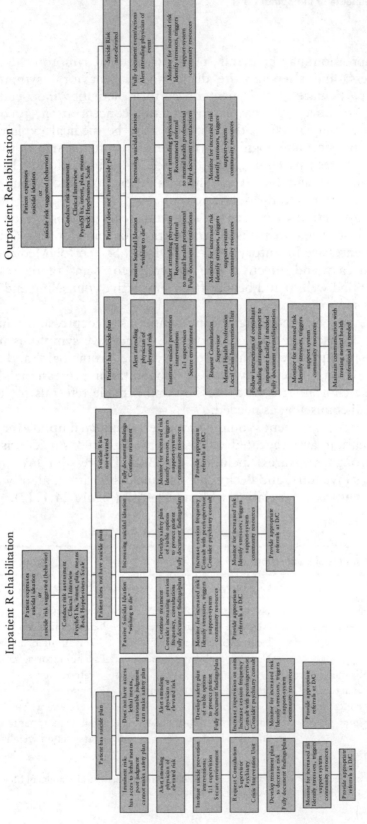

Figure 24.1. Suicide risk assessment and safety plan.

Anxiety

Anxiety symptoms can range from nervousness and sleep difficulty to panic or catastrophic reactions. Signs of panic attacks include accelerated heart rate, trembling, sweating or hot flashes, sensation of shortness of breath, chest pain, dizziness, nausea or gastrointestinal distress, derealization, fear of losing control or dying, and paresthesias. Other symptoms of anxiety include restlessness, psychomotor agitation, ruminative worry, catastrophization, and avoidance of anxiety-provoking stimuli. The Beck Anxiety Inventory (BAI) can help quantify specific anxiety symptoms and may help measure progress.

TREATMENT

Psychologists utilize a variety of interventions and techniques to ameliorate or contain symptoms and promote independence. The premise of rehabilitation psychology is an approach that focuses on education and teaching adaptive behaviors to deal with the problems of living, specifically designed for a disabled person in an able-bodied community, and return to the world outside of the hospital. The primary goal of counseling is to develop a patient's sense of control over a life that is characterized by a loss of independence and master the new rules that govern how his or her body functions. Because the patient's perception of his or her identity is frequently damaged, part of the task is redeveloping a sense of self and control in the face of challenging physical limitations (5).

Learning how to relate to others after SCI presents a significant challenge to many patients, especially if social and recreational activities are limited by transportation and accessibility. Patients are concerned about how others will perceive them and whether their peers and strangers will accept them. This is especially true for single patients who find dating and developing romantic relationships difficult because they feel that they are no longer desirable or have little to offer a partner.

Rehabilitation psychologists help disabled individuals learn how to develop a peer group that includes people who are able bodied as well as those who are physically challenged. Additionally, psychologists empower patients to teach others how to relate to them and how to respond to general misunderstandings and stereotypes some able-bodied people may hold about disabled persons. Through psychological counseling, individuals are able to redefine their sense of self into one that incorporates their disability without being consumed by it.

Psychological treatment of pain is built on the premise that a patient has the ability to control his or her level of "suffering." It has been argued that suffering is largely influenced by psychosocial variables in an individual's life; therefore, interventions need to be focused on addressing these psychosocial issues as well as the patient's emotional and behavioral reactions to pain (11). Cognitive-behavioral treatment (CBT) along with pharmacologic intervention and education has been shown to be highly effective in managing chronic pain

Table 24.3

Commonly Used Antidepressant Medications

Medication name	Indications	Dosage	General side effects	Potential SCI side effects	Drug interactions
Type: SSRI					
Sertraline (Zoloft)	Variety of depressive and anxiety disorders	50–200 mg/daily	Nausea, diarrhea, decreased appetite, headaches, insomnia, sweating, anxiety, dry mouth, fatigue, dizziness, tremor; may trigger mania in bipolar patients	May interfere with effectiveness of spasticity medications	May lead to mild elevations of TCAs and anti-arrhythmics
Fluoxetine (Prozac)		20–80 mg/daily; also available in delayed-release—once-weekly capsules			**Potential discontinuation syndrome** Fluoxetine may cause increased sedation and psychomotor impairment when used with benzodiazepines
Paroxetine (Paxil)		10–80 mg/daily			
Escitalopram (Lexapro)		10–30 mg/daily			
Type: Miscellaneous					
Venlafaxine (Effexor)	Depressive disorders: major depression, dysthymia, bipolar	75–375 mg/daily	Nausea, diarrhea, decreased appetite, headaches, insomnia, sweating, anxiety, dry mouth, fatigue, dizziness, tremor		May lead to serotonergic syndrome when used with monoamine oxidase inhibitors (MAOIs)
Bupropion (Wellbutrin)		75–450 mg/daily			
Trazodone (Desyrel)	Depressive disorders: insomnia	Depression: 200–600 mg/daily Insomnia: 25–200 mg qhs		May interfere with effectiveness of spasticity medications	Trazodone may potentiate the effects of other sedating medications
Duloxetine (Cymbalta)	Depressive disorders, chronic pain	20–60 mg bid			

	Indications	Dosage	Adverse effects	Clinical notes	Interactions
Type: Tricyclic (TCA)	Depressive and anxiety disorders; chronic pain; insomnia			May help manage neurogenic pain syndrome	Can lead to toxicity when used with Fluoxetine or Paroxetine
Amitriptyline (Elavil)		Depression: 150–250 mg/day	Dizziness, dry mouth, sleep disturbance, weight gain, sexual dysfunction		
		Chronic pain: 25–300 mg qhs	Adverse drug effects: anticholinergic effects, orthostatic hypotension		
Nortriptyline (Pamelor)		25–150 mg.day			
Type: Tetracyclic	Depressive disorders	15–45 mg qhs	Weight gain, dry mouth, fatigue, dizziness, orthostatic hypotension		Low liability of drug interactions
Mirtazapine (Remeron)					

Note: Information is based on average dosage; initial dosage may need to be lower and titrated to therapeutic level to reduce potential side effects or when treating elderly patients.

Source: Data retrieved from Albers, Hahn, and Reist: Handbook of Psychiatric Drugs, Laguna Hills, CA, 2005, Current Clinical Strategies Publishing.

symptoms in SCI patients. Specific CBT strategies including cognitive restructuring and decatastrophizing have been linked to improving self-efficacy and management of chronic pain. Other techniques include relaxation training, guided imagery, and biofeedback.

Education on the secondary medical issues associated with SCI along with supportive and problem-focused counseling improves patients' self-efficacy and sense of empowerment. As patients become more knowledgeable and gain mastery of their bodies, they tend to catastrophize less and employ proactive strategies to prevent potentially disabling secondary conditions.

Individuals with premorbid psychiatric disorders often require specialized psychological services. Psychopharmacological interventions need to be monitored closely since patients may respond differently to psychotropic medication after SCI. Behavioral treatment plans that focus on maintaining motivation and treatment compliance are usually necessary. This population requires extensive case management for discharge placement and outpatient services.

Depression

Psychopharmacologic interventions, especially selective serotonin reuptake inhibitor (SSRI) antidepressants, can help alleviate symptoms of depression and should be used when depressive symptoms interfere with motivation and participation in rehabilitation (Table 24.3).

Anxiety

Many patients respond well to cognitive behavioral strategies (relaxation techniques, guided imagery) (Table 24.4). Psychopharmacologic intervention (anxiolytics) may also assist in containing acute anxiety symptoms. Commonly used anxiolytics include short-acting benzodiazepines (Ativan, Xanax) and long-acting benzodiazepines (Klonopin, Valium). Physicians should use caution when prescribing short-acting benzodiazepines for extended periods of time because of their high risk of abuse. Long-acting benzodiazepines may also be useful in treating tone and spasticity in SCI patients. Anxiolytics can have a significant sedating effect and lead to changes in mental status in older patients and those taking multiple medications.

Patient Safety

1. Given the high prevalence of depression and increased risk of suicide in this population, it is important for clinicians to assess and reassess at initial and follow-up clinical visits.

Table 24.4

Relaxation and Guided Imagery Instructions

Guided imagery is convenient and simple. It involves a combination of breathing and relaxation techniques that can help you quickly and easily reduce tension in your body and manage stress. There are a number of CDs and cassette tapes available in most local bookstores to assist you with these techniques.

Recommend time: 0–15 minutes/session
Frequency: 2–3 times/week

1. Get into a comfortable position (lying down, sitting in a chair, lights dimmed or shut off, eyes closed, distractions from external noise removed). Some may feel more comfortable with soft music (nature sounds, classical music) in the background.
2. Use diaphragmatic (deep breathing/belly breathing) to take in as much air through your nose as you can. Hold it for 3 seconds and slowly exhale through your mouth. Focus on breathing in calm and tranquility and breathing out stress/pain. Practice inhaling/exhaling several times, breathing relaxation into each part of your body. Start with your head and work toward to your toes. With each inhale; breathe relaxation and comfort into each part of your body. With each exhale release any tension, stress, or pain.
3. Once relaxed, begin to envision yourself in the most relaxing environment you can imagine. For some it may be a sandy beach on a tropical island with the sun gently warming your skin, or floating in the cool, clear waters with the smell of the sea in the air; for others it might a snowcapped mountain with a cool winter breeze brushing across your face and the smell of pine in the air.
4. As you imagine the scene, try to involve all of your senses. How does it look? How does it feel? What does it smell like? What do you hear?
5. Continue to practice your breathing and visualization, going deeper and deeper into a state of relaxation. In this state, all of your stresses, pain, and difficulties are far away. Stay in this state as long as you like. When you are ready to come back to reality, count back from twenty (continuing to breathe deeply). As you come back, tell yourself that when you get to "one" you will be at peace, calm, alert, refreshed and ready to enjoy the rest of your day.

2. Abrupt discontinuation or rapid titrating down (>10 mg increments) of SSRIs can result in SSRI siscontinuation ayndrome. Symptoms may start within 48 hours and include severe flu-like symptoms: headache, diarrhea, nausea, vomiting, chills, dizziness, and fatigue. Insomnia, agitation, impaired concentration, vivid dreams, depersonalization, irritability, and suicidal thoughts may also occur. Symptoms can last from one to several weeks.
3. Cognitive impairment can be common after SCI and can adversely affect both medical and psychological treatments. Clinicians should assess for cognitive impairment in SCI patients.

Patient Education

1. Anger management: Empathic listening, normalizing, teaching effective coping and communication strategies and verbal deescalation techniques are often effective interventions in managing expressions of anger (Table 24.5).
2. Adjustment after SCI:
   a. Identify patient's coping styles and resources. Discuss other difficult events they have encountered and how they got through them.
   b. Rehabilitation and adjustment occurs in stages and overtime: "Try to be patient with yourself and understand that physical and emotion healing comes with time."
   c. Seek support of family and friends: "Family and good friends don't evaluate your worth by what you are physically capable of doing."
   d. Watch for overgeneralizations, catastrophizations, and misattributions: "Doing things differently than before does not mean that you cannot do them or do them worse than you used to."
   e. Alert the patient that professional help is available and asking for it not a sign of weakness.

Table 24.5

Anger Management Strategies

COSTS
- Educating patient on the physical, emotional, interpersonal, and individual costs of anger

TRIGGERS
- Identifying and understanding triggers of anger and its perceived payoffs

TRACKING
- Keep an anger log (stressor, triggers, anger rating, behavior/response, outcome)

TECHNIQUES
- Relaxation techniques (see relaxation/guided imagery instructions)
- Written contract: 24-hour commitment to "act" calm
- What to do when you get angry:
  o Delay any response; notice the emotion, accept it
  o Act the opposite (smile instead of frown, speak softly rather than loudly, relax instead of tighten, disengage rather than attack, empathize rather than judge)
- Manage anger distortions:
  o Blaming
  o Catastrophizing
  o Global labeling
  o Misattributions
  o Overgeneralization
  o Demanding/Commanding

For specific exercises, see McKay M, Rogers R. The Anger Control Workbook. Oakland, CA: New Harbinger, 2000.

REFERENCES

1. McKinley W, Santos K, Meade M, Brook K. Incidence and outcomes of spinal cord clinical syndromes. J Spinal Cord Med 2007; 30(3):215–224.
2. Elliott TR, Herrick SM, Witty TE, et al. Social support and depression following spinal cord injury. Rehabil Psychol 1992; 37:37–48.
3. Heinemann AW. Spinal cord injury. In: Goreczny AJ, ed. Handbook of Health and Rehabilitation Psychology. New York: Plenum Press, 1995.
4. Gill M. Psychosocial implications of spinal cord injury. Crit Care Nurs Q 1999; 22(2):1–7.
5. Moore AD, Patterson DR. Psychological intervention with spinal cord injured patients: promoting control out of dependence. SCI Psychosoc Process 1993; 6:2–8.
6. Krause JS. Skin sores after spinal cord injury: relationship to life adjustment. Spinal Cord 1988; 36:51–60.
7. Fullerton DT, Harvey RF, Klein MH, Howell T. Psychiatric disorders in patients with spinal cord injury. Arch Gen Psychiatry 1981; 38(12):1369–1371.
8. Kennedy P, Marsh N, Lowe R, et al. A longitudinal analysis of psychological impact and coping strategies following spinal cord injury. Br J Health Psychol 2000; 5:157–172.
9. Rohe DE, Krause JS. The five-factor model of personality: findings in males with spinal cord injury. Assessment 1999; 6:203–214.
10. Fichtenbaum J, Kirshblum S. Psychological adaptation to spinal cord injury. In: Kirshblum S, Campagnolo DI, DeLisa JS, eds. Spinal Cord Injury Medicine. Philadelphia: Lippincott Williams & Wilkins, 2002.
11. Widerstrom-Noga EG, Felipe-Cuervo E, Yezierski RP. Chronic pain after spinal cord injury: interference with sleep and daily activities. Arch Phys Med Rehabil 2001; 82:1571–1577.

25 | Neuropsychiatric Sequelae of the Brain-Injured Adult

Monique Tremaine
Kimberly McGuire

Traumatic and acquired brain injuries have lasting physical, cognitive, emotional, behavioral, and psychosocial consequences that require intervention beyond acute stages. The extent of physical and neuropsychological involvement will vary based on preinjury factors such as health and psychological coping style as well as postinjury factors such as degree of impairment and financial and supportive resources. Timely and consistent intervention should be multidisciplinary in scope and include oversight from neurology, physiatry, neuropsychology, and physical, occupational, speech, and cognitive rehabilitation therapies to ensure an optimal return to community and functional environments. Apart from medical stabilization and survival, successful recovery from a brain injury should be measured by level of personal acceptance of injury and ability to reintegrate into the community in a way that is meaningful to the survivor.

Traumatic brain injury (TBI) can result from any sudden impact to the brain resulting in temporary or long-term neurologic, cognitive, or functional impairment. At least 1.4 million people in the United States sustain a TBI annually, resulting in 50,000 annual fatalities and 235,000 hospitalizations. Motor vehicle accidents and falls are the most common causes of TBI, accounting for 48% of reported injuries, while assault accounts for 11% of injuries (1). Notably, the incidence of combat-related brain injuries has recently received increased attention.

According to the literature, males are about three to four times more likely to sustain a TBI than females, although this figure may be inflated due to underreporting of TBI in female victims of domestic violence. TBI is most common in persons between the ages of 15 and 24 and in persons over age 75. Alcohol is associated with up to half of all reported accidents.

Cerebral vascular accident (CVA; stroke) is a disease with substantial physical and psychosocial implications. Stroke has a prevalence of 2.6% in the U.S. population, amounting to approximately 5.7 million individuals. Stroke occurs in approximately 700,000 individuals annually in the United States, and about two thirds of individuals will receive rehabilitation services. Stroke tends to affect men at younger ages and women at older ages and is the number three cause of death in the United States, behind heart disease and cancer (2).

Approximately 400,000 people have been diagnosed with multiple sclerosis (MS) in the United States (3). Symptoms often begin to appear in people in their twenties and thirties, with a mean age of 32 for symptom onset. Women are more commonly affected than men. MS occurs with increased frequency in higher latitudes and is more common in Caucasians (3). Cognitive dysfunction in MS occurs in approximately 50–60 % of individuals, and impairment is unpredictable in terms of onset and severity (4,5).

Brain injuries can be broadly divided into two groups: traumatic (TBI) and acquired (CVA, MS). In traumatic brain injury, diffuse axonal injury (DAI) rather than focal injury will have the most global effect on cognition. Individuals with mild TBI may not seek medical attention and are often released from emergency services upon negative radiologic findings. As many as 50% of patients with concussion may develop postconcussion symptoms (6). The diagnosis is often made within a week to 3 months of the initial trauma (see Table 25.1). Formal diagnosis may be complicated by an interaction between physiologic and psychological factors. These symptoms are often first reported to the primary care physician. Moderate (GCS = 9–12) to severe (GCS 3–8) traumatic brain injury often results in a cascade of primary phenomena associated with diffuse axonal injury such as hematoma and cerebral edema, which can result in increased intracranial pressure (ICP).

Cognitive impairment is often associated with stroke and will present somewhat differently based on the location of the stroke. Left hemispheric stroke typically results in expressive or receptive language impairment, but may also affect more global skill areas such as memory, attention, and executive functioning. Right hemispheric stroke tends to result in nonverbal impairment such as impairment of visual attention and spatial reasoning, flattening of the emotional response to self and others, as well as impairment in memory, auditory attention, and executive functioning.

Table 25.1

Symptoms Commonly Reported in Postconcussion Syndrome		
Physical	Emotional	Cognitive
Headache	Irritability	Poor concentration
Neck pain	Mood swings	Memory deficits
Dizziness	Anxiety	Mental fatigue
Vertigo	Depression	Misplacing items, forgetting appointments, names, etc.)

Table 25.2

Typical Areas of Cognitive Impairment in Multiple Sclerosis

Working memory	Acquisition of information	Attention and processing speed	New learning/ episodic memory	Executive functioning
Inability to hold information for 15–20 seconds for further processing	Impaired ability to encode and consolidate information for storage in the brain	Impaired sustained and divided attention Slower processing speed	Poor recent memory	Impaired planning, anticipation, self-monitoring Impaired shifting cognitive set in response to environmental demands

As stated earlier, cognitive dysfunction in MS occurs in approximately 50–60 % of individuals, and similar to other symptoms of MS, cognitive impairment is unpredictable in terms of onset and severity (5). It is important to remember that an individual's intellect is not affected by the cognitive impairment. Brain functions such as attention and concentration that are required for behavioral efficiency and activation of the intellect are most affected.

Cognitive impairment in MS tends to be in the areas of working memory, information, acquisition, divided and sustained attention, information processing speed, new learning, and executive functioning. Table 25.2 provides details regarding the functions of these cognitive areas.

ANATOMY AND PHYSIOLOGY

Often, both traumatic and acquired brain injury will involve a disruption of the neural circuitry connecting the primitive limbic centers, or emotional centers, of the brain with the more evolved neocortex and, specifically, the frontal lobes of the brain. The intricately webbed nerve tracts and fiber bundles of the frontal lobes allow us to plan for the future, anticipate its outcomes, strategize, and alter our strategies when they fail. These pathways allow us to organize information from the internal and external environment and to formulate responsive, goal-directed behavior. Our ability to self-regulate and monitor behavior, decide when to act and when to hold back, evaluate the perspective of another, and empathize and cooperate with others is essential to our survival. These abilities were the latest to develop in human evolution and, unfortunately, the most vulnerable to cerebral insult or injury. These critical cognitive abilities are collectively known as executive functioning and are typically associated with the frontal lobes of the brain.

Cognitive sequelea of brain injury are often associated with impairment of the frontal lobes. Frontally mediated connections with specific posterior cortical, thalamic, limbic, and basal ganglia structures play a critical role in the expression of complex behavioral patterns. Disruption of frontal systems can result from a number of factors, including disruption within cortical frontal pathways, disruption of pathways connecting lower brain structures with the frontal lobes, white matter lesions disrupting frontal connections, direct contusion, countercoup injury, shearing forces, cardiovascular lesions disrupting the flow of blood and oxygen to the brain, and diffuse axonal injury resulting from traumatic brain injury, which indiscriminately effects multiple frontal networks and pathways.

PATIENT ASSESSMENT

Organic syndromes resulting from brain injury can be as unique and diverse as the individuals who sustain them. While there are a number of common symptomatic presentations following brain injury, the cognitive and behavioral changes following injury are highly individualized and are the sum of multiple pre- and postinjury factors. When assessing the brain-injured patient, one must consider that the postinjury behavioral presentation does not exist in isolation of preinjury personality, coping style, pathology, family structure, age, level of education, intelligence, and lifestyle habits. These previously existing factors will interact with the type and severity of brain injury, the localization of greatest impact, and the subjective experience of cognitive sequelea.

Upon evaluation of the brain-injured patient, an awareness of these preinjury factors can be useful. It is also useful to adjust the communication style to fit the cognitive and demographic level of the patient (see Table 25.3).

In milder injuries and pathologies it may be difficult to distinguish cognitive versus psychological symptoms. Patients may offer a vague description of symptomatolgy that may not be useful in differential diagnosis. Significant

Table 25.3

Tips on Communicating with Brain-Injured Adults

For milder injuries	For moderate to severe injuries
Ask clear, concise, and directive questions	State your name and why you are there
Avoid open-ended questions	Reorient the patient to place and situation
Speak slowly, pausing between concepts or ideas	Speak in a soothing manner to avoid agitation
Ask the patient to repeat any instructions or directives to ensure understanding	Do not allow more than one person to speak at a time
Redirect confrontive or hyperverbose patients	Try to reduce any external noise or distraction (TV, open doors)
Validate the patient's experience	Try not to reason or rationalize with a patient who is confused or disoriented
	State what you are doing and why in a step-by-step manner
	Allow the patient appropriate time to respond
	Give only one command or directive at a time

radiologic findings such as hemorrhaging and ischemic changes are valuable in assessing whether there has been a brain injury, but in the case of TBI much of the damage occurs at the cellular level and is not readily detected by magnetic resonance imaging (MRI) or computed tomography (CT). Any significant loss of consciousness or posttraumatic amnesia may be useful in differential diagnosis. Additional studies such as electroencephalogram (EEG) may also be useful if the patient is describing seizure-like activity. Also, if there has been an unexplained deterioration in cognitive status, it may be useful to conduct a metabolic study.

To examine cognitive or mental status, some physicians use a screening tool such as the Mini Mental Status Evaluation, which will evaluate very basic orientation, attention, memory, and visual spatial skills. It is important to note that this is only a screening tool that will detect injury at more moderate to severe levels. A brief but careful interview may help clarify diagnostic issues. Psychological testing, such as the Beck Depression Inventory–Fast Screen is useful in detecting disorders of depression and is helpful because it does not have a focus on vegetative symptoms. If these screening measures are administered early on and mood disorders are detected, they can be appropriately treated in an effort to maximize the recovery process (see Table 25.4).

Should the patient endorse any of the cognitive or psychological symptoms listed in Table 25.5, they should be referred for a neuropsychological evaluation. A neuropsychological evaluation will more thoroughly assess an individual's strengths and weaknesses in various brain processes, such as attention, concentration, receiving information (input), processing information, output of information, memory, problem solving, and executive functioning (e.g., planning, organizing, divided attention, multitasking). A careful evaluation will compare the patient's current level of functioning with estimated preinjury level of intellectual, psychological, cognitive, and adaptive functioning. The evaluation should be conducted by a licensed neuropsychologist. This level of training and expertise allows cofactors such as depression, anxiety, and/or fatigue to be discerned from actual cognitive deficits related to brain injury. Based on the results of the evaluation, recommendations for further intervention can be made. Referring a patient for a neuropsychological evaluation is not meant to replace other treatments but to complement and assist with treatment recommendations.

TREATMENT

The focus of an *inpatient* rehabilitation setting can easily highlight improving physical function without consistent incorporation of the neuropsychological and social factors. Therefore, an interdisciplinary team approach is essential in the recovery process from TBI, stroke, and MS exacerbations (see Tables 25.5 and 25.6). Families are not often equipped to manage patients with cognitive and psychological dysfunction, as they often lack an understanding of the cognitive deficits and psychosocial adjustment issues that patients face. It is

Table 25.4

Diagnostic Interview for Differential Diagnosis of Cognitive Versus Psychological Sequelae

History	Cognitive	Emotional
Date of injury	Have you noticed any changes in your thinking?	Have you noticed any personality or mood changes since the injury?
Field Glasgow Coma Scale (GCS)	**Attention/Executive Dysfunction** Ensure basic orientation is intact	**Depression** Are you any more or less emotional than before/apathetic?
Duration of loss of consciousness or altered consciousness	Have you resumed your daily routine? Do you have any difficulty multitasking? Do you have difficulty focusing when you are reading? Does your attention wander in conversation?	Has your mood changed? Do you have episodes of angry behavior? Have you had any feelings of hopelessness or despair?
Posttraumatic amnesia	Do you frequently lose or misplace personal items? Do you lose track of what you are doing? Are you less organized?	Do you cry more frequently? Do you have thoughts of suicide?
Acute intervention	Have you gotten lost while driving? Do you have any difficulty getting motivated? Do you say things that you shouldn't say?	**Anxiety** Do you feel nervous much of the time? Are you fearful of the worst happening?
Radiological findings: CT, MRI, EEG, brain SPECT	**Language** Has your voice changed?	Does worry keep you awake at night? Do you have frequent physical symptoms?
Seizures	Do you have trouble finding words or names?	
Mental status upon awakening	Do you have difficulty organizing your thoughts when speaking?	
Physical status upon awakening	Do you speak too much or too little?	

Beck Depression Inventory–Fast Screen

Interview family

Metabolic studies

Multiple Sclerosis Neuropsychological Questionnaire (MSNQ); MS-specific, self and informant versions

Assess for substance abuse

Memory
Are you forgetting to take medications?
Are you forgetting appointments?
Do you forget conversations?
Do you have any difficulty getting motivated?
Do you say things that you shouldn't say?
Do you ask repetitive questions?

Physical
Have you lost your sense of taste or smell?
Do you have headaches, vertigo, or nausea?
Has your vision changed?
Do you hear ringing sounds in your ears?
Do you have difficulty sleeping?
Do you sleep more or less than before?

Posttraumatic Stress
Are you having nightmares?
Are you having obsessive thoughts about the accident?
Do you frequently attempt to recall memory lost at the time of the accident?
Does anger at persons involved in the incident preoccupy you?

Obsessive-Compulsive
Are you experiencing recurrent and distressing thoughts and images?
Are your worries incongruent with real life problems or irrational?
Are you unable to suppress these thoughts?
Do you engage in repetitive behaviors that serve no purpose?

Table 25.5

Interdisciplinary Team Approach: Disciplines and Areas of Specialty

Speech therapy	Occupational therapy	Physical therapy	Multidisciplinary cognitive therapy	Psychology and neuropsychology
Expressive and receptive language deficits Reading, writing Dysphagia Memory books, planners	Fine motor impairment Visual spatial impairment Activities of daily living Medication management Hand therapy	Ambulation Vestibular therapy Assistive physical devices Spasticity management	Higher-order cognitive skills such as functional problem solving, reasoning, memory, executive functioning Vocational counseling Predriving evaluation Case management for access to community and federal resources Interest and skill development Introduction to assistive devices, palm pilots, planners	Psychosocial adjustment Individual psychotherapy Family therapy Neuropsychological evaluation

Table 25.6

Pertinent History and Physical Examination Questions for Patients with MS and Stroke

1. Has the patient been sleeping well? Difficulty falling asleep? Difficulty staying asleep? Awakens from sleep feeling rested? History of sleep problems? Awakens during the night with worrying thoughts?
2. Has the patient been having difficulty following conversations?
3. Does the patient decline social invitations due to cognitive impairments?
4. Have family or friends stated that they have noticed changes in the patient's interactions with them?
5. Ask about substance abuse or use currently or historically.
6. (MS specific): Is the patient using supplements, vitamins, or marijuana to assist with pain and/or appetite management?
7. Ask about depression, anxiety, and suicidal thoughts.

important to educate the patient and caregiver(s) on the cognitive and behavioral changes following TBI, stroke, and MS exacerbations to maximize the recovery process, prevent further injury, and facilitate a successful transition to the community (see Table 25.7).

Often patients will exhibit a healthy amount of denial. It is important to not confront the denial directly, especially if it is cognitive denial. Cognitive denial

Table 25.7

Important Information to Disseminate to Patients and Caregivers: MS and Stroke

Multiple sclerosis	Stroke
Number of lesions does not always correspond with level of cognitive and/or physical decline	Reduce stimuli
Depression and fatigue are common	Limit visitors to two at a time during the acute recovery phase
This is an unpredictable disease process	Turn TV off while talking with patient during the acute recovery phase
This disease is degenerative in nature	Allow extra time for responses from the patient
The patient will not die from MS	Do not always provide the answers for the patient—instead try to guide the process for them to find the answer
Frequent vague suicidal thoughts common	

can be healthy if it motivates an individual to participate in treatment recommendations. For example, a patient with MS who has recently experienced a decline in ambulation and is in need of a walker might make a statement such as: "I know I will get back to walking without any walker [assistive device]." This belief [even if factually untrue] motivates the individual to participate in learning to ambulate with the walker; therefore, it would *not* prove beneficial to confront this type of denial. Behavioral denial can be more problematic. For example, if this same patient with MS made the above-mentioned statement and decided to *not learn* to ambulate with a walker because he or she was going to recover to the point of ambulating without an assistive device, this type of denial interferes with effective treatment and progress. Therefore, if behavioral denial is interfering with the recovery process, the patient can be referred for psychological intervention.

Cognitive rehabilitation (CR) that is neuropsychologically driven, evidence based, and holistic in practice can assist patients to navigate the stages of recovery, return to productive living, and improve quality of life. CR serves to augment the natural healing process and promote the reemergence of cognitive skills, as well as to provide skilled training in adaptive strategies across naturalistic and functional settings. Special attention should be paid to behavior management, social skills training, improving insight and awareness, and, ultimately, long-term psychosocial adjustment. CR should utilize a client-, family-, and rehabilitation team–centered approach to combine clinical expertise and compassionate care to assist clients with brain injury in resuming meaningful and productive lives (see Table 25.8).

Table 25.8

Recommendations for the Compensation and Improvement of Cognitive Impairments

Activities of Daily Living
- Keep the environment free of distraction
- Rely on structure, routine, and consistency
- Use a planner to plan a weekly schedule
- Break up tasks into small parts
- Rehearse common tasks and social interactions
- Take frequent rest periods throughout the day
- Weekly schedule should include activities of daily living (ADLs), rest periods, cognitive activities
- Use a stopwatch system/pillbox to remember medications
- Use visual cues for ADLs (checklists for sequencing steps)
- Gradually introduce more challenging settings such as shopping malls, family gatherings

Cognitive Activities
- Card games (rummy)
- Word search puzzles
- Legos games
- Computer games such as "Brain Age" by Gameboy
- Reading
- Audit a college or community class

PSYCHIATRIC SYNDROMES

It is important to address cognitive impairment, yet it is often the psychosocial aspects of TBI, stroke, and MS that tend to be more disabling for patients. Psychiatric symptoms often accompany traumatic and acquired brain injury, with depression being the most common. There is debate as to whether the injury itself can result in depression or whether the depression is the result of the injury. Post–brain injury personality disturbance can therefore be divided into three basic categories as follows: (1) neuropsychologically mediated disturbances as a direct consequence of brain injury, (2) adjustment disturbances as an indirect effect of brain injury, and (3) exaggeration of preexisting personality and psychiatric disturbance (7). See Table 25.9 to assist in identification and treatment of psychiatric syndromes.

Neuropsychological disturbances occurring as a direct result of organic impairment tend to have a sudden onset and symptoms and may not congruent with mood. One such syndrome is pseudobulbar affective syndrome (PBA), also known as involuntary emotional expression disorder (IEED), which affects a small percentage of individuals with MS and CVA. The symptoms are uncontrollable laughter and/or crying that appear to have little or no relationships to current mood or events. PBA/IEED differs from major depressive disorder (MDD) in that symptoms of PBA/IEED are often sudden, unpredictable, and contrary to the individual's mood (8).

Table 25.9

Mental Health Considerations in Individuals Diagnosed with Multiple Sclerosis

Mental health diagnosis	Lifetime prevalence (%)	Symptoms/Diagnostic criteria	Treatment recommendations
Major depressive disorder	42–50	1. Significant changes in appetite 2. Significant changes in weight 3. Significant changes in sleeping patterns 4. Isolative 5. Feelings of worthlessness, hopelessness, or helplessness 6. Recurrent thoughts of dying 7. Depressed mood on more days than not 8. Diminished interest in previously pleasurable activities 9. Difficulty focusing and concentrating	Combination of antidepressants and psychotherapy
Involuntary emotional expressive disorder/pseudo-bulbar affect	10	Uncontrollable laughter and/or crying that have little to no relationship to events	Psychotropic medications Type SSRI Citalopram (Celexa) Escitalopram (Lexapro) Sertraline (Zoloft) Fluoxetine (Prozac) Paroxetine (Paxil)
Anxiety disorders	36	Worrying thoughts Racing thoughts Increased heart rate Increased sweating rate	Psychotherapy Psychotropic medications (e.g., Apralozam [Xanax], Lorazepam [Ativan], or SSRIs)
Bipolar disorder	15	Abnormally elevated mood along with periods of depression	Combination of psychotherapy and psychotropic medications
Psychosis	Unavailable	Auditory, visual, or tactile hallucinations in the absence of dementia or delirium	Antipsychotic medications

Note: Medications highlighted in this table are those that are often prescribed. There are additional medications that physicians might choose to prescribe.

Depression

Organically mediated depression is commonly associated with stroke. MDD will present as apathy and refusal to participate in therapeutic treatments. Major depression is diagnosed with a greater frequency immediately following a left hemispheric stroke, particularly in patients with left frontal lesions (9). Studies indicate that depression in patients with left frontal lesions had improved at 2-year follow-up, indicating organicity, whereas stroke patients who were not initially depressed showed a deterioration in mood state at 2-year follow-up, indicating adjustment difficulty (10). Poststroke depression can be a result of cerebral insult, psychosocial adjustment issues that arise afterward, or a combination of both factors. The National Institute of Mental Health estimates that 10–27% of individuals will experience a MDD and 15–40% will experience some symptoms of depression within 2 months after a stroke (11). It is important to assess the size and location of the stroke as well as the individual's psychiatric history when considering a diagnosis of poststroke depression. Assessing an individual's ability to cope with stressful situations will also help in accurately diagnosing and treating poststroke depression.

Other studies have also attempted to correlate depression in relation to brain region in TBI populations with some suggestion that depression occurs to a greater extent in TBI persons with left dorsolateral frontal lesions/basal ganglia lesions and TBI persons with parietal-occipital and right hemispheric lesions (12).

While there is some suggestion of injury-induced depression, multiple factors contribute to depression, including neurochemical factors, cognitively mediated search and selection mechanisms to explore alternative solutions to problems, negative and inaccurate beliefs about the self, particularly with regard to wholeness, and what might be considered a normal adjustment reaction to a life-changing event. Symptoms of depression that arise as a result of psychological or social adjustment to the situation tend to have an identifiable trigger, such as individuals being concerned about their decreased independence, the role changes they are experiencing in their personal lives, etc. Often such symptoms occur in the months or years following the CVA or TBI or MS diagnosis. For example, brain injury patients did not report greater levels of depression than orthopedic controls at 6 months postinjury, though report of depression in brain injury populations increased at 1-, 2-, and 3-year follow-up (13).

Adjustment Reactions

Adjustment reactions tend to occur when insight into behavior, deficit, and life consequences begins to emerge. Most people build their goals, interests, and even personality around cognitive skills and abilities. When people find themselves unable to process, retain, and retrieve information in the way they are accustomed, they may feel compromised and ineffective, leading to a loss of perceived self-sufficiency and self-esteem. This is often the cause of depression in individuals with MS who typically are challenged with an uncertain future regarding disease progression.

It is generally suggested in the literature that individuals with neurologic disorders are at increased risk for suicide, and the increased risk is correlated with depression, social isolation, feelings of hopelessness or helplessness, cognitive impairment, moderate physical disability, recent loss(es), younger age (under 60), and psychiatric history (14) (see Chapter 24).

Preexisting Personality and Psychiatric Disturbances

Individuals with preexisting personality and psychiatric disturbance may fail to regulate pathology following acquired or traumatic brain injury, resulting in an exaggeration of premorbid conditions. This is often the case in postconcussion syndrome and mild TBI. This may be a result of suppression of primitive coping and defensiveness and inability to utilize more sophisticated defense mechanisms, resulting in a flooding of previously controlled pathology as a consequence of injury.

These patients should be referred for pharmacologic intervention. It is equally critical that such patients be referred for neuropsychological evaluation to determine the nature and extent of cognitive and psychological involvement. Immediate psychological and behavioral intervention may prevent chronic cognitive and behavioral dysfunction. For example, prior to injury, obsessive-compulsive disorder (OCD) personality traits may have contributed to organization and overall individual success; following brain injury, such individuals may be unable to disengage from repetitive, mundane, and dysfunctional behaviors in exchange for more adaptive behaviors.

To the untrained observer, the above-mentioned syndromes are often mistaken for psychiatric symptoms. This can lead to misdiagnosis, prescription of improper medications, and misjudgment of character. Conversely, preexisting psychiatric symptoms may become exaggerated. Finally new psycho-diagnostic syndromes such as depression and posttraumatic stress may emerge. Careful assessment and diagnosis can eliminate such confusion.

Patient Safety

1. Patients with brain injury should be screened for suicidal ideation and depression.
2. Patients with preexisting personality and psychiatric disturbances may fail to regulate pathology following acquired or traumatic brain injury, resulting in an exaggeration of premorbid conditions.

Patient Education

Persons with mild traumatic brain injury or concussion may not immediately seek emergency attention and often follow up with their family physician. In some cases, the chemical and structural process that follows a concussion may result in a cascade of events, resulting in further damage. Persistence of symptoms such as vomiting, worsening headache, ringing in the ears (tinnitus), drowsiness, unequal pupil size, and increasing disorientation may be a sign of increasing intracranial pressure. Consequently, worsening symptoms in the 24- to 72-hour period after the event warrant immediate medical attention. These symptoms should be discussed with patients.

Patients and families should also be informed about potential behavioral changes and management techniques as well as safety and supervision needs, particularly those with more moderate to severe cognitive deficits. Many patients will need medical clearance before returning to driving and work. In more moderate injuries, 24-hour supervision may be required for safety. Patients with severe injuries may not benefit from intensive rehabilitation settings and may be better served by adult day treatment or in home services. Families should be provided with basic information on managing disruptive behaviors at home (see Table 25.10).

It is important to stress that the patient stay mentally engaged and active. Structure and repetition are key to successful recovery. Encourage the patient and caregiver to use a weekly planner to plan a schedule of activity with intermittent rest periods. Included should be basic activities of daily living plus 3–4 hours of cognitive activity per day. See Table 25.10 for tips for in-home cognitive activities.

Table 25.10

Managing Disruptive Behaviors at Home and in the Community

	Confabulation	Disinhibition	Aggression	Apathy
Avoid arguing or rationalizing			x	
Provide distraction	x	x	x	
Give step-by-step directives			x	x
Speak in soothing tones			x	x
Correct erroneous information	x	x		x
Avoid open-ended questions	x		x	x
Provide feedback on behavior	x	x	x	x
Avoid labels such as lazy, rude, stubborn	x	x	x	x
Do not take behavior personally	x	x	x	x

Table 25.10 (*Continued*)

Attempt to manage your anxiety when dealing with the patient	x	x	x	x
Frequently reorient the patient	x		x	
Keep environment free of distraction			x	
Avoid talking to the patient in a condescending manner	x	x	x	x
Agree on a nonverbal signal such as a hand gesture that will alert the patient to inappropriate behavior	x	x		

REFERENCES

1. Centers for Disease Control and Prevention. January 2006 Update: Traumatic Brain Injuries in the United States: Emergency Department Visits, Hospitalizations, and Deaths. Centers for Disease Control and Prevention, 2006.
2. American Heart Association. Heart Disease and Stroke Statistics—2008 Update. Dallas, TX: American Heart Association. 2008.
3. National Multiple Sclerosis. Multiple Sclerosis Information Sourcebook. Prognosis, 2006. Retrieved January 2, 2007, from www.nationalmssociety.org.
4. DeLuca J. What we know about cognitive changes in multiple sclerosis. In: LaRocca N, Kalb R, eds. Multiple Sclerosis: Understanding the Cognitive Challenges: New York: Demos Medical Publishing, 2006.
5. LaRocca N, Sorensen P. Cognition. In: Kalb RC, ed. Multiple Sclerosis, 3rd ed. New York: Demos Medical Publishing, 2004.
6. Bazarian J, Atabaki S. Predicting postconcussion syndrome after minor traumatic brain injury. Acad Emerg Med 2001; 8(8):788–795.
7. Prigatano G. Personality disturbances: theoretical perspectives. In: Principles of Neuropsychological Rehabilitation. New York: Oxford University Press, 1999:118–147.
8. LaRocca N. Stress and emotional issues. In: Kalb RC, ed. Multiple Sclerosis, 3rd ed. New York: Demos Medical Publishing, 2004.
9. Robinson R, Price T. Post-stroke depression disorders: a follow-up study of 103 patients. Stroke 1982; 13:635–641.
10. Robinson R, Bolduc P, Price T. A two-year longitudinal study of post-stroke depression: diagnosis and outcome at one and two years. Stroke 1987; 18:837–843.
11. National Institute of Neurological Disorders and Stroke, www.ninds.nih.gov/disorders/stroke/poststrokerehab.htm, retrieved Dec 31, 2007.
12. Federoff J, Starkstein S, Forrester A, et al. Depression in patients with acute traumatic brain injury. Am J Psychiatry 1992; 149:918–923.
13. Godfrey H, Partiridge F, Knight R. Course of insight disorder and emotional dysfunction following closed head injury: a controlled cross sectional follow up study. J Clin Exp Neuropsychol 1993; 15(4):503–515.
14. Arciniegas DB, Anderson CA. Suicide in neurologic illness.
15. Curr Treatment Options Neurol 2002; 4:457–468.

26 | Respiratory System

Miroslav Radulovic
Gregory Schilero
Michael La Fountaine
Marvin Lesser

Compromise of respiratory function is a frequent consequence of neurologic disease. Although underlying pathophysiologic mechanisms of neurologic diseases are inherently different, the subsequent respiratory impairment(s) can be uniformly characterized as a consequence of impaired neural control of the respiratory system, resulting in respiratory muscle weakness, ineffective cough, and susceptibility to infections. Factors contributing to respiratory infection include aspiration, immobility, and malnutrition. However common these events are across neurologic diseases, there are still unique aspects to specific disorders that need to be given special consideration.

Respiratory complications, excluding pulmonary embolism, are the leading cause of death during the first year following spinal cord injury (SCI) and the third leading cause thereafter (1). Respiratory complications during the acute hospitalization phase following injury have been reported to be as high as 84% for C1–C4 levels of injury (LOI), 60% for C5–C8 LOI, and 65% for thoracic levels. Respiratory complications place a great socioeconomic burden on the affected individuals, caregivers, and health-care system.

The most common respiratory complications following SCI are pneumonia, atelectasis, and respiratory failure (2). Individuals with multiple sclerosis (MS), because of the muscle weakness and relative inactivity, may have significant compromise of pulmonary function in the absence of perceived symptoms and overt clinical findings. In these individuals respiratory complications become more prominent with the progression of the disease, and in the terminal stage mortality often results from bulbar weakness, leading to aspiration pneumonia and respiratory failure. In the Danish Multiple Sclerosis Registry study (3) respiratory failure and pneumonia were the most frequent underlying causes of death among patients with MS. The Sepsis Occurrence in Acutely Ill Patients (SOAP) study (4) revealed that individuals with acute brain injury (stroke or traumatic brain injury [TBI]) developed ICU-acquired sepsis and respiratory failure more frequently than other patients, with higher mortality rates and longer duration of stay in the hospital. In addition, the majority of neurologic disabilities associated with

335

immobility places this group at higher risk for development of venous thromboembolic disease.

This chapter addresses the pathophysiology of respiratory dysfunction in individuals with neurologic diseases, explores standard approaches to the diagnosis and treatment, and highlights the specific treatment considerations for common disabilities presenting with respiratory impairment.

ANATOMY, PHYSIOLOGY, AND PATHOPHYSIOLOGY

The principal function of the respiratory system is to provide continuous gas exchange for oxygen uptake and carbon dioxide removal at the alveolar/capillary interface. The respiratory system also plays a critical role in acid-base balance, water balance, heat regulation, blood filtration, and speech. It also performs important endocrine functions.

Neural Control of Breathing

Breathing is primarily an involuntary process under control of respiratory centers located in the medulla and pons. The medulla contains two respiratory centers: the dorsal respiratory group, consisting mainly of inspiratory neurons, and the ventral respiratory group, containing both inspiratory and expiratory neurons. The pons contains the apneustic and pneumotaxic centers responsible for the control of intensity of breathing and regulation of tidal volume and respiratory rate, respectively. The respiratory centers receive constant feedback from chemoreceptors sensitive to CO_2 and O_2 concentrations.

Mechanics of Breathing

The mechanics of breathing require coordinated movements of the respiratory muscles. In order to generate flow, a pressure gradient is required between the airway opening and terminal lung units. During spontaneous breathing, inspiratory flow is achieved upon contraction of the inspiratory muscles, principally the diaphragm, which results in expansion of the thoracic cavity and generation of subatmospheric pressure in the alveoli. Expiration is mainly a passive process driven by the inwardly directed elastic recoil of the lungs and chest wall. When demand for ventilation increases as with exercise (periods of increased physiologic demand), expiration becomes an active involving requiring coordinated contractions of the abdominal wall muscles and internal intercostals.

The Respiratory Muscles

Respiratory muscles can be divided into (a) inspiratory muscles—diaphragm, external intercostals, and accessory muscles including the scalene, sternocleidomastoid, trapezius, and pectoral muscles—and (b) expiratory muscles (during periods of increased demand or stress)—internal intercostals, the abdominal muscles (rectus abdominis, obliques, transversus abdominis), and diaphragm. Innervation of the respiratory muscles is through motor neurons arising from different levels of spinal cord.

The Airways

The respiratory tract extends from the mouth and nose to the alveoli and can be divided into the upper and lower airways. The primary role of the upper airway (mouth and nose) is to filter airborne particles and to humidify and warm the inspired gas. The principal function of the lower airway (trachea, bronchial tree, and alveoli) is to transport air via bulk flow through conducting airways (trachea and bronchi to the level of terminal bronchioles) and to facilitate gaseous diffusion at the level of the transitional and respiratory zones (respiratory bronchioles, alveolar ducts, and alveolar sacs). The airway epithelium contains specialized cells responsible for a variety of functions, the foremost of which include barrier and immune function, mucociliary clearance, and surfactant production. The epithelium is subtended by a smooth muscle layer, the contraction or relaxation of which affects tone and caliber (bronchomotor tone).

Parasympathetic (cholinergic) neurotransmission carried via efferent vagal pathways leads to contraction of airway smooth muscle and thus airway narrowing (bronchoconstriction) and represents the dominant autonomic influence upon resting bronchomotor tone, as well as a stimulus for mucus gland secretion. Bronchodilation can also occur through relaxation of airway smooth muscle via binding of circulating catecholamines to airway β_2-adrenoreceptors and, although of debatable functional significance, via sympathetic neurotransmission to airways arising from the upper six thoracic nerve roots. Endogenous and exogenous factors such as airway stretch, inhaled irritants, and cytokine release by resident inflammatory cells can also affect airway tone and caliber.

Respiratory Impairment Following SCI

The extent of the respiratory impairment following SCI directly depends upon level and completeness of injury. Injuries at the L1 level or below have no documented effects on respiration. Thoracic level injury is associated with variable degrees of paralysis of intercostals and abdominal muscles, which has the greatest impact upon expiratory muscle function, particularly the ability to cough. Therefore, there is as LOI becomes more rostral and injury becomes more complete, progressive attenuation of ventilatory force and cough generation. Individuals with C5–C8 LOI have additional accessory respiratory muscles compromised including the scalenes and pectoralis major. Inability to generate an effective cough to clear respiratory secretions is a major reason why some individuals initially require supportive ventilation following acute injury. Poor trunk posture stemming from interrupted postural muscle innervation will affect quiet respiration due to suboptimal positioning of the diaphragm in persons with higher cord lesions. The diaphragm is the major inspiratory respiratory muscle, its contraction accounting for approximately 65% of the achieved vital capacity (VC). Motor innervation of the diaphragm is supplied by the phrenic nerves arising from the third, fourth, and fifth (C3–C5) cervical spinal nerve roots. Injuries at the C3–C4 level result in diaphragmatic weakness which often necessitate the need for ventilatory support following acute injury. Of those requiring ventilatory support, approximately 80% of the patients will be weaned successfully. A complete injury at the C2 level results in total loss of diaphragmatic function and is incompatible with spontaneous respiration.

Individuals with chronic tetraplegia and high paraplegia (HP) exhibit a restrictive ventilatory deficit due to respiratory muscle weakness and paralysis. Pulmonary function tests (PFTs) reveal resultant decreases in all lung volumes and increases in residual volume (RV), the latter due to expiratory muscle weakness. The extent of restrictive deficit is correlated with the level and completeness of injury. Studies of individuals with chronic tetraplegia have shown that in addition to restrictive physiology, many exhibit obstructive airway physiology commonly seen in individuals with asthma. The majority also exhibit airway hyperresponsiveness (exaggerated bronchoconstriction) following inhalation of methacholine (an acetylcholine analogue), histamine, and aerosolized distilled water (5). Studies using body plethysmography to measure specific airway conductance (sGaw) in persons with tetraplegia, have confirmed the presence of baseline airway narrowing (bronchoconstriction) with restoration of normal airway caliber following bronchodilator administration (6). It is postulated that these findings are due to unopposed cholinergic innervation of airways due to interruption of sympathetic innervation.

Respiratory Impairment in Multiple Sclerosis

MS can produce a variety of respiratory abnormalities because of the multifocal nature of central nervous system (CNS) involvement. The prevalence of respiratory muscle dysfunction in patients with moderately severe MS is high. Studies have demonstrated that up to 98% of the patients eventually develop respiratory muscle weakness to some extent, as determined by measurement of maximal static inspiratory and expiratory pressures (MIP; MEP) (7). Expiratory muscle weakness affecting the abdominal and intercostals muscles is often more pronounced and explained by the ascending nature of the paralysis in MS. The diaphragm, which receives innervation from high cervical spinal nerves, is expected to be affected last. Surprisingly, severe muscle dysfunction may be accompanied by little or no decrement in lung volumes. Clinically, as long as MIP remains above 40% predicted, the decrease in VC is relatively small.

There appears to be a correlation between the extent of respiratory impairment and the degree of disability as assessed by the Expended Disability Status Score (EDSS) (8). The VC and forced expiratory volume in one second (FEV_1) are normal in ambulatory patients (EDSS <7), but are reduced in wheelchair-bound and particularly in bedridden patients. Among different spirometric indices, the forced vital capacity (FVC) and maximal voluntary ventilation (MVV) were found to correlate best with the level of disability as assessed by EDSS. The FEV_1/VC ratio remains unaffected in the majority of such individuals, implicating a purely restrictive impairment due to respiratory muscle weakness. This is supported by positive findings of correlation between maximum static pressures and VC in the advanced stages of disease.

Due to the variable course of MS there appears to be poor correlation between respiratory impairment and duration of the disease. Severe respiratory dysfunction typically occurs in advanced-stage MS but can also complicate acute relapses earlier in the natural course of the disease. Typically, these patients can develop acute respiratory failure presenting with reduced FVC, hypoxemia, hypercapnia, or even respiratory arrest. In addition, abnormalities of respiratory control have been reported in individuals with MS during acute exacerbations. Paralysis of voluntary breathing, paroxysmal hyperventilation, paralysis of automatic respiration (Ondine's curse), and apneustic breathing (sustained deep inspiration lasting several seconds followed by rapid exhalation driven by the elastic recoil of the lung) have been described in these patients. Nocturnal desaturation is also commonly observed.

Respiratory Impairment Following Acute, Severe Brain Injury (TBI and Stroke)

Pulmonary complications following acute severe brain injury are common and often lead to poor outcome in affected individuals. Neurologically injured patients may require hemodynamic support to maintain adequate cerebral perfusion. The Traumatic Coma Databank report which evaluated extracranial complications of severe TBI in defining outcomes and reported respiratory failure as the most common complication surpassing cardiovascular disorders, coagulopathy, and sepsis. Each of these complications had an independent negative effect on outcome. A post hoc analysis of the SOAP study revealed that neurologic patients (41% with TBI and 50% with stroke) developed ICU-acquired sepsis and respiratory failure more frequently than nonneurologically injured patients (9). In addition, mortality rates and length of ICU stay were higher in the neurologically injured group.

In individuals with TBI, pulmonary complications can be divided into those directly related to trauma (flail chest, pneumothorax, and hemothorax) and those related to subsequent neurologic impairment such as respiratory failure, aspiration pneumonia, neurogenic pulmonary edema, and complications related to prolonged tracheal intubation. Klingbeil found that close to 40% of patients with TBI required tracheostomy, but with careful airway management and rehabilitation, the majority of the patients recovered sufficiently to allow decannulation (10).

Following acute stroke, a significant number of individuals will develop one or more respiratory complications. Abnormal respiratory patterns are often seen in patients with acute stroke but bear little or no prognostic significance.

The exception is tachypnea with respiratory alkalosis, which is associated with a poor outcome. As in other individuals with neurologic disease, pneumonia is common in the acute phase following neurologic injury, but also remains the most prevalent rehospitalization diagnosis for up to 5 years following stroke. Among the nearly 5% of patients with stroke who develop pneumonia during the acute phase of the disease, aspiration related to dysphagia and/or cough ineffectiveness due to decreased consciousness underlie approximately 60% of the events. Patients requiring ICU management and nasogastric tube feeding appear to be at higher risk. Management is focused toward airway protection and aspiration prevention. Endotracheal intubation and mechanical ventilation may be indicated for progressive neurologic deterioration, seizures with status epilepticus, or development of pulmonary edema. The rate of intubation is higher in individuals with stroke due to intracerebral hemorrhage as compared to individuals sustaining an ischemic stroke. The need for intubation alone is associated with a poor outcome.

PATIENT ASSESSMENT

History

Assessing the severity of respiratory a dysfunction in individuals with neurologic disease can be quite challenging. Neurologic disorders that present with abrupt injury to the neurons involved in the control of respiration can lead to acute respiratory failure as an initial presentation (acute cervical spinal cord injury, stroke, etc). Other conditions can have a more chronic and insidious course. It is important to remember that neurologic disease often limits mobility, thus precluding early recognition of breathlessness or dyspnea as an initial presentation of affected respiratory function. Pronounced fatigability and diminished awareness of the need to cough are often seen in MS and may mask subjective pulmonary symptoms. Furthermore, significant cognitive dysfunction or limited communication ability are often present in individuals with brain injury and can limit the utility of interview, patient education, and compliance. High clinical suspicion should be employed, and subjective symptoms of respiratory dysfunction should be actively sought.

To date no validated questionnaires have been developed for assessment of respiratory function in individuals with neurologic impairments. Interviews should be tailored to the individual and reflect their level of disability and the potential effects upon respiratory function. The following should be addressed: (a) presence of shortness of breath, (b) presence of wheezing (whistling noises in the chest), (c) episodes of cough, (d) sputum production, (e) difficulty clearing phlegm from the chest (effectiveness of cough), and (f) experience of fatigue.

In addition to identifying pulmonary symptoms, further efforts should be made to clarify under what conditions symptoms occur (at rest, in supine vs. seated vs. standing positions, during physical exertion, during activities of daily living such as transfer to the bed in wheelchair-bound individuals etc.), if symptoms are more prominent during a particular time of day (associated with sleep disruption, worse upon awakening, progressive across the day, etc.), and to quantify the frequency of the episodes (e.g., multiple times a day, several times a week).

Past medical history should focus on:

- Preexisting respiratory diseases (e.g., presence of asthma, chronic obstructive pulmonary disease [COPD]).
- Degree of respiratory dysfunction at the time of initial presentation (during acute phase of SCI, TBI, or following acute stroke) or the degree of respiratory compromise during MS exacerbations.
- Previous history of respiratory failure requiring endotracheal intubation and mechanical ventilation, the length of intubation, and presence of complications.
- Etiology of past episodes of respiratory failure (due to respiratory muscle weakness, aspiration, ventilator-associated pneumonia, adult respiratory distress syndrome, neurogenic pulmonary edema, pulmonary embolism, etc.).
- Frequency and etiology of respiratory complications during chronic stable phases of the underlying neurologic disease (chronic SCI, TBI, and stroke patients post rehabilitation period, MS patients during remissions, etc).

A high index of suspicion for obstructive sleep apnea (OSA) is needed for all individuals with underlying neurologic disabilities. Appropriate screening is needed. This is particularly important in individuals with tetraplegia and those with cofounding risk factors such as morbid obesity, increased neck circumference, tobacco use, male gender, and in older individuals. Many different screening tools have been developed. One example is Berlin Questionnaire (Figures 26.1 and 26.2)

A social history should be taken to determine if factors are present that can exacerbate or further promote respiratory impairment such as tobacco use, environmental exposure to noxious respiratory stimuli, alcoholism (which increases the risk of aspiration), and substance abuse, particularly via the inhalation route (e.g., marijuana or crack cocaine).

Physical Exam

The structural examination of the thorax can provide important information regarding the impact of underlying neurologic conditions upon respiratory function. By observation of the breathing cycle, the clinician can gain a better understanding of respiratory physiology. Globally restricted motion of the rib cage during either inhalation or exhalation may suggest underlying respiratory muscle weakness. Use of accessory muscles, particularly the abdominal muscles, for active or labored exhalation are potential signs of impending respiratory failure. Paradoxical rib cage movement of the upper portion of the chest (inward movement of the rib cage with inspiration) can sometimes be observed in persons with tetraplegia due to differential paralysis of intercostal muscles while diaphragmatic function is retained. Underlying pneumonia or atelectasis may lead to reduced respiratory excursion over the affected area. Percussion can yield flatness (pleural effusion) or dullness (consolidation or atelectasis).

B E R L I N   Q U E S T I O N N A I R E

Height (m) _____ Weight (kg) _____ Age ____ Male / Female

Please choose the correct response to each question.

CATEGORY 1

1. **Do you snore?**
___ a. Yes
___ b. No
___ c. Don't know

If you snore:

2. **Your snoring is:**
___ a. Slightly louder than breathing
___ b. As loud as talking
___ c. Louder than talking
___ d. Very loud – can be heard in adjacent rooms

3. **How often do you snore?**
___ a. Nearly every day
___ b. 3-4 times a week
___ c. 1-2 times a week
___ d. 1-2 times a month
___ e. Never or nearly never

4. **Has your snoring ever bothered other people?**
___ a. Yes
___ b. No
___ c. Don't Know

5. **Has anyone noticed that you quit breathing during your sleep?**
___ a. Nearly every day
___ b. 3–4 times a week
___ c. 1–2 times a week
___ d. 1–2 times a month
___ e. Never or nearly never

CATEGORY 2

6. **How often do you feel tired or fatigued after your sleep?**
___ a. Nearly every day
___ b. 3–4 times a week
___ c. 1–2 times a week
___ d. 1–2 times a month
___ e. Never or nearly never

7. **During your waking time, do you feel tired, fatigued or not up to par?**
___ a. Nearly every day
___ b. 3–4 times a week
___ c. 1–2 times a week
___ d. 1–2 times a month
___ e. Never or nearly never

8. **Have you ever nodded off or fallen asleep while driving a vehicle?**
___ a. Yes
___ b. No

If yes:

9. **How often does this occur?**
___ a. Nearly every day
___ b. 3–4 times a week
___ c. 1–2 times a week
___ d. 1–2 times a month
___ e. Never or nearly never

CATEGORY 3

10. **Do you have high blood pressure?**
___ Yes
___ No
___ Don't know

Figure 26.1. Berlin Questionnaire.

The questionnaire consists of 3 categories related to the risk of having sleep apnea. Patients can be classified into High Risk or Low Risk based on their responses to the individual items and their overall scores in the symptom categories.

Categories and scoring:
Category 1: items 1, 2, 3, 4, 5.
Item 1: if 'Yes', assign **1 point**
Item 2: if 'c' or 'd' is the response, assign **1 point**
Item 3: if 'a' or 'b' is the response, assign **1 point**
Item 4: if 'a' is the response, assign **1 point**
Item 5: if 'a' or 'b' is the response, assign **2 points**
Add points. **Category 1 is positive if the total score is 2 or more points**

Category 2: items 6, 7, 8 (item 9 should be noted separately).
Item 6: if 'a' or 'b' is the response, assign **1 point**
Item 7: if 'a' or 'b' is the response, assign **1 point**
Item 8: if 'a' is the response, assign **1 point**
Add points. **Category 2 is positive if the total score is 2 or more points**

Category 3 is positive if the answer to item 10 is 'Yes' OR if the BMI of the patient is greater than 30kg/m2.
(BMI must be calculated. BMI is defined as weight (kg) divided by height (m) squared, i.e., kg/m2).

High Risk: if there are 2 or more Categories where the score is positive

Low Risk: if there is only 1 or no Categories where the score is positive

Figure 26.2. Scoring Berlin Questionnaire. (Adapted from Table 2 from Netzer NC, Stoohs RA, Netzer CM, Clark K, Strohl KP. Using the Berlin Questionnaire to identify patients at risk for the sleep apnea syndrome. Ann Intern Med 1999; 131(7):485–491.)

Auscultation might reveal focal signs of consolidation, such as bronchial breath sounds, or be decreased with atelectasis or pleural effusion. Ultimately, careful auscultation, percussion, and palpation of all lung fields should be integral parts of the examination. Inspection of the upper airways and measurement of neck circumference can yield important information regarding increased risk for OSA. Respiratory rate, oxygen saturation, and breathing patterns should also be recorded.

Diagnostic Tests

Pulmonary Function Tests
Complete pulmonary function testing includes performance of spirometry and measurement of full lung volumes and static respiratory pressures. Restrictive

respiratory pattern defined by decreases in FVC, FEV_1, forced mid-expiratory flow rate ($FEF_{25-75\%}$) with unchanged FEV_1/FVC ratio as well as decreases in total lung capacity (TLC), VC, expiratory reserve volume (ERV), functional residual capacity (FRC) and increase in RV are commonly observed. Degree of impairment as measured by static respiratory pressures (MIP and MEP) is directly correlated to the degree of respiratory muscle weakness. In individuals with SCI due to greater affection of the expiratory muscles, MEP is decreased significantly as compared to MIP. Individuals with profound respiratory muscle weakness are often unable to meet the American Thoracic Society (ATS) criteria for acceptability and reproducibility. Kelley et al., in their longitudinal follow-up of individuals with chronic SCI, found that individuals who were unable to meet ATS standards had the most abnormal pulmonary function (11). Loosening the standard to exclude two common causes of test failure in SCI (excessive back-extrapolated volume [EBEV] and failure to exhale maximally for the minimum of 6 seconds) increased the number of subjects who were able to produce three efforts that met ATS acceptability criteria to 92%. It is our opinion that such modified standards are applicable in all individuals with neurologic disabilities.

Chest X-Ray

Physical examination can be limited in these patients due to difficulties delineating the effect of the underlying neurologic condition on respiratory function and possible superimposed processes. Therefore a clinician should have a high level of suspicion and utilize the chest x-ray as a relatively simple and safe diagnostic study to rule out underlying structural or infectious process. This is specifically true for patients presenting with symptomatic dyspnea not previously observed, increased secretions with difficulty in clearance, and other clinical or laboratory findings suggestive of respiratory infection.

Computed Tomography

Computed tomography (CT) can be employed to further look at the underlying pathologic process in the lungs. Pulmonary angiography is occasionally necessary if there is a suspicion of pulmonary embolism.

Arterial Blood Gases

There are no specific arterial blood gas (ABG) abnormality associated with neurologic disabilities. ABG is a test that measures the amount of oxygen (PaO_2) and carbon cioxide ($PaCO_2$) in the blood, as well as the acidity (pH). A stepwise approach in interpreting an ABG is advised. This helps delineate whether the underlying impairment in gas exchange and acid-base balance is primarily due to respiratory or metabolic in abnormalities and if the process is acute or chronic.

Normal ABG on room air: pH = 7.3–7.45; PaO_2 of 80–100; $PaCO_2$ of 35–45; HCO_3 of 22–26 (calculated); SaO_2 of 95–100%.

- Step 1: Assess the pH value. If normal, a normal or compensated state exists. Assess whether acidosis or alkalosis is present.
- Step 2: Assess hypoxemia state. If the PaO_2 is <60 mmHg, hypoxemia state exists.
- Step 3: Analyze the CO_2. $PaCO_2$ < 35 mmHg is termed respiratory alkalosis or hypocarbia and is seen with alveolar hyperventilation. $PaCO_2$ > 45 mmHg is termed respiratory acidosis or hypercarbia and is the sign of ventilatory impairment or failure. Determine whether this is acute or chronic state (whether compensation occurred by looking simultaneously at PH value, PCO_2, and HCO_3).
- Step 4: Assess the metabolic component. If HCO_3 is <22 mEq/liter, metabolic acidosis is present. If HCO_3 is >28 mEq/liter, metabolic alkalosis exists.

Acid-Base Status Disturbances

- Acute respiratory failure (acute respiratory acidosis): pH , $PaCO_2$, HCO_3 normal.
- Chronic respiratory failure (compensated respiratory acidosis): pH or normal, $PaCO_2$, HCO_3.
- Acute hyperventilation (acute respiratory alkalosis): pH , $PaCO_2$, HCO_3 normal.
- Chronic hyperventilation (chronic respiratory alkalosis): pH , $PaCO_2$, HCO_3.
- Acute metabolic acidosis: pH , $PaCO_2$ normal, HCO_3.
- Chronic metabolic acidosis: pH or normal, $PaCo_2$, HCO_3.
- Acute metabolic alkalosis: pH , $PaCO_2$ normal, HCO_3.
- Chronic metabolic alkalosis: pH or normal, $PaCO_2$, HCO_3.

TREATMENT

Prevention

Respiratory function in individuals with neurologic disabilities requires assessment on a regular basis. We recommend annual pulmonary function testing as a sensitive method for capturing further decline in respiratory function. Due to high prevalence of OSA, all individuals with neurologic disability should be actively screened. Smoking cessation is crucial. Weight loss, lifestyle modifications, assisted cough techniques, abdominal binding, as well as respiratory muscle training may be required.

Medications

Bronchodilators are reserved for individuals with symptomatic complaints and for those with underlying pulmonary conditions such as COPD or asthma. Both anticholinergic agents and β_2-agonists can be used (Table 26.1).

In our opinion due to underlying unopposed cholinergic tone as an underlying mechanism of bronchoconstriction in tetraplegia, anticholinergic agents are the drugs of choice. In individuals with MS, β_2-agonists might be more beneficial, particularly because of the limited immunomodulatory effects on interleukin-12, believed to be important in MS.

Respiratory Failure

Respiratory failure is commonly seen in individuals with underlying neurologic disorders either at initial presentation (acute cervical SCI, acute stroke, or TBI), during exacerbations of neurologic disease (MS), or due to intervening acute respiratory illnesses such as atelectasis or pneumonia. A mainstay of the therapy is early recognition of impending respiratory failure and provision of adequate ventilatory support through invasive (endotracheal intubation and mechanical ventilation) or noninvasive measures (continuous positive airway pressure [CPAP] or bilevel positive airway pressure [BiPAP]).

Initial assessment of patients presenting with moderate to severe respiratory distress should include ABG, routine laboratory studies, and chest x-ray (as previously outlined). In addition, continuous monitoring of oxygenation and end-tidal CO_2 to assess the quality of gas exchange should be initiated. Further monitoring of the pulmonary function is achieved by serial respiratory muscle strength assessment of by measurement of VC or maximal negative inspiratory force (NIF). In individuals with acute SCI, decrease in VC to less than 15 ml/kg or the fall in NIF below -20 cmH_2O are both indications for intubation and mechanical ventilation. The decision to intubate the patient needs to be made without delay, especially if there is prolonged respiratory distress, rising PCO_2 and falling PH, none or only minimal improvement in respiratory function with noninvasive measures, or if there is a high risk for aspiration that will further impair respiratory function.

Determination of the underlying pathophysiology is crucial in guiding further treatment including mechanical ventilation. The Consortium for Spinal Cord Medicine clinical guidelines for Respiratory Management Following Spinal Cord Injury supports the use of a protocol that includes increasing ventilator tidal volumes and relatively low peak inspiratory pressures (PIP), to prevent development, or to assist resolution of existing atelectasis. Tidal volumes are titrated upward while monitoring the airway pressures until the atelectasis/pneumonia is resolved on chest x-ray and the patient is afebrile. This protocol is reserved only for well-defined patient subgroups in whom respiratory muscle weakness is the main cause of respiratory failure. In the presence of underlying primary pulmonary processes or general trauma because of the high frequency of acute lung injury and/or adult respiratory distress syndrome, low tidal volume ventilation protocols should be implemented to prevent barotrauma to the lungs. Barotrauma refers to occurrence of extra-alveolar air during mechanical ventilation due to alveolar overdistention and consequent rupture.

In addition to adequate ventilatory support, vigorous measures to assist the clearance of secretions from the airways are necessary. Commonly employed

Table 26.1

Medications Commonly used in the Treatment of Respiratory Disease

Name	U.S. Brand Names	Class	Dose	Common side effects	Contraindications
Albuterol sulfate	AccuNeb®; ProAir™ HFA; Proventil® HFA; Proventil®; Ventolin® HFA; VoSpire ER®	Short-acting β₂-agonists	Metered-dose inhaler (MDI): 2 puffs every 4–6 hours prn. Nebulization: 1.25–5 mg every 4–8 hours prn	Tachycardia, flushing, dizziness, rush, dry mouth, tremor	Hypersensitivity to albuterol, adrenergic amines, or any component of the formulation
Lev-albuterol	Xopenex HFA™; Xopenex®	Short-acting β₂-agonists	MDI: 2 puffs every 4–6 hours. Nebulization: 0.63 mg 3 times/day at intervals of 6–8 hours	Tremor, headache, dizziness, tachycardia (<3%), pharyngitis	Hypersensitivity to levalbuterol, albuterol, or any component of the formulation
Salmeterol	Serevent® Diskus®	Long-acting β₂-agonists	Inhalation, powder: One inhalation (50 μg) twice daily (~12 hours apart)	Headache, dizziness, rush, flu-like symptoms	Hypersensitivity to salmeterol, adrenergic amines, or any component of the formulation; need for acute bronchodilation
Formoterol	Foradil® Aerolizer™; Performist™	Long-acting β₂-agonists	Foradil®: 12 μg capsule inhaled every 12 hours via Aerolizer™ device. Performist™: 20 μg twice daily	Palpitations, anxiety, diarrhea, nausea, bronchitis, pharyngitis possible increased risk of stroke (March 2008)	Foradil®: Hypersensitivity to formoterol, or any component of the formulation
Ipratropium bromide	Atrovent® HFA; Atrovent®	Anticholinergic agent	Nebulization: 500 μg (one unit-dose vial) 3–4 times/day with doses 6–8 hours apart. MDI: 2 inhalations 4 times/day, up to 12/24 hours	Bronchitis, upper respiratory tract infection, palpitations, nausea, dyspnea	Hypersensitivity to ipratropium, atropine (and its derivatives), or any component of the formulation
Tiotropium	Spiriva®	Long-acting anticholinergic	Powder for oral inhalation (18 μg/capsule): once a day	Xerostomia, upper respiratory tract infection, sinusitis possible increased risk of stroke (March 2008)	Hypersensitivity to tiotropium, derivatives or any component of the formulation (contains lactose); not for use as an acute bronchodilator

methods are frequent suctioning, assisted coughing, chest physiotherapy, and positioning. Mobilization and aggressive management of secretions prevents further complications. Manually assisted cough techniques such as "quad cough" or abdominal thrust have been shown to be more effective than standard suctioning. Active measures to prevent development of pneumonia, atelectasis, and aspiration should be employed. Attempt to wean the patient from ventilatory support should be attempted early if indicated clinically. Consider using progressive ventilator-free breathing (PVFB) over synchronized intermittent mandatory ventilation (SIMV). Empiric coverage followed by targeted antimicrobial therapy based on susceptibility testing should be initiated as soon as possible if underlying pneumonia is suspected. Use of bronchodilator therapy can also add to symptomatic relief.

Data from individuals with SCI reveal that following initial insult, recovery of respiratory function occurs in two distinctive phases. Within the first 3–5 months there is a relatively rapid increase in spirometric indices of VC, inspiratory capacity (IC), TLC, and inspiratory and expiratory airflow along with a decrease in FRC. The second stage is characterized by gradual improvement in VC with consecutive decrease in FRC, while TLC and ventilatory indices remain unchanged. Although data are very limited, it appears that respiratory muscle training using resistive devices accelerates the speed and extent of recovery.

Bacterial Pneumonia

Development of pneumonia is a frequent complication among patients with neurologic diseases, leading to increased mortality, need for mechanical ventilation, and prolonged rehabilitation. Physical findings are often masked by underlying neurologic impairment, requiring a high level of clinical suspicion. Fever, leukocytosis, and altered levels of consciousness are common initial presentations, prompting proper clinical workup and initiation of adequate empiric treatment. Risk of aspiration, the need for mechanical ventilation, colonization of the airways with resistant bacterial strains, prolonged use of antibiotics, frequent use of steroids blunting immune response, and prolonged hospitalization need to be part of the decision-making process prior to the initiation of empiric antibiotic coverage. Early recognition and timely institution of such regimens is the mainstay of clinical management, particularly in individuals with severe respiratory distress. The reader is referred to Chapter 7 of this book for the assessment and treatment of pneumonia.

Pulmonary Embolism

It is well known that neurologic disability predisposes individuals to the development of deep vein thrombosis (DVT) and pulmonary embolism (PE) through prolonged immobilization, decreased mobility, and possibly through underlying systemic inflammatory response. Pulmonary angiography is a "gold standard" for the diagnosis of PE, but CT angio is more commonly used. Diagnosis of PE should be actively sought in patients with otherwise unexplainable dyspnea, pleuritic pain, cough, tachypnea, tachycardia, or fever. Defining the clinical suspicion for PE can guide further diagnostic approach. There are several tools for initial assessment of the clinical probability of PE, including the modified Wells Criteria (Table 26.2). Based on the Wells Criteria, high probability of a PE is defined as a score of greater than 6; moderate probability as 2–6, and low probability as less than 2.

Chest x-ray, arterial blood gas analysis, electrocardiogram (EKG) and routine laboratory tests have a very limited role in the diagnosis of PE. D-dimer, a degradation product of cross-linked fibrin, has good sensitivity and a negative predictive value, but poor specificity. In individuals with low clinical probability, normal D-dimer is associated with 99% likelihood of not having PE. VQ scan is an acceptable alternative, particularly if IV contrast is to be avoided.

In patients presenting with PE, initial care should be focused on stabilizing the patient, providing adequate respiratory support based on the level of distress, and maintaining hemodynamic stability. If massive PE is present, mechanical ventilation and pressor support is often needed. Patients with severe initial presentation and hemodynamic instability despite vigorous supportive measures should be evaluated for thrombolytic therapy or considered for embolectomy if thrombolysis is contraindicated or unsuccessful.

In addition to supportive measures, initiation of PE-directed therapy should be considered. Anticoagulation needs to be initiated in all individuals with high clinical suspicion with no strong contraindication to therapy pending further diagnostic workup. Initiation of empiric anticoagulation in patients with low to moderate suspicion should be based upon risk-vs.-benefit assessment. Individuals with neurologic impairment and risk of potentially life-threatening bleeding, particularly in the CNS, need to be carefully assessed. Initial choice of anticoagulation depends on this assessment. If there is an increased risk of bleeding or hemodynamic instability, we recommend use of intravenous unfractionated heparin.

Table 26.2

Modified Wells Criteria

Clinical symptoms of DVT (leg swelling, pain with palpation)	3
Other diagnosis less likely than pulmonary embolism	3
Heart rate > 100	1.5
Immobilization (>3 days) or surgery in the previous 4 weeks	1.5
Previous DVT/PE	1.5
Hemoptysis	1
Malignancy	1
Probability	Score

In a hemodynamically stable patient with low potential for serious hemorrhage, use of subcutaneous low molecular weight heparin is preferred. In confirmed cases, long-term anticoagulation therapy needs to be initiated based on existing criteria for duration of treatment and risk of bleeding. In selected patient groups with PE and high risk of bleeding, placement of inferior vena cava (IVC) filters may decrease mortality and the number of recurrent PE episodes, but may in turn increase the incidence of recurrent deep venous thrombosis (DVT).

Neurogenic Pulmonary Edema (NPE)

NPE infrequently occurs among patients with stroke or TBI, particularly if there is an adjacent subarachnoid hemorrhage. As in other forms of pulmonary edema, the underlying pathophysiologic mechanism is rapid filling of alveolar spaces with fluid. It is characterized by sudden onset and progression following neurologic insult. Physical examination can reveal the presence of bilateral rales with consecutive worsening hypoxia and respiratory distress. Chest x-ray typically reveals bilateral interstitial infiltrates with alveolar involvement. Therapy is directed toward respiratory supportive measures including mechanical ventilation with positive end expiratory pressure (PEEP) and treatment of the underlying neurologic condition. Dobutamine, osmotic diuresis, loop diuretics, and α-adrenergic blockers have all been successfully used in the treatment of this condition.

Sleep Apnea

Sleep apnea is a serious and potentially life-threatening condition commonly seen in individuals with neurologic disabilities. Impaired CNS control of breathing predisposes such individuals to the development of central sleep apnea (CSA) characterized by repetitive episodes of apnea in the absence of respiratory effort. OSA is distinguished from CSA by obstruction of the pharyngeal airway despite persistent respiratory efforts leading to repetitive episodes of apnea and/or hypopnea (a decrement in airflow of at least 50%). Both CSA and OSA may be associated with significant falls in oxygen saturation and disruption of the normal sleep architecture. Terms commonly used to quantify the severity of OSA include the apnea index (AI), which represents the number of apneic episodes per hour of sleep, and the apnea–hypopnea index (AHI) which represents the sum of apnea/hypopnea episodes per hour of sleep. As per the American Academy of Sleep Medicine Task Force guidelines, OSA can be categorized as mild (AHI < 15), moderate (15 < AHI < 30) or severe (AHI > 30). Failure to recognize and treat OSA may lead in the long term development of hypertension, coronary artery disease, myocardial infarction, pulmonary hypertension, stroke, and cognitive impairment. The incidence of OSA in individuals with neurologic disorders is higher than in the general population, especially if there is underlying involvement of the nerves controlling the muscles of the upper airways as seen in SCI, parkinsonism, stroke, or myasthenia gravis.

Although nocturnal desaturation may occur in both conditions, OSA does not seem to be more prevalent in persons with MS than in the general population. In individuals with SCI, four cross-sectional screening studies yielded a prevalence of OSA ranging from 22 to 62% based upon an AHI > 15 events per hour of sleep (12). Individuals with cervical SCI appear to be particularly affected. When considering OSA in individuals with stroke, it is important to note that these two diseases share common risk factors and that the noted higher prevalence rates may be coincidental rather than causative. Limited data however, suggest that stroke may predispose to or exacerbate sleep apnea in affected individuals. OSA following stroke is often characterized by minimal complaints of daytime sleepiness and a tendency to spontaneously improve over time. Sleep disturbances due to leg spasms, pain, immobility, nocturia, or use of medications are common in neurologic disorders, making it more challenging to screen for OSA based upon sleep-related symptoms. Possessing an understanding that neurologic disorders and OSA can coexist and potentially exacerbate each other is of utmost importance when clinically assessing such individuals.

Patient Safety

1. Sleep apnea is a serious and potentially life threatening condition—especially in adults with SCI. Failure to recognize it may lead to the development of hypertension, coronary artery disease, myocardial infarction, pulmonary hypertension, and stroke.
2. Respiratory failure is commonly seen in individuals with underlying neurologic disorders either at initial injury or due to secondary events that impair respiratory function. If strong clinical suspicion of impending respiratory failure is present, it is important to provide early adequate ventilatory support through either invasive or noninvasive interventions.

Patient Education

Patients and their caregivers should be educated on the following:
1. Normal respiratory anatomy and physiology and the impact of the neurologic disease on the patient's respiratory system

2. Symptoms of pneumonia, pulmonary embolism, and impending respiratory failure and instructions on when and where to seek medical assistance
3. Management of secretions and basic chest physiotherapy
4. Medications prescribed for the respiratory system, including indications, dosage, common side effects, significant side effects, and potential drug–drug interactions.

REFERENCES

1. DeVivo MJ, Black KJ, Stover SL. Causes of death during the first 12 years after spinal cord injury. Arch Phys Med Rehabil 1993; 74(3):248–254.
2. Jackson AB, Groomes TE. Incidence of respiratory complications following spinal cord injury. Arch Phys Med Rehabil 1994; 75(3):270–275.
3. Koch-Henriksen N, Bronnum-Hansen H, Stenager E. Underlying cause of death in Danish patients with multiple sclerosis: results from the Danish Multiple Sclerosis Registry. J Neurol Neurosurg Psychiatry 1998; 65(1):56–59.
4. Vincent JL, Sakr Y, Sprung CL, et al. Sepsis in European intensive care units: results of the SOAP study. Crit Care Med 2006; 34(2):344–353.
5. Grimm DR, Arias E, Lesser M, Bauman WA, Almenoff PL. Airway hyperresponsiveness to ultrasonically nebulized distilled water in subjects with tetraplegia. J Appl Physiol 1999; 86(4):1165–1169.
6. Schilero GJ, Grimm DR, Bauman WA, Lenner R, Lesser M. Assessment of airway caliber and bronchodilator responsiveness in subjects with spinal cord injury. Chest 2005; 127(1):149–155.
7. Smeltzer SC, Skurnick JH, Troiano R, Cook SD, Duran W, Lavietes MH. Respiratory function in multiple sclerosis. Utility of clinical assessment of respiratory muscle function. Chest 1992; 101(2):479–484.
8. Mutluay FK, Gurses HN, Saip S. Effects of multiple sclerosis on respiratory functions. Clin Rehabil 2005; 19(4):426–432.
9. Mascia L, Sakr Y, Pasero D, Payen D, Reinhart K, Vincent JL. Extracranial complications in patients with acute brain injury: a post-hoc analysis of the SOAP study. Intensive Care Med 2008; 34(4):720–727.
10. Klingbeil GE. Airway problems in patients with traumatic brain injury. Arch Phys Med Rehabil 1988; 69(7):493–495.
11. Kelley A, Garshick E, Gross ER, Lieberman SL, Tun CG, Brown R. Spirometry testing standards in spinal cord injury. Chest 2003; 123(3):725–730.
12. Young T, Palta M, Dempsey J, Skatrud J, Weber S, Badr S. The occurrence of sleep-disordered breathing among middle-aged adults. N Engl J Med 1993; 328(17):1230–1235.

27 Neurologic Disability and Its Effect on Sexual Functioning

Norma Parets
Audrey J. Schmerzler

The need for sexual expression is inherent in all human beings. The presence of a neurologic dysfunction/disability does not lessen or abate that need. However, too often both the patient and the healthcare professional are uneasy discussing a subject that, at best, often carries with it embarrassment and misinformation. A positive correlation between sexual expression and adaptation to a disability has long been observed in successful community reintegration.

For the patient, the area of sexuality may be one of the most profound concerns after injury but is seldom acknowledged. Both patient and healthcare professional are hesitant to address this issue due to embarrassment, religious and cultural beliefs, lack of time and other stressors, as well as a basic lack of knowledge regarding sexual functioning in the presence of neurologic losses.

The physical effect of neurologic loss on sexual function includes sensory changes, bowel and bladder issues, spasticity, and changes in motor function, including loss of flexibility. At the same time, specific disabilities may require specific precautions, such as instructing a person with cardiovascular accident (CVA) to avoid pressure on a subluxed shoulder or the danger of autonomic dysreflexia for a person with spinal cord injury (SCI) undergoing rectal probe ejaculation (RPE).

Cognitive losses, which can include short- and long-term memory loss, issues with judgment, lack of awareness of boundaries, and disinhibition, are all areas that should be acknowledged and addressed when dealing with sexual functioning in this population.

This chapter will educate and reassure the healthcare professional that this is a topic that is as crucial for this patient population as any other. But this topic needs to be approached with sensitivity and respect for all parties concerned.

PATIENT ASSESSMENT

PLISSIT Model

A useful tool in discussing sexuality is the PLISSIT model (1), which breaks down this emotionally charged topic into manageable components: permission, limited information, specific strategies, and intensive therapy.

- Permission entails assuring the patient that it is okay to have sexual feelings. Patients may not be ready to verbalize or address these concerns immediately after injury; sometimes staff needs to be the initiator of the discussion.
- Limited information refers to providing factual information within the patient's comfort level and in a manner that is accessible to the individual patient. For example, a female may wonder if she can conceive following a spinal cord injury. A simple answer of yes reassures the person that they are still a sexual being.
- Specific suggestions and strategies refer to the need to individualize suggestions to the specific disability. An example of this is advising a person with multiple sclerosis (MS) to engage in sexual activity when his or her antispasmodic medication is at its optimal level, thereby decreasing discomfort and increasing flexibility.
- Intensive therapy reminds the healthcare professional that certain individuals will need more intensive and specialized interventions. A male may need a referral to a neuro-urologist to ensure successful impregnation of his partner.

Of course, the healthcare professional must have insight into his or her level of comfort and the influence of religious and cultural factors, which can interfere with an effective interaction with the patient. The healthcare professional must be aware of this possibility and guard against it.

In addition to the usual questions asked during the history and physical, the patient's sexual history, including sexual preference, age at which he or she became sexually active, age of menarche, and number of viable pregnancies should also be part of the admission process. Table 27.1 illustrates additional areas of concern. Having this knowledge allows the healthcare professional to tailor the discussion to meet each individual's needs.

Table 27.1

Previous Sexual Function History

	Male	Female
Previous sexual function	Any previous problems with sexual function, e.g., erectile dysfunction	Any previous problems with sexual function
	Able to achieve erection with or without medication?	Number of partners
	Number of partners	Heterosexual or same sex relationship
	Heterosexual or same sex relationship	Age of menarche
	A history of sexually transmitted disease (STD)	Regular or irregular periods
		Number of pregnancies
		Number of living children
		Any problems with delivery

Drugs That Effect Sexual Functioning

The effects of medications on sexual functioning should never be overlooked. Many of the drugs (Table 27.2) that a patient takes on a daily basis may have the potential to adversely effect his or her sexual function by decreasing libido, increasing vaginal dryness, increasing fatigue, altering consciousness, and/or affecting the ability to achieve an erection.

Adjustment Issues and Sexual Function

Who we are and how we think of ourselves in relation to others is all put into question in the face of neurologic loss. The need for assistive devices, such as wheelchairs and walkers, the loss of bowel and bladder control, or the inability to express oneself verbally all may have an adverse effect on self-image and self-esteem. Fear of being rejected, no longer being loved, or not being able to please one's partner may interfere with accepting and adjusting to neurologic loss. Societal attitudes also play a big part in self-acceptance. Society has a long way to go before it can look at the person apart from the wheelchair.

TREATMENT

The healthcare professional can employ many different means to present and discuss information regarding sexuality, including written material, videos (2), open discussion, role playing, and even humor. In this area the role of peer mentoring should not be overlooked. Sexuality information should be included in staff orientation programs to rehab programs.

Healthcare professionals should look for opportunities to raise the subject of sexuality and be sensitive to the patient's readiness to engage. This topic should

Table 27.2

Sexual Side Effects of Commonly Taken Medications

Medication	Effect
Antidepressants	Decreased interest in sex
	Decreased arousal and erectile dysfunction
	Ejaculatory dysfunction
	Decrease vaginal lubrication
	Delayed orgasm
Antihypertensives	Difficulty achieving and/or maintaining an erection
	Decreased vaginal lubrication
Antiulcer medications	Low desire
	Erectile dysfunction
	Inability to reach orgasm
Alcohol/Recreational drugs	Difficulty achieving and/or maintaining an erection
	Decreased lubrication; takes longer to reach orgasm

be addressed early in the hospital stay. Consider having a section regarding sexuality on the admission history and physical forms.

Of course, all discussions on sexuality should take into account the patient's level of comfort, cultural background, and educational level. Healthcare professionals must recognize that people learn differently and use different terms for genitalia and sexual activity. Good techniques to encourage discussion are the use of open-ended questions, repetition and clarification of what was said, and allowing sufficient response time.

Spinal Cord Injury

Sexual functioning in the presence of a SCI can be severely compromised. Sexual satisfaction cannot be predicted based upon level or completeness of injury. There are many ways to experience sexual satisfaction; intercourse is just one way. Persons with SCI can experience heightened sensations in previously unexplored areas of their body, e.g., nipples and/or ear lobes. It is not unusual for a person with a complete injury to state that the area of the body where the sensation stops becomes highly sensitive and if the partner licks, bites, or nibbles at that place he or she can experience orgasm-like sensations.

The male with SCI may have difficulty achieving and/or sustaining an erection, producing ejaculate, and inseminating his partner.

Erections

Following a SCI reflex activity depends on the completeness versus incompleteness of the injury as well as whether the SCI is an upper motor neuron or lower motor neuron injury (Tables 27.3 and 27.4). There are two types of erections: reflexogenic (touch) and psychogenic. Reflex erections are initiated by noncortical stimulation and occur through a reflex arc at S_{2-4} spinal segments (3). They can be achieved either through external (touch) or internal (full bladder) stimulation. In a person with an upper motor neuron injury, reflex erections occur independently of the brain and are not under psychological control. For example, when a nurse places a Texas catheter on a patient, he may have an erection; this is a reflex reaction to touch, and if this occurs the nurse should not be embarrassed or offended. This is an opportunity for the nurse to educate

Table 27.3

Ability to Achieve Erection Following SCI: Complete vs. Incomplete Injury

	Complete injury	Incomplete injury
Erection (reflexogenic)	Possible unless injury occurs at S_{2-4} segments	Yes if injury is UMN
Erection (psychogenic)	Possible if lumbar (L_2 and below) or sacral injury	Possible

Table 27.4

Expected Sexual Dysfunctions Following Complete SCI

	T10–L1 segments and above	L2–S1 segments	S2–S4 segments
Genital sensations	Lost	Lost: vague feelings possible	Lost
Erection (touch)	Yes (sacral segments intact)	Possible	No
Erection (mental)	No: fibers coming to T10–L1 interrupted	Possible: may be getting signals at T10–L1	Possible: because T10–L1 segments intact

the patient as well. A psychogenic erection is initiated by cortical brain stimulation involving a combination of visual, auditory, and olfactory information that the person perceives as erotic.

Achieving and Maintaining an Erection

A number of devices are available to assist the individual with a SCI to achieve and then maintain an erection. Penile implants and vacuum devices are two of the older methods in use. The penile implant is a surgically implanted rod or saline-inflatable pump device. Risks of this device include scarring, infection, erosion of the rod, malfunction, and priapism. The vacuum device involves an external device that works by negative pressure to increase blood flow to the penis, resulting in an erection. Risks include bruising and constriction. Some of the newer methods include injectable and/or oral medications. The injectable medications work by increasing blood flow to the penis. They are given with a small needle and syringe and injected into the base of the penis. Either the patient or his partner can be responsible for injecting the medication. Oral medications such as sildenafil, vardenafil, and tadalafil are administered orally prior to sexual activity. However, they do not work unless manual stimulation of the penis occurs. Side effects of these medications (some more than others) include hypotension, visual disturbances, stuffy nose, and headache. Regardless of the method used to achieve erection, a tension ring is usually placed at the base of the penis to help maintain the erection. This ring should not be left in place more than 20 minutes to prevent damage.

Ejaculation and Fertility

Although ejaculation and erection are mediated through similar areas of the spinal cord, it is important to note that one can function in the absence of the other.

Even though a male may be able to ejaculate, he may not be able to impregnate his partner through intercourse. In this case a neuro-urologist should be consulted. The neuro-urologist can suggest and/or employ the most effective method to obtain the sperm. The neuro-urologist and the patient work closely with an obstetrician to coordinate the female's cycle to optimize success.

Some of the common methods used to obtain semen in a person with SCI include:

- Masturbation.
- Vibratory stimulation—there are special vibrators on the market to assist in obtaining semen. In general it has been found that the higher the level of injury, the more effective this method. An example of a commonly used vibrator is the Ferti Care.
- Electro-ejaculation— this method involves the insertion of a rectal probe as well as manual stimulation of the penis to obtain semen. In general it has been found that the lower the level of injury, the more effective this method. One of the major concerns using this method is the possibility of autonomic dysreflexia.
- Aspiration—this is the insertion of a needle to aspirate sperm.

Women with SCI can be become pregnant; fertility is rarely compromised. When pregnancy occurs, issues that need to be addressed include medications that cross the placenta and changes to bowel and bladder routines. A serious concern is confusing autonomic dysreflexia with preeclampsia. With autonomic dysreflexia, a contraction results in increased blood pressure; as the contraction subsides, the blood pressures returns to normal. In preeclampsia, the blood pressure remains elevated continuously.

Multiple Sclerosis

Issues specific to MS and sexual functioning include muscle weakness, fatigue, and bowel and bladder dysfunction, cognitive losses resulting in difficulties with concentration and attention span, as well as spasticity. Fatigue, one of the hallmarks of MS, is one factor resulting in a lack of sexual interest. Another may be pain. Spasticity, pain, and sensory loss can interfere with positioning. Use of pillows and timing of medications can decrease the effects of pain and spasm activity. Often trial and error will help to determine the best position as well as the best time to engage in sexual activity.

Issues of erection and ejaculation for the male and lubrication and sensation for the female are similar to those experienced by persons with SCI, and treatment is similar for both patient populations.

Stroke

Fear that sexual excitement can bring about another stroke is of paramount importance in this population. Other areas that need to be addressed include right brain damage, which may alter attention span, judgment, and planning, making previous patterns of sexual activity difficult or impossible. The side effects of medications, particularly those for high blood pressure, may affect sex drive and performance. Depression, which often follows stroke but is often overlooked, dulls sex drive. A frank discussion and education regarding sexual activity is necessary. Patients and partners need to be educated on issues affecting sexual activity post stroke (4). These may include:

- Awareness of change in body image (hemiparesis, facial droop, drooling)
- Need for positioning aids, including pillows, to support hemiparetic limbs
- Timing to minimize medication side effects and maximize medication benefits
- Avoiding sexual activity after large meals and alcohol consumption
- Setting aside private uninterrupted time

Traumatic Brain Injury

Some general concerns for this patient population include depression, which often occurs concurrently with injury and medication side effects. The healthcare professional should look at the medications prescribed and be cognizant of the possible side effects that can adversely interfere with sexual function. For individuals with traumatic brain injury (TBI), the area of the brain affected (Table 27.5) can determine the area of concern. If the brain injury occurs in the pituitary gland and fertility is an issue an endocrinological workup should be considered.

Persons with TBI also pose cognitive challenges that can interfere with sexual performance. These include reduced memory and organizational skills, lack of interest, distractibility, and disinhibition. Education includes instructing the patient and his or her partner to find a quiet and distraction-free environment. While longstanding partners may have subtle signals and cues to initiate sexual activity, these signals may no longer be perceived by the person with a TBI. The partner needs to be aware of this and not rely on previous

Table 27.5

Area of Brain Injury and Possible Effect on Sexuality

Area of brain injury	Effect on sexuality
Brain stem	Decreased libido
Hypothalamus	Decreased initiation
	Hormonal regulation
Frontal lobe	Sexual apathy
	Loss of initiative
Pituitary gland	Infertility
	Decreased secondary sex characteristics
Temporal Lobe	Diminished responsiveness

Medical Management of Adults with Neurologic Disabilities

cues and habits, but be more concrete in expressing needs and wishes. If patients are disinhibited and/or masturbate in public, the healthcare professional must be consistent and nonjudgmental when redirecting inappropriate sexual behavior.

Patient Safety

Patient safety can never be overemphasized. Some highlights include:
1. Having a disability does not preclude a person from getting a sexually transmitted disease/AIDS. Safe sex should be practiced at all times, and, religious beliefs permitting, a condom should be worn.
2. Penile implants can erode the skin. If this should happen, a physician should be consulted immediately.
3. The use of oral medications to achieve an erection could result in priapism. An erection that lasts more than 4 hours requires medical attention.
4. Females with spinal cord injuries at thoracic 6 and above are susceptible to autonomic dysreflexia (AD). In the pregnant patient, AD is often confused with preeclampsia. The treatment for AD associated with pregnancy is very different than the treatment for preeclampsia. It is strongly advised that females with SCI who want to get pregnant consult with an ob-gyn that is familiar with spinal cord injury.

Patient Education

Sexual activity may require some planning—for example, bowel and bladder routines have to be taken care of before engaging in sexual activity and/ or medication administration may have to be timed to enable sexual performance. Some additional suggestions are listed in Table 27.6.

Touch is also a wonderful way express feelings. The patient should be encouraged to pay attention to the parts of his or her body where pleasurable sensations may be heightened. Tha patient should communicate to his or her partner about what feels good and what doesn't. He or she should be reminded that mutual satisfaction may take some time. The use of humor and an open mind cannot be overemphasized. Answers to commonly asked questions about sexuality in adults with neurologic disabilities are listed in Table 27.7.

An issue that should be emphasized with all patient populations is the risk of sexually transmitted disease(s) and unwanted pregnancy. All sexually active individuals should practice safe sex and protect against unwanted pregnancies with appropriate birth control methods.

Table 27.6

Suggested thing to do Before Engaging in Sexual Activity

1. Choose a time when both partners are feeling rested, relaxed, and when privacy is guaranteed.
2. Pay attention to personal hygiene and grooming.
3. Patients on a bowel and bladder routine should be advised to complete the routine prior to engaging in sexual activity. They should also be advised to have towels available in case of any accidents.
4. Avoid excessive alcohol as it can have an effect on the ability to achieve or maintain an erection.
5. Avoid a heavy meal or wait a couple of hours after eating. This will allow time for the food to be properly digested.
6. Persons with mobility issues should try different positions or use pillows to support weak or paralyzed limbs. (For diagrams of different positions, the educational pamphlet "Chronic Low Back Pain and How It May Affect Sexuality" is available at http://www.ukhealthcare.uky.edu/patiented/booklets.htm)
7. A vibrator can result in pleasant sensations as well as assist with ejaculation (in some injuries).
8. Females with dryness/difficulty with lubrication should use a water-soluble lubrication jelly or over-the-counter moisturizers to make intercourse more comfortable.

Table 27.7

Answers to Commonly Asked Question About Sexuality in Adults with Nuerologic Disabilities

1. Will people view me as a sexual person?
   Answer: How people view you depends upon how you present yourself.
2. When should I discuss with my partner what I can and cannot do sexually?
   Answer: That depends on the nature of your relationship. If you are in a relatively new relationship, discussing the possibility of an accident should not take place until you are more familiar with each other. You need to decide how the relationship is going and how you feel your partner will respond.
3. How soon after my bowel and/or bladder routine can I engage in sexual activity?
   Answer: once you are sure that your bowel and/or bladder are completely empty, you can engage in sexual activity. The reason you don't want to engage in sexual activity before a scheduled bowel and/or bladder routine is in order to decrease the likelihood of an accident. It is always helpful to keep towels, a washcloth, and/or chux nearby in case an accident does occur.
4. Can I have sex with a Foley in place?
   Answer: It is possible to engage in intercourse with a Foley in place. Females can tape it to the leg or on the abdomen to keep it out of the way. Males can fold it over and place a condom over it.
5. Can I have an erection?
   Answer: Each person is affected differently by his disability. The ability to have an erection is based on a number of different things, e.g., type of injury, area of injury, completeness vs. incompleteness of the injury, as well as medications. The best way to find out is to touch yourself or have your significant other stimulate you to see if you can achieve an erection. The same goes for ejaculation; the best way to find out is through trying.

REFERENCES

1. Hoeman SP, ed. Rehabilitation Nursing: Process and Application, 4th ed. St. Louis: Mosby, 2007.
2. Alexander CJ, Sipski ML. Sexuality Reborn: Sexuality Following Spinal Cord Injury [video-tape]. West Orange, NJ: Kessler Institute for Rehabilitation, 1993.
3. Zedjlik, C.P. Management of Spinal Cord Injury. 2d ed. Boston: Jones and Bartlett, 1992.
4. Kautz DD. Hope for Love: Practical Advice for Intimacy and Sex after Stroke. Rehabil Nurs 2007; 32(3):95–103.

28 | Sleep Disorders

Brian D. Greenwald
Rosanna C. Sabini

Sleeps serves the purpose of restoring, reviving, and rejuvenating. Sleep disorders are commonly associated with neurologic illness. Too much, too little, or nonrefreshing sleep are all seen. Through a complex orchestration the brain initiates and maintains sleep. Therefore, injury or disease of the brain, including psychiatric illness, can have effects on sleep. Multiple organ systems are affected by sleep—in particular, the musculoskeletal and respiratory systems. Impairments in these systems can impact sleep quality and quantity.

In the general population chronic insomnia is an underrecognized and undertreated problem that affects between 10 and 15% of the population, with an increased frequency in women and the elderly (1). Chronic insomnia is often associated with a wide range of adverse conditions, including mood disturbances, difficulties with concentration and memory, as well as some cardiovascular, pulmonary, and gastrointestinal disorders. Previously, insomnia had been viewed as a sleep disturbance that was transient due to situational disturbances or that was chronic secondary to medical or psychiatric disorders. Insomnia is now increasingly recognized as a chronic disorder that for some patients may require chronic treatment.

Related complaints of sleep impairment include fatigue, irritability, depressed mood, poor concentration and memory, and impaired performance. Insomnia is also associated with increased healthcare costs and decreased quality of life. In the general population persistent insomnia increases the risk for future psychiatric disorders, particularly mood and anxiety disorders, as well as medical conditions, such as hypertension and diabetes mellitus.

Sleeping difficulties are relatively common complaints after traumatic brain injury (TBI). The relationship between excessive daytime somnolence (EDS) and TBI is complex, and the causes for EDS are multiple. Disordered sleep can have adverse behavioral, physical, and cognitive consequences. Insomnia, or difficulty initiating or maintaining sleep, is reported with a frequency of 27–70% or higher in those with higher frequencies early postinjury (2,3).

363

As with TBI, patients often complain of poor sleep quality after stroke, and it is not uncommon for stroke victims to develop insomnia. In the past 20 years there have been several studies looking at the link between sleep-disordered breathing (SDB) and stroke. Rates of SDB in acute hospitalization of stroke has been shown to be as high as 60–70% and continue to be as high as 50% in the year-after-stroke phase.

Studies have also shown that there is a high correlation between sleep apnea and cardiovascular disease. Risk factors for SDB and stroke share many commonalities. Smoking, high body mass index, high cholesterol, and alcohol use can all be predictors of stroke and SDB. Recently research has been investigating the possibility that SDB may lead to stroke. Presence of sleep disorders after stroke may have a significant negative impact on functional outcome.

Sleep disorders are fairly common in people with multiple sclerosis. One study on sleep disorders in people with multiple sclerosis (MS) found that 36% suffered from some form of sleep disorder (4). Some postulate that stress, spasticity, inactivity, and increased need to go to the bathroom also contribute to broken sleep patterns in people with MS.

Sleep apnea is common in persons with SCI, among whom an estimated 9–45% have the disorder (5). Incidence is higher in persons with tetraplegia. Weakness of respiratory muscles may contribute to the problem, especially in persons with tetraplegia, because the muscles cannot easily interrupt episodes of apnea. Obesity and male gender are also relatively common in this population, both known risk factors for sleep apnea.

Abnormalities in melatonin secretion as well as pain and bowel and bladder programs also lead to sleep fragmentation. The use of sedating antispasticity medications such as baclofen is also considered a potential risk factor. Nasal congestion is also common in SCI due to disruption of the autonomic nervous system, and this further obstructs the airway.

In patients with spinal cord injury and multiple sclerosis, sleep impairment is considered a key cause of the high prevalence of fatigue. In the MS population age, sex, and degree of disability did not bear any direct relation to sleep disorders. The only symptom of MS the study found that had a direct relationship to problems with sleep was depression (4). Other studies on fatigue and sleep disorders in people with MS found that there was a significant correlation between fatigue in MS patients and disrupted sleep or abnormal sleep cycles. The secondary consequence of fatigue exacerbates the physical and/ or psychologic impairments in these patients.

ANATOMY AND PHYSIOLOGY

Despite the fact that sleep affects the whole body, sleep is initiated and maintained by the brain. The homeostatic drive to maintain the circadian rhythm of sleep and wakefulness is maintained by brain. Not surprisingly, therefore, an injury to the brain from any source can have an impact of sleep and wakefulness.

The suprachiasmatic nucleus is the body's master clock, coordinating the body's internal 24-hour time sequences with the 24-hour terrestrial cycle. One basic system that governs overall arousal level is the ascending reticular activation system, which extends from the medulla through the pons. The initiation of sleep bout is partly or mostly initiated by nuclei in the forebrain (actually more active at night than during daytime). The forebrain cholinergic system tends to inhibit sleep. The non–rapid eye movement (REM) cycle during sleep is regulated by pontine nuclei. Noradrenergic, and serotonergic systems together cross-regulate a cholinergic pontine system that normally produces REM sleep. The pons has rostral efferents to make rapid eye movements, but also has caudal efferents to suppress limb movements during active dreaming. The thalamus plays an important role as the site of generation of sleep spindles within its reticular nucleus but also coordinates with the prefrontal systems and an intrinsic cortical slow rhythm to produce slow waves and K complexes. The histamine system in the posterior hypothalamus assists with maintaining wakefulness and alertness. A recently discovered system in the lateral hypothalamus uses the alerting neurotransmitter orexin and plays a role in sleep–wake regulation to prevent narcolepsy-like sleep pathologies. Undoubtedly there are more brain regions whose ability to regulate sleep-related behaviors and experiences we do not yet fully understand.

PATIENT ASSESSMENT

Insomnia in general is defined as a disturbance in sleep initiation, maintenance, or restorative properties of sleep. Primary insomnia is sleeplessness that is not attributed to a medical, psychiatric, or environmental cause. The most common sleep disorders are discussed in Table 28.1. The International Classification of Sleep Disorders categorizes sleep disturbances as follows:
- Dyssomnias—intrinsic sleep disorders arising from bodily malfunctions. This includes sleep apnea, restless legs syndrome, and periodic limb movement disorder.
- Parasomnias—disorders of arousal or sleep stage transition. These include sleep-walking, bruxism, and sleep terrors.
- Sleep disorders due to medical and psychiatric disorders. Disorder types include endocrine (thyroid disease, diabetes); pulmonary (asthma, COPD); gastrointestinal (gastro-esophageal reflux); pain; psychiatric (anxiety, depression); cardiac; and neurologic (movement disorders).

To adequately assess and treat sleep disorders, a comprehensive history and physical exam are needed (Table 28.2).

History of a sleep problem should include whether the problem is falling asleep, staying asleep, early morning awakening, or a combination. Hypersomnia and nonrestful sleep should also be evaluated. Past medical history including previous history of sleep problems and treatments should be reviewed (Table 28.3).

Table 28.1

The Most Common Syndromes Contributing to Sleep Disorders

- Insomnia: Difficulty falling asleep or staying asleep or having nonrestorative sleep.
- Narcolepsy: Falling asleep spontaneously.
- Sleep–wake schedule disturbance: The schedule for sleeping and being awake is different from the desired schedule, but the time spent sleeping is normal.
- Restless legs syndrome: Urge to move the legs because they feel uncomfortable, especially at night or lying down.
- Bruxism: Grinding or clenching teeth.
- Sleep apnea: Blockage of breathing when sleeping, causing loud snoring and frequent awakenings.
- Periodic limb movement disorder: Involuntary movement of extremities during sleep that causes arousal of which the individual is unaware.
- Sleepwalking: Walking or performing other activities while sleeping and not being aware of it.

Table 28.2

Key Parts of History and Physical Exam

- Past medical history including history or treatment of sleep disorder.
- Sleep quality and quantity looking for difficulties in falling or staying asleep.
- Degree of daytime tiredness.
- Review all medications, including over the counter, and other potential stimulant use (caffeine).
- Calculate body mass index to evaluate obstructive sleep apnea risk (weight (kg)/[height (m)]^2).
- Vitals signs
- Affect, thyroid, heart, lungs, musculoskeletal exam.

Table 28.3

Conditions Commonly Associated with Sleep Disorders

- Obesity
- Endocrine (thyroid disease, diabetes)
- Pulmonary (asthma, COPD)
- Gastrointestinal (gastro-esophageal reflux)
- Pain; psychiatric (anxiety, depression)
- Cardiac; neurologic (movement disorders)

Insomnia Questionnaires

The Pittsburgh Sleep Quality Index (PSQI) is a self-administered questionnaire measuring sleepiness and sleep quality. A global PSQI score of greater than 5 is a sensitive and specific measure of poor sleep quality. The PSQI is commonly used in the general population and has previously been validated in for use in a TBI population (2).

The Epworth Sleepiness Scale (ESS) (Table 28.4) is a self-administered eight-item questionnaire that was validated as a good screening test for sleep-disordered breathing. A score of ≥10 indicates significant sleepiness. The ESS has previously been used in TBI research (6).

Objective Measures of Sleep

The mean sleep latency test (MSLT) is a sleep disorder diagnostic tool generally done the day after polysomnography. It is used to measure the time it takes from the start of a nap period to the first signs of sleep. The test is based on the idea that the sleepier one is, the faster he or she will fall asleep. It can be used to test for narcolepsy and to distinguish between physical tiredness and true excessive daytime sleepiness. Its main purpose is to serve as an objective measure of sleepiness. The test consists of four or five 20-minute naps that are scheduled about 2 hours apart. During the test electroencephalogram (EEG), muscle activity, and eye movements are recorded. The entire test normally takes about 7 hours.

Nocturnal polysomnography (NPSG) is an overnight objective evaluation of sleep disturbance. During sleep the following bio-parameters are monitored: eye movement, EEG, muscle movement via EMG, respiration, heart rate and rhythm, blood oxygen levels, and continuous audiovisual monitoring. NPSG is most commonly used to diagnose obstructive sleep apnea. It is often considered

Table 28.4

Epworth Sleepiness Scale

How likely are you to doze off or fall asleep in the following situations?

Use the following scale for each situation
0 = no chance of dozing
1 = slight chance of dozing
2 = moderate chance of dozing
3 = high chance of dozing

Situation	Chance of dozing
Sitting and reading	
Watching TV	
Sitting in a public place (e.g., theater)	
As a passenger in a car for an hour	
Lying down to rest in the afternoon	
Sitting and talking to someone	
Sitting quietly after lunch without alcohol	
In a car, while stopped for a few minutes in traffic	

Score of ≥10 indicates significant sleepiness.
Source: Johns MW. A new method for measuring daytime sleepiness: The Epworth Sleepiness Scale. Sleep 1994; 17:703–710.

the criterion standard for diagnosing, determining the severity of the disease, and evaluating various other sleep disorders (see Table 28.1). NPSG can offer the clinician objective evidence if a sleep disorder is the cause of excessive daytime sleepiness and therefore guide treatment.

Actigraphy uses a portable device, commonly shaped like a watch, to evaluate sleep–wake patterns and establishes circadian rhythms by assessing movement. It is most commonly used as part of a comprehensive sleep evaluation. Patients wear the actigraph over multiple days and keep a sleep and rest diary. Actigraphy may be useful in circadian rhythm disorders and to evaluate the effectiveness of the treatment of sleep disorders.

TREATMENT

Evaluation and treatment of sleep disorders may require a multidisciplinary team. Many of these treatments, including respiratory aides, are beyond the scope of this chapter. Limited research exists on specific treatments for sleep disorders after neurologic injury. Sleep hygiene and pharmacologic and psychologic treatments are discussed below.

Sleep Hygiene

Many sleep disturbances are acquired over time due to poor sleep habits. Prior to initiating any other sleep treatment, a review of sleep hygiene and education about sleep hygiene is critical (Table 28.5). If this is not effective, the treatment options discussed below may be added.

Pharmacologic Treatment: Prescribed

Antidepressants, antipsychotics, and other psychotropic agents may have predictable desirable or undesirable effects on sleep and waking (Table 28.6) (7). In patients treated for comorbid psychiatric conditions, it may be possible

Table 28.5

Sleep Hygiene

- Avoid caffeine, nicotine, and alcohol in the evening.
- Exercise regularly in the late afternoon but not 3 hours before bedtime.
- Avoid napping during the day.
- Make sure there is not too much light or noise in bedroom.
- If you can't sleep for more than 30 minutes, get out of bed and do something relaxing or boring till you feel sleepy.
- Go to bed and get up the same time each day.
- Avoid bright light before going to bed.
- Avoid going to bed hungry or having a heavy meal before going to bed.

to prescribe these medications to take advantage of their sedating or alerting effects. Selected antidepressants and antipsychotics have been prescribed on an off-label basis solely to promote sleep. The moderately long elimination half-life of many of these medications increases the risk for undesired next-morning or daytime sedation following bedtime use. Antidepressants often recommended to promote sleep include trazodone, amitriptyline, doxepin, and mirtazapine. The report from the 2005 NIH State-of-the-Science Conference on chronic insomnia highlighted the safety concerns and lack of supportive data in the use of these medications to treat insomnia (1).

Currently, two general classes of medications are approved by the U.S. Food and Drug Administration (FDA) for the treatment of insomnia: benzo-diazepine receptor agonists (BZRA) and selective melatonin receptor agonists. Knowledge in regard to the physiology of sleep–wake cycle regulation and the respective pharmacologic characteristics of these medications predicts the beneficial sleep-related effects, potential undesired daytime sedation, and other possible adverse effects (8).

BZRA medications are modulators of GABA responses at the GABAA–receptor complex. The BZRA hypnotics available in the United States include five medications with a basic benzodiazepine structure and four formulations of newer nonbenzodiazepine hypnotics.

The five benzodiazepine BZRA hypnotics range in half-life from hours (tri-azolam) to days (flurazepam and quazepam). The longer–half-life medications may result in residual daytime effects, and the serum levels may accumulate until a steady state is reached when taken on a nightly basis. All of these benzo-diazepine hypnotics have standard immediate-release pharmacokinetics.

The four BZRA nonbenzodiazepine hypnotics include three immediate-release formulations (eszopiclone, zaleplon, and zolpidem) and one extended-release formulation (zolpidem extended-release). The elimination half-lives range from the ultrashort zaleplon at about 1 hour to eszopiclone at approxi-mately 6 hours. Accordingly, these compounds have a reduced risk for residual next-day sedation. The extended-release zolpidem formulation is designed to maintain a higher serum level of the medication throughout the early and middle portions of the night, but allows a sufficiently rapid decline later during the night to avoid residual sedation the following morning.

The most predictable adverse effect of the BZRA hypnotics is residual daytime sedation, especially with the longer half-life medications. Although generally well tolerated, other potential undesired effects of these medications include headache, dizziness, nausea, diarrhea, anterograde amnesia, sleepwalk-ing, and confused behaviors during the night.

Ramelteon is a nonsedating selective melatonin receptor agonist and the only non-BZRA approved for the treatment of insomnia. It is selective for the MT1 and MT2 melatonin receptor subtypes, high concentrations of which are located in the suprachiasmatic nucleus. The approved indication is for the treatment of insomnia characterized by difficulty with sleep onset. Ramelteon

Table 28.6

Pharmacology of Sleep

Drug	Typical dose	Impact on sleep	Indication for insomnia	Side effects and adverse effects	Drug–drug interactions
Benzodiazepines	Varies by drug	↓ Sleep latency, ↑ TST, ↓ NA	Generally not recommended	Rebound insomnia, altered sleep architecture, dependence, tolerance, amnesia, paradoxical aggression	May increase effect of other sedatives. Modafinil may prolong effect of benzodiazepine.
Zolpidem	5–10 mg	↓ sleep latency, ↑ TST, ↓ NA, ↑ sleep efficiency[a]	Sleep initiation; less useful for sleep maintenance; approved for short-term use	Amnesia and impaired motor skills while drug is active, possible rebound insomnia, rare somnambulism; somnolence, dizziness	May increase effect of other sedatives.
Zolpidem extended-release	6.25–12.5 mg	Same as zolpidem, but with improved sleep maintenance	Sleep initiation and sleep maintenance; approved for short-term use	Similar to zolpidem, headache	May increase effect of other sedatives.
Zaleplon	5–10 mg	↓ sleep latency	Sleep initiation; little impact on sleep maintenance due to short half-life; approved for short-term use	Less likely to cause next-day impaired psychomotor skills	Cimetidine may increase zaleplon levels.

Drug	Dose	Sleep effects	Indication	Adverse effects	Interactions
Eszopiclone	1–3 mg	↓ sleep latency, ↑TST, ↑ sleep efficiency, ↑ depth an quality of sleep	Sleep initiation and maintenance; approved for long-term use	Amnesia and impaired motor skills while drug is active, noting relatively long half-life; bitter taste, dry mouth, dizziness, and somnolence	Avoid admin with high-fat meals. Azole antifungals, clarithromycins, protease inhibitors, erythromycins, and fluvoxamine can increase eszopiclone levels.
Trazodone	25–250 mg	↓ sleep latency, ↑TST	Sleep initiation and/or maintenance, particularly for those with depression	Dizziness, dry mouth, nausea, blurry vision, drowsiness, hypotension, rebound insomnia, psychomotor impairments, potential QT prolongation.	MAOIs, azole antifungals, protease inhibitors, warfarin, and fluvoxamine can increase trazodone levels.
Mirtazepine	15–30 mg	↓ sleep latency, ↑TST, ↑ sleep efficiency	Sleep initiation and/or maintenance, particularly for those with depression	Drowsiness, dry mouth, ↑ appetite, weight gain, dizziness Impaired driving performance following initial dosing.	MAOIs, triptans, and SSRIs may increase risk of serotonin syndrome. May decrease efficacy of central α_2 agonists
Ramelteon	8 mg	↓ sleep latency, ↑TST	Sleep initiation and/or maintenance; approved for long-term use	Drowsiness, fatigue, and dizziness; contraindicated for those with severe hepatic dysfunction; use with caution in those with moderate hepatic dysfunction	Azole antifungals, barbiturates, carbamazepine, cipro, clarithromycins, protease inhibitors, phenytoin, oral contraceptives and fluvoxamine can increase ramelteon levels.

TST, total sleep time; NA, nocturnal awakenings.
aSleep efficiency = TST/time in bed.

has been shown to have no abuse potential and, therefore, is classed as a non-scheduled medication by the U.S. Drug Enforcement Agency.

The prescribing guidelines for ramelteon include evening use approximately 30 minutes prior to bedtime. It is available in a single 8-mg dose. Although there is no evidence of psychomotor or cognitive impairment with ramelteon, hazardous activities should be avoided following the dose due to anticipated sleepiness. Adverse effects may include somnolence, dizziness, and fatigue. Due to the possibility of elevated ramelteon blood levels, it should not be used by people with moderate-to-severe hepatic impairment or those taking fluvoxamine.

Pharmacologic Treatment: Over the Counter

All of the regulated over-the-counter sleep aids contain antihistamines. Most have diphenhydramine as the active ingredient. Although these readily available medications may enhance sleep onset and maintenance, there is minimal evidence in regard to their use in the treatment of insomnia. Additionally, there are important safety considerations. The most common difficulty with the antihistamine sleep aids is residual next-morning sedation following bedtime use due to the relatively long half-lives. Diphenhydramine also has anticholinergic activity that can result in confusion, delirium, and urinary retention (1).

Pharmacologic Treatment: Herbs

Among these unregulated substances is an assortment of homeopathic and dietary supplement preparations marketed as sleep aids or used as folk remedies. These include products containing valerian, hops, lavender, skullcap, chamomile, passion flower, kava kava, melatonin, and others. There is an absence of compelling efficacy evidence in the treatment of insomnia, and few studies have examined potential pharmacologic effects related to sleep (1). A major challenge is that the plant preparations often contain a large number of separate molecules, and it is unclear which single molecule or combination of active ingredients might influence sleep. One potential problem with this general class of substances is that their use may delay sleep-disordered individuals from seeking help from healthcare professionals. Generally these substances are regarded as safe, although FDA has issued a warning with regard to kava-containing preparations and severe liver injury.

The current understanding of the effects of endogenous melatonin on the suprachiasmatic nuclei (SCN) and the influence on the sleep–wake cycle would predict possible benefits of exogenous melatonin in enhancing sleep onset. Although melatonin has been widely used as a sleep aid, data from meta-analyses have not supported the efficacy of over-the-counter melatonin used as a bedtime insomnia treatment. However, melatonin may be therapeutic in applications involving circadian rhythm disorders.

Psychologic Treatments

In clinical practice hypnotic medications remain the most frequent treatment for insomnia. Side effects and risk of dependence are concerns with these medications. The neurologically impaired group may have a greater risk of adverse effects. Recent efforts have been devoted to the development of behavioral treatments for insomnia (9).

Behavioral insomnia treatment options include stimulus control (associating the bed, bedroom, and bedtime stimuli with sleep rather than with frustration, anxiety, or tension), relaxation techniques, sleep restriction (limiting the time spent in bed to the actual total time spent sleeping), cognitive behavioral treatments (identify, challenge, and alter a set of dysfunctional beliefs and attitudes about sleep), and sleep hygiene (Table 28.4). Cognitive behavioral therapy has been shown to be successful and even superior to pharmacologic treatment in the general population. Cognitive behavioral therapy has also been shown to be useful in TBI patients. The combination of stimulus control, sleep restriction, cognitive therapy, and sleep hygiene education produced improvements in sleep onset, awakenings, and efficiency.

REFERENCES

1. National Institutes of Health. National Institutes of Health State-of-the-Science Conference statement on manifestations and management of chronic insomnia in adults, June 13–15, 2005. Sleep 2005; 28:1049–1057.
2. Fichtenberg NL, Zafonte RD, Putnam S, Mann NR, Millard AE. Insomnia in a post-acute brain injury sample. Brain Injury 2002; 16:197–206.
3. Mahmood O, Rapport LJ, Hanks RA, Fichtenberg NL. Neuropsychological performance and sleep disturbance following traumatic brain injury. J Head Trauma Rehabil 2004; 19: 378–390.
4. Stanton BR. Sleep and fatigue in multiple sclerosis. Multiple Sclerosis 2006; 12:481–486.
5. Burns SP, Kapur V, Yin KS, Buhrer R. Factors associated with sleep apnea in men with spinal cord injury: a population-based case-control study. Spinal Cord 2001; 39:15–22.
6. Castriotta RJ, Wilde MC, Lai JM, Atanasov S, Masel BE, Kuna ST. Prevalence and consequences of sleep disorders in traumatic brain injury. J Clin Sleep Med 2007; 3:349–356.
7. Flanagan SR, Greenwald BD, Weiber S. Pharmacological treatment of insomnia for individuals with brain injury. J Head Trauma Rehabil 2007; 22:67–70.
8. Jones BE. Basic mechanisms of sleep-wake states. In: Kryger MH, Roth T, Dement WC, eds. Principles and Practice of Sleep Medicine. Philadelphia: Elsevier, 2005:136–153.
9. Medline Plus sleep disorders: http://www.nlm.nih.gov/medlineplus/sleepdisorders.html.

29 | Spasticity

Rosanna C. Sabini
Steven R. Flanagan

Spasticity is defined as an involuntary, velocity-dependent increase in resistance to passive range of motion (ROM). It is caused by diseases of the central nervous system (CNS), including cerebral palsy (CP), multiple sclerosis (MS), stroke, and acquired brain and spinal cord injuries (SCIs) (1,3–7). Spasticity can present with positive symptoms (hyperreflexia, emergence of primitive reflexes [e.g., Babinski], loss of autonomic control, contractures, and clonus) and negative symptoms (fatigue, loss of dexterity, weakness, and paralysis) (1,3–7).

Spasticity is known to affect more than half of CP, MS, and SCI populations, interfering with their mobility and activities of daily living (ADL) (1,4). By impairing motor control, restricting joint ROM, and causing muscle shortening, spasticity can complicate caregiving and hinder patient positioning and hygiene. In addition, secondary complications can develop, which include skin ulcerations, sleep disorders, breathing and swallowing difficulties, muscle contractures, joint subluxations or dislocations, long bone fractures, and peripheral neuropathy (1,3–7). However, spasticity is not always detrimental and at times may improve function in an otherwise weakened limb. For example, spasticity can be used to one's advantage by using a leg positioned in extension as a splint to allow one to stand, ambulate, and transfer. In addition, spasticity may assist in maintaining muscle bulk and preventing osteoporosis. Therefore, successful management is based on formulating an individualized program that first assesses its impact on function, comfort, and joint ROM. It is then followed by a well-thought-out treatment plan to reduce spasticity, when appropriate, with the goal of enhancing patient's independence and quality of life.

The goal of this chapter is to provide an overview of the causes, assessment, and treatment of spasticity and emphasize key patient safety and patient education points.

ANATOMY AND PHYSIOLOGY

Spasticity, which is part of the upper motor neuron (UMN) syndrome, is a sensorimotor phenomenon caused by an injury to the CNS (excludes the anterior horn cells) (1,3–7). Injuries can arise from trauma, hemorrhage, infarction, demyelination, inflammation, infection, or neoplasm. Initially, such lesions often manifest with a period of muscle flaccidity (3–6). But as the recovery process ensues, the CNS reorganizes and leads to abnormal patterns of neuronal activation and involuntary muscle hyperactivity (likely secondary to neural sprouting) (3–6). There is a loss of descending inhibitory influences from the brain and hyperexcitability of the α-motor neurons and spinal interneurons, all leading to increased stretch reflexes and muscle tone (3–6). If left untreated, properties and functions of muscle can change into contractures and fibrosis, further inhibiting functional activities (3–6).

PATIENT ASSESSMENT

History and Physical Examination

The interdisciplinary team in rehabilitation is ideal in providing an individualized spasticity treatment plan for maximizing function and minimizing side effects. As with any patient encounter, history and physical examination are the key components to an accurate diagnosis and treatment (Table 29.1). One of the most important questions to ask a patient is: "Does your spasticity

Table 29.1

Pertinent History Questions and Physical Examination Points for Spasticity

History Questions
- When did your spasticity begin?
- How frequent and severe is your spasticity?
- What are the aggravating and alleviating factors?
- What spasticity treatments have you tried and how successful were they?
- Does your spasticity interfere with your daily activities or lifestyle?
- What medications are you taking and what other medical illnesses do you have?
- What is your current living situation?
- Do you require assistance for everyday activities? If yes, how much assistance is required and who helps you?

Physical Examination Points
- Mental status—level of consciousness, orientation, recent and remote memory, attention and judgment, calculations, agnosia, apraxia
- Speech—aphasia and dysarthria
- Cranial nerves I–XII
- Coordination—finger to nose, heel-knee-shin, rapid alternating movements, tandem gait
- Reflexes—deep tendon, superficial and primitive, clonus
- Motor—adventitious movements, strength, muscle bulk, and tone at each joint
- Sensory—pinprick and light touch, proprioception, vibratory sense, two-point discrimination and localization
- Gait—balance, walking, toe-and-heel walk, postural reflexes
- Spasticity—muscle co-contraction, rigidity, and velocity induced resistance to passive ROM using the Ashworth, spasm frequency, and Tardieu scales

or spasms interfere with your daily activities or lifestyle?" Not all spasticity requires treatment, and a patient may prefer to preserve spasticity in one location of their body to perform certain tasks. Women, for instance, may want to keep elbow flexor tone to hold their purse, or others may prefer lower extremity tone to pivot transfer and ambulate (3). In addition, patient compliance is very important because some medications, if not taken as directed, can lead to medical emergencies (e.g., Baclofen withdrawal).

After eliciting a comprehensive medical history, a complete physical should include a detailed neurologic, musculoskeletal, functional examination and quantitative measurement of spasticity.

Measurement

Spasticity is measured using severity and frequency scales. The most commonly used are the Modified Ashworth Scale (4,5,7,8) (Table 29.2), the Spasm Frequency Scale (4,7) (Table 29.3), and the Tardieu Scale (2) (Table 29.4). One or all the scales can be used for treatment; but to effectively monitor progress, the same scales should be used consistently.

Table 29.2

Modified Ashworth Scale

Grade	Description
0	No increase in muscle tone
1	Slight increase in muscle tone, manifested by a catch and release or by minimal resistance at the end of motion when the affected part(s) is moved in flexion or extension
1+	Slight increase in muscle tone, manifested by a catch, followed by minimal resistance throughout the remainder (less than half) of the range of movement (ROM)
2	More marked increase in muscle tone through most of the ROM, but affected part(s) easily moved
3	Considerable increase in muscle tone, passive movement difficult
4	Affected part(s) rigid in flexion or extension

Source: Refs. 4,5,7,8.

Table 29.3

Spasm Frequency Scale

Score	Criteria
1	No spontaneous spasms, but vigorous sensory or motor stimulation results in spasms
2	Occasional spontaneous spasms or easily induced spasms
3	Greater than one but fewer than 10 spontaneous spasms per hour
4	Greater than 10 spontaneous spasms per hour

Source: Refs 4,7.

Table 29.4

Tardieu Scale

Score	Criteria
0	No resistance throughout the course of the passive movement
1	Slight resistance throughout the course of passive movement with no clear catch
2	Clear catch interrupting the passive movement, followed by release
3	Fatigable clonus (lasting <10 seconds when maintaining the pressure)
4	Unfatigable clonus (lasting >10 seconds when maintaining the pressure)
5	Joint is immovable

Measurement of spasticity is performed with the patient lying supine, head midline, and at three different velocities: V1 (speed slower than limb falling under gravity), V2 (speed equivalent to limb falling under gravity) and V3 (speed faster than limb falling under gravity).
Source: Ref 2.

TREATMENT

Successful spasticity treatment encompasses a patient's functional goals, medical condition and prognosis, spasticity onset, location and severity, cognitive and functional abilities, and availability of both social and economic supports. Treatment options include rehabilitation (ice, electrical stimulation, ROM exercises, stretching, casting), medications (oral, intrathecal), injections (phenol, botulinum toxin), and surgical interventions (discussed later). Untreated, spasticity can cause pain, interfere with functional skills, positioning, hygiene, and overall patient care (1,3–8). Based on an individual's goals, frequent assessments are needed for appropriate management to determine treatment efficacy. For example, rapidly evolving spasticity may require more aggressive dosing of antispasticity medications or early use of interventional procedures to prevent secondary complications (8). Also, a sudden increase in spasticity can be an indicator of noxious stimuli and should be immediately diagnosed and treated (Figure 29.1) (1,3–8).

Rehabilitative Treatment

Education
Teaching the patient and caregivers about spasticity management and treatment early in rehabilitation can maximize functional outcomes and reduce secondary complications. Education should not only focus on proper positioning and stretching, but also emphasize decreasing fatigue and stress. Ill-fitting braces can also exacerbate spasticity, and patients/caregivers need to be instructed on proper application. As mentioned earlier, spasticity worsens with noxious stimuli secondary to urinary retention, constipation, infection, ingrown toenails, pressure ulcerations, deep venous thrombosis, kinked urinary catheters, heterotopic ossification, or fractures. Especially in the cognitively impaired,

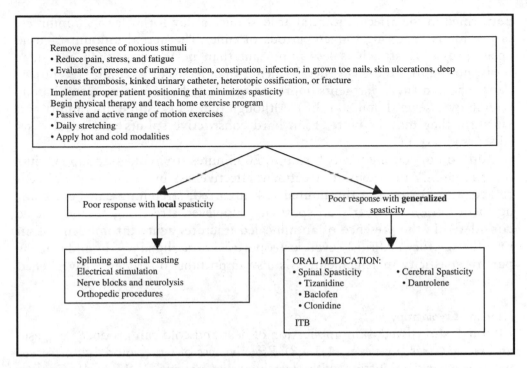

Figure 29.1. Treatment plan for spasticity management.

caregivers need to be aware of such complications, and worsening of their spasticity warrants immediate medical attention.

Positioning
Comfortable, stable, and symmetrical trunk and limb positions should be achieved to decrease spasticity (1,3,4). Physical and occupational therapists can provide appropriate seating systems, foot straps, and back supports to achieve and maintain body positions that minimize spasticity and promote function. Proper limb positioning ideally begins at the time of injury, prior to the development of spasticity, in order to enhance recovery and maintain maximal ROM (8). While positioning is important, prolonged immobility in any position should be avoided because there is an increased risk of developing contractures and pressure ulcers. For example, prolonged sitting in a wheelchair may make it difficult for an individual to lie supine for sleep.

Stretching, Passive Range of Motion, and Strengthening Exercises
Slow and sustained muscle stretching provided by either passive or active assisted ROM is effective in decreasing spasticity and preventing muscle contractures (1,3–5,7,8). Long-term effects positively correlate with the frequency and length of stretch given: the more the better. It is also thought that sustained versus intermittent stretching has increased functional benefit (3). Although there are no specific guidelines, stretching is recommended to be

performed in the affected joint(s) at least once a day for at least 20 minutes, larger joints requiring longer periods of time. The actual amount of time spent providing stretch is less important than performing it on a regular basis, noting that more is generally better than less. For example, recent evidence showed Lycra garments improved spasticity by providing a continuous stretch over several hours (1,3,8). Although they cause some discomfort and warmth, they may be better than hard constrictive splints and serial casts (discussed later) (1).

Addition of cooling packs for up to 20 minutes (to avoid skin injury) during stretching can potentiate treatment effectiveness by reducing the stretch reflex (4,8). Because of the limited risk involved, stretching can be a management option for nearly all spasticity. However, stretching should not be considered in the presence of an unhealed fracture, acute thromboembolism or inflammatory arthritis, severe osteoporosis, or malignancy. In addition, as part of spasticity management, it is also important to strengthen weakened muscles.

Heat and Cryotherapy

Although short-lived, skin application of heat and cold can produce analgesia and reduce stretch reflexes (1,3,4,8). Effectiveness of either modality increases when used in conjunction with stretching and passive ROM (1,4). Cooling can be applied as ice or administered via an evaporative cooling spray (ethyl chloride) to decrease muscle spindle sensitivity, stretch reflexes, and slow nerve conduction velocities (4). Heat can decrease pain through vasodilation and can be applied via hydrocollator packs, ultrasound, paraffin baths, and whirlpool (4). To prevent thermal injuries, especially in patients with sensory and/or cognitive impairments, treatment is limited to 20 minutes (8). If properly educated, patients/caregivers can use these modalities at home along with their daily stretching program.

Splinting and Serial Casting

Splints made of either soft or firm materials can be used to maintain a spastic limb in a maximally stretched or functional position for a prolonged period of time, improving both ROM and function (1,4,5,7,8). Applying a series of plaster casts is indicated in restricted joint ROM to progressively stretch the limb, maximize joint mobility, and prevent joint contractures (4,8). The casts are positioned about 5 degrees from maximal passive ROM to avoid increasing spasticity and then changed every 3–5 days until the maximum range is achieved (4). Appropriate patients include those that can tolerate the casts without excessive sweating or agitation (4). Elbows, wrists, knees, and ankles are the most commonly casted joints, and given their bony prominences, proper fit and monitoring for skin breakdown are essential. Although the maximum ROM that can be achieved limits the effectiveness of serial casting, many clinicians prefer to combine casting with other modalities such as heat, enteral medications, or motor point injections to maximize treatment benefits.

Electrical Stimulation

Transcutaneous electrical nerve stimulation (TENS) devices have been used for the management of spasticity, although their efficacy is debatable (4). Electrical impulses can fatigue spastic muscles and activate antagonist muscles to increase joint ROM and flexibility (1,3,8). In addition, TENS can also help reduce nociceptive pain associated with spasticity (3).

Oral Pharmacotherapy

Oral medications are often considered early in the treatment of spasticity. Currently, FDA has approved four drugs for the treatment of spasticity: diazepam, baclofen, dantrolene, and tizanidine (5). Other medications commonly used as "off-label" for spasticity treatment will also be discussed.

Recommendations regarding which oral medicine to use depend upon whether spasticity is spinal or cerebral in origin. Some medications have generalized side effects, such as sedation or cognitive effects, and are not appropriate for brain-injured patients (Table 29.5). Therefore, treatment is patient dependent, requiring frequent monitoring for side effects and efficacy.

Benzodiazepines

Benzodiazepines, such as diazepam, were historically used first line in the treatment of spasticity because of their ability to inhibit both muscle spasms and hyperreflexia, while increasing passive ROM (3–5). Benzodiazepines bind to GABA-a receptors, which open chloride channels and hyperpolarize the cell membrane, resulting in increased presynaptic inhibition of reflexes (3–5). Studies have shown treatment efficacy in SCI; however, benzodiazepines are not recommended in acquired brain-injured patients because of their potential to impair neurorecovery and cognition, and worsen arousal (3–5,8). This medication class may also be beneficial for treating spasticity with co-existing anxiety disorders or nocturnal spasms (4). Potential side effects include CNS depression, ataxia, behavioral changes, memory dysfunction, fatigue, cognitive impairment and addiction, and withdrawal if discontinued abruptly (3–5).

Baclofen

Baclofen binds to GABA-b receptors, inhibiting calcium influx into presynaptic terminals and release of neurotransmitters involved in mono- and polysynaptic reflex pathways (3–5). Studies have shown that baclofen is more effective in the treatment of spasticity in SCI and MS than acquired brain injury populations (likely secondary to its side-effect profile) (3–5,8). Side effects include confusion, sedation, memory impairment, dizziness, and ataxia, which can worsen a brain-injured patients' condition (1,3–5). Other adverse effects include paresthesias, bronchoconstriction, nausea, and hypotension (1,3–5). In the event that baclofen needs to be discontinued, it must be tapered slowly (over 1–2 weeks) to prevent withdrawal seizures, hallucinations, rhabdomyolysis, multiorgan failure, and death (discussed later) (4). Under certain conditions, baclofen may also be administered intrathecally.

Table 29.5

Oral Pharmacotherapy for Treatment of Spasticity

Medication	Starting and maximum daily dose	Half-life (hr)	Mechanism of action	Side effects	Drug use safety	Comments
Diazepam	2–4 mg 60 mg	20–80	Presynaptic inhibition via GABA-a receptors	Hypotension, ataxia, sedation, somnolence, CNS and respiratory depression, fatigue, impaired cognition and memory. Elderly and debilitated patients are at an increased risk of side effects.	Dantrolene and opioids increase risk of CNS depression. Alcohol can increase toxicity. Contraindicated in hypersensitivity to diazepam. Precautions in liver insufficiency. Avoid abrupt discontinuation.	Potential negative impact on neurorecovery. Recommended in spinal spasticity.
Baclofen	5–10 mg 80 mg[a]	3.5	Active at GABA-b receptors, inhibiting neurotransmitter release and activation of synaptic reflexes	Sedation, somnolence, headache, dizziness, ataxia, constipation, nausea, vomiting, hypotension, agitation, seizures, respiratory depression, bradycardia, mild hypothermia.	Alcohol and sedatives increase CNS depression. Abrupt discontinuation is contraindicated because of withdrawal symptoms (fevers, altered mental status, rebound spasticity, hallucinations, rhabdomyolysis, multiple organ failure, and death). Contraindicated in baclofen sensitivity. Use lower dosages in elderly or renal patients.	Potential negative impact on neurorecovery. Recommended in SCI and MS spasticity.
Dantrolene	25 mg 400 mg	15	Inhibits calcium release at sarcoplasmic reticulum, weakening contraction force	Drowsiness, dizziness, weakness, headache, sedation, fatigue, paresthesias, nausea, constipation, diarrhea, diplopia, visual disturbance.	Diazepam and opioids increase risk of CNS depression. Contraindicated in acute liver disease. Avoid in women and age >30 years (increased risk of hepatocellular disease). Requires frequent LFT monitoring.	Recommended in CP, SCI and cerebral spasticity.

Drug	Dose	Mechanism	Side effects	Precautions/Contraindications	Comments
Tizanidine	4 mg 36 mg	α_2-Adrenergic receptor agonist, inhibits excitatory release	Weakness, somnolence, dry mouth, dizziness, bradycardia, abnormal LFTs, orthostatic hypotension (have patient get up slowly from supine position).	Avoid abrupt cessation (rebound hypertension, tachycardia, and hypertonia). Monitor BP when used with other antihypertensive agents (hypotension). Avoid alcohol use. Precaution in renal and liver disease. Contraindicated w/ use of ciprofloxacin and fluvoxamine or hypersensitivity to tizanidine.	May have negative impact on neurorecovery. Recommended in spinal spasticity.
Clonidine	0.1 mg[b] 0.4 mg[b]	Acts on locus ceruleus, decreasing tonic facilitation; α_2-adrenergic agonist	Weakness, dizziness, syncope, hypotension, bradycardia, dizziness, somnolence, depression, constipation, nausea, dry mouth.	Allergic skin reaction to transdermal. Avoid alcohol, barbiturates, or other sedatives. Avoid abrupt discontinuation (rebound hypertension).	Potential negative impact on motor recovery. Recommended in SCI.
Gabapentin	300 mg 3600 mg	Centrally acting GABA agonist	Somnolence, dizziness, fatigue, ataxia, nystagmus, peripheral edema, myalgia, tremor.	Avoid abrupt discontinuation (status epilepticus). Contraindicated with hypersensitivity to gabapentin. Precaution in renal disease.	Recommended in SCI and MS.

[a] Although not recommended, doses as high as 300 mg have been safely used.
[b] Oral dose is given daily; transdermal dose is given weekly.
Source: Refs. 1,3–5,7,8.

Dantrolene

Dantrolene is different from other medications because it acts directly on the skeletal muscle. By inhibiting the release of calcium from the sarcoplasmic reticulum, it weakens the force of muscle contractions (1,3–5,8). Dantrolene has been shown to have no effect on neural pathways and is frequently recommended in CP, SCI, and acquired brain injury (3–5,8). Although rare, its use is limited by increased risk of liver toxicity, requiring monitoring of liver function tests (LFTs) (1,3–5,8). The greatest risk was found in women over the age of 30 treated with high doses of dantrolene for a prolonged period of time (3–5,8). Usually hepatotoxicity is reversible with discontinuation of the drug (3,4,8). Baseline LFT's should be drawn prior to administration, followed by weekly levels for the first month, progressing from monthly to every 3 months thereafter if stable (3). Other side effects include generalized weakness, sedation, paresthesias, nausea, and diarrhea (1,3–5,8).

Tizanidine

Tizanidine, an imidazoline derivative, is an α_2-adrenergic agonist that reduces spasticity by inhibiting excitatory amino acids (glutamate and aspartate) and facilitating glycine (an inhibitory neurotransmitter) (1,3–5,8). The primary side effect of tizanidine is weakness, but others include fatigue, dry mouth, dizziness, hypotension, and abnormal LFTs (1,3–5,8). Tizanidine is an effective antispasticity treatment for SCI and MS, but may slow recovery in acquired brain-injured patients (3–5,8).

Clonidine

Clonidine is also an imidazoline derivative traditionally used for the treatment of hypertension, but it has been shown to decrease muscle spasms and resistance to stretch (3–5,8). In addition, clonidine decreases tonic facilitation at the locus ceruleus (4,5). Although the side effect profile is similar to tizanidine, clonidine can be administered orally or transdermally, the latter allowing for easier administration and well-balanced drug levels (3–5). However, patients who have sensitivities to adhesives may not tolerate the patch. Currently, use of clonidine is most effective in SCI spasticity and limited in acquired brain injury because of its negative effects on neurorecovery (3,4).

Gabapentin

Gabapentin (an anticonvulsant agent) is a GABA analogue that has demonstrated spasticity reduction in MS and SCI patients (3–5,8). Studies have shown that a minimum dose of 400 mg three times daily is required to improve spasticity (3,5,8). Usually, the dose is slowly titrated based on the desired results and slowly tapered when discontinued. At times, dosages can reach antiseizure levels and may benefit certain patients (3). Side effects are relatively benign and primarily cause somnolence, dizziness, fatigue, ataxia, and nystagmus (3–5). Gabapentin can also be used for the treatment of neuropathic pain (8).

Other Oral Agents

Other agents such as GABA, α-agonists, phenytoin, cannabinoids, and morphine have also been used for the treatment of spasticity; however, they are not routinely recommended, and additional studies are needed to determine their efficacy (3–5).

Neurolytic Pharmacotherapy

Focal or regional interventional treatments are reasonable options for managing spasticity, especially when systemic therapies cause generalized side effects or cognitive impairments (Table 29.6). In the presence of a CNS lesion, chemical neurolysis of motor nerves at the neuromuscular junction creates a lower motor neuron lesion. This lesion can now disrupt the efferent signals from the hyperexcitable anterior horn cells and decrease spasticity (4,5).

Phenol

Phenol is a low-cost and effective agent for treating spasticity. Once injected into a muscle or nerve, phenol disrupts conduction via protein coagulation and necrosis (3–5,8). Phenol has immediate anesthetic effects, with antispasticity effects occurring within 2 days. The effects can last 3–6 months and in some cases may result in permanent spasticity reduction (5,7).

Because phenol targets proteins indiscriminately, vasculature and mixed and/or sensory nerves can also be affected, causing vascular complications, dysesthesias, and sensory loss (3–5,8). Such complications are usually related to clinician experience, concentration used, and the nerve injected (e.g., injection of the median nerve is more likely to cause dysesthesias than injection to the musculocutaneous nerve). Using electromyography (EMG)-guided needling can minimize these effects. If dysesthesias become intolerable, therapy and membrane-stabilizing anticonvulsants or neuropathic agents (e.g., gabapentin) can be used. In some cases, reblockade of the nerve has also been shown to relieve symptoms (3).

Other phenol side effects include pain at injection site, excessive weakness and loss of beneficial spasticity, swelling, edema, bleeding, and deep venous thrombosis (3–5). If absorbed systemically, phenol can cause nausea, CNS depression, convulsions, and cardiovascular instability; however, these are uncommon since dosages used are well below toxic levels (diluted 2–7%) (3–5).

Phenol has been used for CP and acquired brain injury–related spasticity (3–5,8). Despite its positive impact, using phenol too early is controversial because neurolysis in the early stages of recovery may scar muscle tissue and impair future recovery (8).

Botulinum Toxins

Chemoneurolysis with botulinum toxins is approved for the treatment of certain dystonias. With a low side-effect profile, they have also been successfully

Table 29.6

Injectional Pharmacotherapy for Treatment of Spasticity

Medication	Dosage	Duration	Mechanism of action	Side effects	Comments
Phenol	2–7% aqueous solution	Immediate onset, lasting 3–6 months[a]	Chemically disrupts nerves by denaturing protein.	Dysesthesias, vascular complications, skin discomfort.	Cost is minimal, longer effect, experience determines effectiveness.
Ethanol	25–100% solutions	Immediate onset, lasting 3–6 months[a]	Chemically disrupts nerves by denaturing protein.	Dysesthesias, vascular complications, skin discomfort.	Cost is minimal, longer effect, easy to obtain, less toxic than phenol.
Botulinum toxin A (Botox)	30–200[b] Units	Onset 2–3 days, lasting up to 2–6 months	Inhibits release of acetylcholine at neuromuscular junction.	Unwanted weakness, local swelling, headache, weakness, flu-like symptoms, dry mouth, self-limited dysphagia (if injected in neck muscles), pain at injection site.	Expensive, efficacy in spasticity proven in studies performed. Contraindicated in hypersensitivity to botulinum toxin A or infection at injection site.
Botulinum toxin B (Myobloc)		Onset 2–3 days, lasting up to 2–6 months	Inhibits release of acetylcholine at neuromuscular junction.	Unwanted weakness, local swelling, headache, weakness, flu-like symptoms, dry mouth, self-limited dysphagia (if injected in neck muscles), pain at injection site, arthralgia.	Expensive, efficacy in spasticity limited by few studies available. Contraindicated in hypersensitivity to botulinum toxin B or infection at injection site.

[a]Effects can last up to 18 months, depending on proximity of delivery and concentrations used.
[b]Average dose per muscle, larger muscles requiring higher doses.
Source: Refs. 1,3–5,7,8.

used as an off-label treatment for spasticity (3–5,8). When botulinum toxin is injected into muscles, it denervates the neuromuscular junction by inhibiting acetylcholine release and decreasing the force of muscle contraction (1,3–5,8). Even though botulinum toxins diffuse through muscle membranes, they are best administered under EMG or electrical localization, especially when injected into small muscles that are difficult to isolate (1,4,7).

Of the seven serotypes available, botulinum toxin A has been the most widely studied. Botulinum toxin A has demonstrated effectiveness in improving ROM, tone, gait, and self-reported disability (3–5). Botulinum toxin B is also commercially available and has been used to treat spasticity; however, studies are limited. Choosing either toxin is discretionary, and there is no specific formula that equates their dosages.

Botulinum toxin B has a slightly longer duration of action and is dispensed in premixed, nonrefrigerated vials. In contrast, type A requires refrigeration and dilution with nonpreserved sterile saline prior to its use, which loses its potency after approximately 4 hours. Studies have also shown that with botulinum toxin A use, antibody formation against the toxins can develop in 3–5% of patients, requiring increased dosages to obtain similar efficacy (1,3–5). Because type B does not cross react with type A toxins, it may be an alternative to those who develop antibodies to type A (1,3,5). The risk of developing antibodies can be decreased if injections are scheduled at least 3 months apart and the lowest effective dosages are used to achieve maximal function (1,3).

Dosages for botulinum toxin A typically range from 30 to 200 Units per muscle (7), where the higher the dose injected, the greater the degree of weakness is expected (3). In addition, larger muscles usually require higher doses to achieve the desired effect (3). Therefore, the treatment must be individualized to a patient's weight, number of muscles being treated, muscle size, and severity of spasticity (5). Effects are usually seen 2–3 days postinjection and can last up to 3–4 months, with additional injections typically necessary thereafter (1,3–5).

A major concern with botulinum toxin is its cost, limiting its use in some patients. However, use may prevent secondary complications and prove to be cost-effective in the long-term (4). Contraindications to botulinum include a history of sensitivity to the toxin, concomitant use of aminoglycosides and spectinomycin antibiotics, and neuromuscular diseases such as myasthenia gravis or Lambert-Eaton syndrome (4,5).

Surgical Intervention

Most spasticity can be managed with a combination of physiotherapy, modalities, and pharmacotherapy. When these methods provide inadequate spasticity control and do not successfully improve functional ROM, tone, positioning, or ADL, more invasive treatments are available to achieve an improved quality of life.

Neurosurgical Procedures: Intrathecal Baclofen (ITB)

When the oral form of baclofen reaches maximal doses and side effects are intolerable, intrathecal administration is a useful alternative. Baclofen delivered intrathecally allows targeted delivery of GABA-mediated inhibition close to its area of action. The end results are use of significantly smaller doses and reduction of negative effects on cerebral physiology and neurorecovery. ITB has been shown to improve spasticity in CP, MS, SCI, and acquired brain injury populations by decreasing painful spasms, improving ROM, functional ADLs and quality of life (3–5). If used, the benefits should outweigh the risks because it is a costly procedure and requires patient and/or caregiver compliance. Timing ITB therapy is dependent upon the evolution of spasticity and success with previously implemented noninvasive treatments. ITB is indicated in the presence of severe spasticity (Ashworth Grade 3 or worse) that compromises functional activities such as hygiene or mobility (4). In addition, the patient/caregiver must be compliant with treatment follow-up to avoid medical complications. Contraindications to an intrathecal pump placement include presence of systemic infections and a history of an allergic reaction to baclofen (4).

To determine if ITB is a possible treatment option, an initial test dose of 50 µg of baclofen is administered via lumbar puncture, with changes in muscle tone assessed throughout the day (3–5). If the trial succeeds in reducing spasticity by one grade on the Ashworth Scale, the pump can be placed. If the initial test dose is unsuccessful at decreasing spasticity, the trial is repeated using 100 µg.

When the patient has passed the screening trial, an implantable pump is placed in the subcutaneous tissue of the abdominal wall with a catheter connected to the subarachnoid space. The catheter tip is usually placed between the spinal levels of T8 and T10 to reduce lower extremity spasticity (3). However, recent evidence suggests that spasticity can be reduced in both upper and lower limbs when the catheter is placed at higher spinal levels, and has been safely administered to levels as high as C4 (3).

The initial ITB dose is usually twice the amount of test dose used. For example, if the patient responded to a test dose of 100 µg, the pump is programmed to deliver 200 µg of baclofen over 24 hours (3,4). Based on the patient's response, dosages can be easily modified using external telemetry. Some patients may require several days or weeks to achieve a satisfactory response, requiring dosage increase of 10–20% (no more than 50 µg per day) (4), typically provided no sooner than 2–3 days between adjustments to allow sufficient time to assess its clinical effect. In the interim, it is critical that the oral baclofen not be abruptly discontinued during this process. Although there is no dosage conversion formula from oral to intrathecal baclofen, the medication should be slowly tapered to prevent withdrawal symptoms.

Depending on the reservoir capacity and dosage given, the pump needs to be refilled on a regular basis (~2–3 months). Using sterile technique, this is achieved by injecting the medication transdermally through the pump's access port. Pumps also have built in audible alarms that alert the patient when the battery is failing (~4- to 7-year life span, requiring replacement of the pump) or the medication reservoir volume has reached a predetermined low level. Both instances require immediate intervention to avoid withdrawal symptoms. Baclofen withdrawal can also occur if the catheter disconnects or is damaged (diagnosed with indium infusion studies and x-rays) (3,4). Baclofen overdose, although less frequent, is also a medical emergency. Infection at the surgical site (usually seen postoperatively with fevers and confirmed with laboratory studies) is another complication of ITB, which can extend to the catheter tip and cause meningitis if not properly treated. In addition, dislodgement of the catheter can cause cerebral spinal fluid (CSF) leakage and spinal headaches (4).

Orthopedic Procedures

Orthopedic procedures should be considered when less invasive spasticity treatments have failed. Limb function in the presence of spasticity can be optimized with joint fusions and muscle and tendon lengthening procedures (3–5). In addition, spastic muscles can be used in areas of weakness to displace forces and allow proper positioning or motion of limbs. Specifics of these procedures are beyond the scope of this book. Details of such procedures, such as the split anterior tibial transfer (SPLATT), can be found in surgical references (4).

Emergencies in Spasticity

Emergencies in spasticity primarily stem from the medications used in its treatment, namely benzodiazepines and intrathecal baclofen. Overdose of benzodiazepines can cause sedation and coma, which worsens with use of alcohol or drugs. Seizures similar to those of alcohol withdrawal can also occur with sudden discontinuation of benzodiazepines, especially if a patient has been taking the medication for a long period of time (4).

Baclofen withdrawal and overdose are common emergencies that can occur because of ITB malfunction or improper dosing. Infusion of the wrong drug concentration is most often due to clinician error and therefore dosing warrants caution. Clinicians need to ensure that the proper concentration of baclofen is infused during pump refill and that the appropriate bridging dose is provided if the drug concentration is changed. The instructions for programming bridging doses are easily accessed by the programmer. Symptoms of withdrawal are evident when there is an abrupt and unexpected increase in spasticity and is usually secondary to medication change. Other symptoms include pruritis without rash, diaphoresis, hypotension, hyperthermia, agitation, confusion, seizure, rhabdomyolysis, and multiple organ failure (3–5). Withdrawal is usually treated with high-dose baclofen while the pump is reprogrammed. Symptoms of baclofen overdose can be seen within an hour of medication change and include somnolence, seizures, bradycardia, nausea, hypotonia, respiratory failure, and coma (4). Removing the medication from the catheter access port (with appropriate kit available and training in performing this procedure) and providing mechanical ventilation, if needed, should be immediate. In addition, respiratory side effects can be reversed with administration of physostigmine (0.5–1 mg intravenously) (4).

Although extremely rare, botulinum toxins can cause dysphagia, typically occurring from overdosage or when injected in proximity to cervical musculature. Some studies have reported mild to severe dysphagia, requiring feeding tubes. Therefore, it is important to make the patient aware of this and that clinicians follow the recommended botulinum toxin dosaging guidelines.

Patient Safety

The following are important patient safety considerations to remember when treating spasticity:

- Positioning: Avoid prolonged sitting or flexed positions such as pillows under knees to prevent contractures.
- ROM or stretching: Aggressive therapy can lead to fractures in osteopenic or osteoporotic bones.
- Heat and cold therapies: Prevent thermal injuries by protecting the skin, especially if there is sensory loss or a cognitive impairment in the patient.
- Splinting and casts: Frequently check the patient's skin for the presence of breakdown.
- Oral medications: Patient should avoid operating heavy machinery or engaging in activities that require mental alertness while under the influence of the medications with that affect cognition.
- Benzodiazepines/baclofen: Titrate medications slowly to avoid medical emergencies.
- Neuroablation: Injecting phenol with EMG guidance can diminish dysesthesias and other complications.

Patient Education

Patients, their families, and caregivers should be educated as to the causes, effects, and complications of spasticity with material at an appropriate educational level. This material should also take into account language barriers and cognitive impairments. Education should also be provided on medications used to treat spasticity, titration schedules, common side effects, and significant adverse events (e.g., avoiding abrupt discontinuation of baclofen). For patients receiving ITB, education should be provided on the signs, symptoms, and dangers of baclofen withdrawal and overdose.

REFERENCES

1. Barnes MP. Spasticity: a rehabilitation challenge in the elderly. Gerontology 2001; 47:295–299.
2. Boyd RN, Graham HK. Objective measurement of clinical findings in the use of botulinum toxin type A for the management of children with cerebral palsy. Eur J Neurol 1999; 6(suppl 4): 23–35.
3. Elovic E, Bogey R. Spasticity and movement disorder. In: DeLisa JA, Gans BM, Walsh NE, eds. Physical Medicine and Rehabilitation: Principles and Practice. Philadelphia: Lippincott, 2005:1427–1446.
4. Gelber DA, Jeffery DR, eds. Clinical Evaluation and Management of Spasticity. Totowa, NJ: Humana Press, 2002.
5. Nance PW, Maythaler JM. Spasticity management. In: Braddom RL, ed. Physical Medicine and Rehabilitation. 3rd ed. Philadelphia: WB Saunders, 2006:651–665.
6. Petropoulou KB, Panourias IG, Rapidi CA, Sakas DE. The phenomenon of spasticity: a pathophysiological and clinical introduction to neuromodulation therapies. Neurochir Suppl 2007; 97(1):137–144.
7. Stein J. Spasticity. In: Frontera WR, Silver JK, eds. Essentials of Physical Medicine and Rehabilitation. Philadelphia: Hanley & Belfus, Inc., 2002:743–746.
8. Zafonte R, Elovic EP, Lombard L. Acute care management of post-TBI spasticity. J Head Trauma Rehabil 2004; 19(2):89–100.

30 | Substance Abuse

Loran C. Vocaturo

Substance abuse in the neurologically disabled population poses significant physical and emotional health risks. Not only have alcohol and drug use been strongly implicated as causal factors of spinal cord injury (SCI) and brain injury (BI; traumatic and acquired), but continued postinjury abuse has proved to have significant long-term negative effects on neurologically disabled patients (1). The implications for negative rehabilitation outcomes and postinjury adjustment problems among neurologically disabled patients are great and require special attention. Rehabilitation professionals must consider the role of alcohol and drug use in their assessment and treatment of these patients.

It has been estimated that 1 in 10 American adults suffers from alcohol abuse and related disorders. Alcohol abuse is the second leading cause of disability in the United States, costing the U.S economy in excess of $220 billion dollars per year. Individuals with co-existing neurologic disabilities are at an even greater risk of developing a substance-related disorder. It is estimated that over 4 million Americans with physical disabilities also suffer from addictive illness (1).

While epidemiologic studies have shown that intoxication is often present at the time of injury, less is known of the exact prevalence of substance abuse in the neurologically disabled population (2). In adults with SCI the prevalence of alcohol use and marijuana use is 21% and 11%, respectively, whereas in multiple sclerosis (MS) patients it is 14% and 14–16%, respectively. The prevalence of alcohol use in adults with traumatic brain injury (TBI) has been reported to be as high as 47%. The information on alcohol and drug abuse among acquired brain injury patients is limited; however, drug misuse has been implicated in cerebral vascular accidents (e.g. ischemic and hemorrhagic stroke). Similarly, little is known about the extent and patterns of alcohol and substance abuse in patients with MS. Cannabis, however, has been reported to be a drug used by MS patients primarily to alleviate symptoms of pain and spasticity. What seems to be more common with MS patients is the use of high doses of nonprescription medications (i.e., vitamin supplements). Clinicians should inquire about the use of nonprescription medications and advise patients of the potential adverse effects and risks of supplements.

In older adults the risk and effects of substance abuse is complicated by a number of factors (Table 30.1). Seventy-five percent of people over 65 and older use medications for common medical conditions that are part of the normal aging process along with medications for concomitant neurologic disabilities. Many older adults also drink alcohol, often to medicate emotional states caused by isolation, limited daily and social activities, or failing health. Because older adults may be receiving medical care from a number of different physicians, coordination of their care is often limited. The possibility of medication interactions and adverse effects when combined with alcohol and other drugs puts older patients are at an even higher risk for catastrophic results. It is imperative that healthcare professionals obtain a comprehensive list of a patient's medications, screen for alcohol and drug abuse, and educate patients about the potential risks as part of routine healthcare visits(3).

Risk factors unique to neurologically disabled patients in addition to those of the general population may predispose them to substance misuse. In the general population, family history, comorbid psychiatric disturbance, and personality characteristics have been associated with substance abuse. The sense of vulnerability that is imposed on neurologically disabled patients places them at risk for developing maladaptive coping mechanisms (e.g., substance use). They are particularly vulnerable to employ harmful coping mechanisms because of the devastation traumatic injuries and the long-term implications the loss of independence plays in their daily lives. Understanding this vulnerability not only helps professionals identify potential risk factors but can also be used to plan interventions during initial hospitalization to prevent the development of misuse or relapse.

Although many neurologically disabled patients demonstrate early abstinence from alcohol and drug use after injury, difficulty adjusting to their resulting disabilities, along with limited accessibility and community integration, can lead to depression and anxiety states. Patients may resort to self-medicating these mood states as a way of escaping their reality and emotional distress. Early and late depression after traumatic brain injury, for example, has been linked to substance abuse. Additionally, patients with pre-existing psychiatric disturbance are more likely to resume maladaptive coping mechanisms (i.e., substance misuse) after their injuries. As in the general population, personality styles have also been implicated in coping and substance abuse.

It has been estimated that 37% of individuals with an alcohol abuse problem and 57% of those with other substance abuse disorders will also meet the diagnostic criteria for another psychiatric disorder. The most prevalent of those are personality disorders (antisocial personality disorder, 87%; borderline personality disorder, 60%; and schizophrenia, 47%). In the SCI population, individuals who abuse alcohol and have antisocial personality traits are more likely to have problems coping with their disability.

Table 30.1

Drug Use and Effects

Drug		Usual methods of administration	Possible effects	Effects of overdose	Withdrawal syndrome
Stimulants	Cocaine	Sniffed, smoked, injected	Increased alertness, excitation, euphoria, increased pulse rate and blood pressure, insomnia, loss appetite	Agitation, increased body temperature, hallucinations, convulsions, possible death	Severely depressed mood, prolonged sleep, apathy, irritability, disorientation
	Amphetamines	Oral, injected			
	Methylphenidate				
	Phenmetrazine				
	Other stimulants				
Depressants	Choral hydrate	Oral	Slurred speech, disorientation, staggering, drunken behavior	Shallow respiration, cold and clammy skin, weak and rapid pulse, coma, possible death	Anxiety, insomnia, tremors, delirium, convulsions, possible death
	Barbiturates	Oral, injected			
	Methaqualone				
	Benzodiazepines				
	Alcohol	Oral			
Narcotics	Opium	Oral, smoked	Euphoria, drowsiness, slowed respiration, nausea	Slow and shallow breathing, clammy skin, constricted pupils, coma, possible death	Watery eyes, runny nose, yawning, loss of appetite, tremors, panic, chills and sweating, cramps, nausea
	Morphine	Oral, injected			
	Codeine	Oral			
	Heroin	Injected, smoked			
	Methadone	Oral, injected			
	Other narcotics				
Hallucinogens	LSD	Oral	Visual illusions, hallucinations, altered perception of one's body, increased emotionality	More prolonged episodes that may resemble psychotic states	Not reported
	Psilocybin				
	Mescaline, peyote				
	Amphetamine variants				
	Phencyclidine	Oral, smoked			
Cannabis	Marijuana	Smoked	Euphoria, relaxed inhibitions, increased appetite, impaired memory and attention	Fatigue paranoia, at very high doses a hallucinogen-like psychotic state	Insomnia hyperactivity (syndrome is rare)
	Tetrahydrocannabol	Oral			
	Hashish	Smoked			

Source: Data from Ray O, Ksir R. Drugs, Society, and Human Behavior. St. Louis: Mosby, 1993.

Although the vast majority of traditional, dually diagnosed patients have personality disorders or psychotic disorders, many more patients with mood and anxiety disorders are being considered and are present in the neurologically disabled population. Individuals with substance abuse history and comorbid depression, anxiety, and attention deficit disorder show higher sensitivity to substances and are more likely to use drugs and alcohol to self-medicate mood states. Alcohol and drug abuse are methods of coping with the losses experienced as a result of neurologic disability and serve as an attempt to ameliorate the physical and emotional distress that result from injury or illness. It important to note, however, that continued substance use could induce and exacerbate negative mood states and contribute to poorer adjustment.

Because many neurologically disabled patients experience chronic pain and problems with spasticity, they are at risk of abusing and developing dependence on prescription medications, particularly long-acting anxiolytics (i.e., Valium) and opioid analgesics (i.e., Percocet, Oxycontin). While politically controversial, some patients (illegally) use marijuana to manage spasticity and pain symptoms. Clinically, patients often report more significant pain relief from marijuana use than from prescription medication. Although patients will not develop the physical dependency on marijuana that they would on anxiolytic or opioid analgesics, the potential for other medical and psychological consequences exist.

Physicians can have a difficult time deciding on treatment options if a patient has a substance abuse history and presents with a comorbid psychiatric and substance abuse problem since the medications that may relieve secondary symptoms can contribute to later substance misuses. Longer-acting and alternatively administered medications (e.g., Duragesic patch) may be better pharmacologic choices than short-acting oral or injectable medications for patients with chemical addiction histories or those identified as high risk. Suboxone (partial opioid agonist and opioid antagonist) may also be an excellent alternative for individuals with opioid dependence or those requiring detoxification.

Cognitive impairment resulting from brain injury (traumatic or acquired) is often also manifested by neuropsychiatric and behavioral sequelae. The cognitive, neuropsychiatric, and behavioral sequelae associated with brain injury place patients at risk for substance abuse and other psychiatric disorders. For example, alcohol abuse and mood disorders are common, co-occurring disorders in BI patients. Patients with a history of alcohol abuse are more likely to develop mood disorders, especially in the first year following brain injury. BI patients may abuse alcohol to self-treat affective lability and anxiety. Studies have suggested that BI patients with a substance abuse history demonstrate poorer cognitive improvement, especially on executive functioning tasks, and have poorer vocational outcomes (4). The negative effects of substance abuse on cognition and community reintegration are greater in BI patients who have a co-existing mood disorder.

PATIENT ASSESSMENT

Alcohol- and drug-related problems have been classified in the *Diagnostic and Statistical Manual of Mental Disorders* as substance-related disorders (5). Substance abuse has been conceptualized and generally accepted to be a disease resulting from a biologic vulnerability triggered by a combination of psychological, social, and environmental factors. Although the disease model has dominated the conceptualization and treatment approach for addictive illness, contemporary researchers suggest that substance-related disorders may be better understood by a continuum model along a spectrum of severity (6). Assessment of substance-related disorders should include identification of patterns of misuse, negative life consequences resulting from substance use, and the possibility of substance dependence.

In the absence of confirming information from acute care toxicology reports or knowledgeable family or friends, the assessment of substance abuse is a difficult but necessary component of rehabilitation. By default, the rehabilitation hospital sometimes provides the atmosphere for detoxification from substances. Obtaining reliable information is often problematic because substance use is measured through self-report questionnaires, and patients are generally guarded in disclosing their histories.

Clinical Interview

Rehabilitation hospitals have attempted to address substance abuse risk by routinely screening and providing educational sessions to all patients during acute rehabilitation. The clinical interview is often the most effective way of gathering information about the patient's history. It provides an atmosphere of understanding and support, which allows the clinician and patient to develop a strong therapeutic rapport. Clinicians should utilize their skills and training to identify a patient's premorbid substance use and risk for potential problems. Standardized assessment measures can help clarify the nature, extent, and duration of a patient's substance use history but should not replace a diagnostic interview.

The Structured Clinical Interview for the Spectrum of Substance Abuse (SCI-SUBS) was designed to explore the spectrum of substance use and its clinical correlates (7). This type of supportive structured interview along with a presentation of risks and consequences of substance use after neurologic disability can provide the framework for patients to begin discussing their struggles. Other observable behaviors may also help rehabilitation professionals identify patients with substance abuse difficulties. Patients with substance abuse histories tend to be more noncompliant with treatment recommendations and participate less in rehabilitation. They may demonstrate irritability, outbursts of anger, and medication-seeking behaviors, all of which are common behaviors seen in early abstinence. Because these behaviors may also be the result of cognitive dysfunction, adjustment or mood states, and relief from injury-related physical symptoms, the clinician must consider multiple factors (i.e., psychiatric history, personality factors, coping strategies) before concluding that a substance abuse problem exists.

Substance Abuse Scales

Some popular scales for assessing substance abuse include the CAGE, MAST, and SASSI. The CAGE is an acronym representing the core factors of substance abuse and has been found to be a valid measure of assessing alcohol abuse in the SCI and BI populations (8). It is administered by asking the patient four questions that make up the test's acronym:

1. Have you ever felt you should cut down on your use?
2. Have you ever felt annoyed by someone criticizing your use?
3. Have you ever felt bad or guilty about your use?
4. Have you ever used first thing in the morning to steady your nerves or to get rid of a hangover (eye-opener)?

The Michigan Alcohol Screening Test (MAST) is a 25-item measure widely used to assess alcohol dependence. The Substance Abuse Subtle Screening Inventory is a 93–item measure used to identify substance abuse and dependence. Both the MAST and SASSI-3 are self-report measures that can help identify the patient's perception of current substance use and consequences. Both scales have been found to be reliable measures for SCI and BI patients because they detect individuals "at risk" for abuse and level of contemplation or active recovery (9).

Alcohol and drug screening should be a routine part of the assessment process and incorporated into treatment for patients with substance-related disorders. Adults receiving opioid medications for the management of chronic pain syndromes should be followed by pain specialists and undergo periodic testing with urine toxicology and have signed a pain agreement in their medical records. "Red flags" of potential aberrant use of opioids include lost prescriptions, multiple opioid prescribers, insistence on a particular opioid, and requesting early prescription refills.

Overt signs of substance abuse through standardized assessment or observed intoxication or withdrawal should prompt the clinician to include substance abuse rehabilitation goals in the patient's treatment plan. Sometimes signs of substance abuse are less obvious. Subtle physical, psychological, cognitive, and behavioral signs are listed in Table 30.2.

Substance abuse has a negative impact on rehabilitation participation, rehabilitation outcomes, and long-term adjustment; this has recently received more attention in the literature. In the neurologically disabled population substance abuse has been associated with longer lengths of stay, lower functional gains, secondary medical complications, and overall dissatisfaction and quality of life (10).

Table 30.2

FRAMES Intervention Model

Feedback	Responsibility	Advice	Menu of options	Empathy	Self-efficacy
Personal feedback including: lab tests, log of days of use, measures, of motivation, etc.	Respectfully remind patient that they are ultimately in charge of what happens, including whether or not to change and how	Clear and respectful advice can be an important component in changing harmful lifestyles and enhancing motivation	Provide patient with options of behavior change, goals and methods	Most crucial component	Belief in one's ability to accomplish a task or change
			Increases perception of personal choice and control	Conveys message of being understood and accepted	Provide experiences where patient can experience his/her own ability to make positive changes
	Reinforce whatever responsibility patient has already taken		Promotes intrinsic motivation and optimism	Creates an environment of safety and reduces defensiveness	
				Builds trust and rapport to allow change to happen	Includes the clinician believing and conveying that the patient can change

TREATMENT

Providing at-risk populations with early interventions not only aids the prevention of psychological and behavioral disturbances, but can also help to reduce the duration and severity of disorders. Interventions tailored to substance abuse provide both emotional and physical benefits. With the patient's primary goal of physical recovery along with the common guardedness of individuals with substance abuse disorders, patients are generally not open to substance abuse counseling during inpatient rehabilitation. Most patients are amenable to education, giving the clinician an opportunity to develop rapport and potentially provide the context for further exploration, disclosure, and treatment.

Peer Support

Identifying community resources and encouraging patient participation improves recovery success. Peer support programs (e.g., Alcoholic Anonymous, AA; Narcotics Anonymous, NA) provide an environment where patients with similar concerns can learn and support each other. Individuals in recovery are considered the "experts" in understanding the struggles and difficulties others with chemical addiction face. AA and NA follow the 12-step disease model of addiction and recovery, found to be an effective means of maintaining sobriety and recovery. Patients with neurologic disability can feel "out of place" and therefore be reluctant to attend. While it is important to address issues of accessibility, or, for brain-injured patients, possible behavioral or emotional dysregulation, it is common for patients in early abstinence to try and avoid AA and NA groups. Therefore, it is important for the rehabilitation clinician to identify and address the patient's attempts to deny or minimize the extent of his or her abuse with real physical and cognitive limitations. There has been a growing number of AA and NA meetings for special groups (i.e., women, gay/lesbian, dually diagnosed), but groups addressing the special needs of neurologically disabled patients can be more difficult to secure.

Individual and Family Counseling

While peer support programs are helpful in developing nonusing support networks, sponsors, and a sense of community, they are unable to provide the clinically trained interventions that address the underlying emotional conflicts and personality dynamics that contribute to addiction and relapse. The rehabilitation clinician must be able to identify and confront denial and minimization, enabling behavior and relationships, triggers for relapse, and potential development of cross-addictions. Individual and family counseling are essential components of recovery for all populations and are often preferred by patients over peer support programs. The desire to confine treatment to individual counseling is often the patient's attempt to control treatment and maintain the secrecy of his or her addiction. Given the onset of the disability and understandable distress, family members may excuse continued substance use, lower their expectations, and, in part, enable the patient to continue abusing substances. A rehabilitation clinician who has knowledge of both disability and addiction can provide patients and families with the tools they need to maintain sobriety, manage the emotional distress of adjusting to a neurologic disability, and fully participate in their lives.

Clinicians use a variety of techniques and interventions when treating patients with substance-related disorders. Regardless of the specific strategy employed, developing a strong therapeutic rapport is crucial to promoting a life without substance use and treatment success. Motivational interviewing, coping and social skills training, and community resource behavioral training are common approaches used with the rehabilitation population.

The most widely used brief intervention model is "motivational interviewing," which has been used alone or in conjunction with other treatment modules. For example, feedback, responsibility, advice, menu of options, empathy, self-efficacy (FRAMES) is a specific intervention model (Table 30.3) that uses specific strategies to develop coping skills and improve decision making and management of stressors to address substance abuse (6).

Relapse Prevention

The development and strengthening of coping skills has long been a common treatment goal for rehabilitation clinicians. Problem-focused coping strategies have been linked to more positive adjustment and less use of maladaptive behaviors (e.g., substance use). Individuals must grieve the loss of substance use as a means of coping with interpersonal and situational stressors. Patients who lack an adequate ability to regulate positive and negative mood states or cope with situational and interpersonal stressors often seek to control or numb their emotional pain by using substances. Coping and social skills training focuses on improving listening and conversational skills, identifying and expressing emotions, and giving, receiving, and responding to criticism. This training has been adapted for TBI patients and is highly recommended for those with significant alcohol dependence (11).

The Community Reinforcement Approach (CRA) is a behavioral module that utilizes natural reinforcers (i.e., family, interpersonal relationships, work and leisure activities) in the patient's environment to facilitate change in substance use (6). Rather than endorsing the "abstinence model" of treatment, CRA encourages patients to commit to a "time out" from substance use and then promotes community reinforcement to prevent the future maladaptive use of substances. Although the abstinence model prevails as the preferred treatment for addiction in the United States, the CRA method has been found to be an effective method of treatment and may be a sound alternative for some patients.

Relapse prevention is an integral part of treatment and recovery that should be incorporated into all treatment modalities (Figure 30.1). Relapse-prevention models address the cognitive, behavioral, and lifestyle components of substance abuse and relapse. Understanding relapse as a common, expected, and, at times, predictable part of recovery allows clinicians to help patients modify their thinking, actions, and lifestyles that can contribute to potential relapse.

Table 30.3

Commonly Used Medications, Side Effects, and Drug Interactions

Drug classification	Suggested use	Side effects	Interactions with alcohol	Interactions with other drugs
Opioid analgesics Morphine Codeine Oxycodone Percocet Methadone Meperidine	Raises pain threshold	Dizziness Drowsiness Euphoria Nausea/vomiting Constipation Potential for abuse; physical/ psychological dependence	Respiratory depression; dizziness; drowsiness	Potentially lethal when combined with MAO inhibitors and stimulants
Antibiotics Penicillin Ampicillin Bactrim Ciprofloxacin	Treatment of infections	Rash Hives Nausea/vomiting Gastrointestinal upset	Potentiates effects of alcohol	Barbiturates decreases effects of medication
Tricyclic antidepressants Amitriptyline Nortriptyline	Treatment of depression and/or management of pain symptoms	Gastrointestinal upset Headache Dizziness Drowsiness Sleep disturbance	Increases sides effects of antidepressant; increases depression of central nervous system; potentially lethal	Fluctuation in blood pressure, internal bleeding, sedation
Psychostimulants Modafanil Methylphenidate Dexmethylphenidate	Increases arousal/attention; decreases distractibility	Restlessness Psychomotor agitation Insomnia Loss of appetite Potential for abuse; physical and psychological dependence	Lowers seizure threshold; potentially lethal	Lowers seizure threshold; potentially lethal

Medication	Use	Side Effects	Interactions
Tranquilizers (anxiolytics) Chlordiazepoxide Clonazepam Alprazolam Lorazepam Neuroleptics	Treatment of anxiety and agitation; treatment of increased muscle tone and spasticity	Drowsiness/Fatigue Mental confusion Slurred speech Depression Weight gain Gastrointestinal upset Potential for abuse; physical/psychological dependence	Increases depression of central nervous system; potentially lethal; severe hypotension; sedation	Antidepressants increase sedative effect; potentially lethal when used with stimulants
Antispasmodics Bacoflen Flexeril	Treatment of increased muscle tone and spasticity	Drowsiness Lightheadedness Blurred vision Mental confusion Slurred speech Depression Gastrointestinal upset	Increases depression of central nervous system; decreases judgment; decreases arousal and alertness; respiratory depression	Sedative and hypnotics increase depressant effects
Anticonvulsants Phenytoin Gabapentin Valproate Phenobarbital	Prevention and control of seizures; management of neurogenic pain	Mental confusion Slurred speech Nervousness Bone loss with long-term use	Chronic alcohol use diminishes effects of medication; lowers seizure threshold	Antidepressants may lower threshold for seizures; anxiolytics may potentiate effects of medication
Anticoagulants Warfarin Heparin Dalteparin	Prevents formation of blood clots	Hemorrhage Nose bleeds Bruising	Increases or decreases effects of medication	Increases or decreases effects of medication

Clinical Interview: Open-Ended Questions
- Drug history and current use:
  - Alcohol, drugs, tobacco, prescription medication

- Patterns of use:
  - Types, methods, amount, frequency, duration

- Previous attempts to control, cut back, stop:
  - Including previous treatment

- Negative experiences as result of drug or alcohol use:
  - Jeopardized or lost relationships, jobs, legal problems

Signs of Substance Abuse
- Physical signs
  - Intoxication or withdrawal (see Table 30.1)
  - Disheveled appearance
  - Decline in self-care or personal hygiene

- Psychological and cognitive signs
  - Change in mood (depression, anxiety, psychosis)
  - Mental status changes

- Behavior signs
  - Noncompliance with treatment
  - Recurrent canceled or missed appointments
  - Recurrent requests for emergency appointments—medication seeking
  - Recurrent lost prescriptions
  - Recurrent request for early refills on prescriptions
  - Multiple physicians with multiple prescriptions

Figure 30.1. Substance abuse assessment.

Patient Education

Substance abuse education is used as a primary prevention model with the goal of preventing the onset of the disorder. Providing education on the postinjury risks of alcohol and drug use or when used in combination with prescription medication is a vital component of rehabilitation (Table 30.4). In conjunction with education programs that improve patients' awareness and knowledge of their injuries and disabilities, rehabilitation professionals must also educate patients on the exaggerated and potentially lethal effects substance can have (12). More specifically, rehabilitation professions should educate patients about the quicker and exaggerated effects a substance will have after neurologic impairment, the increased risk for abuse and dependence, secondary medical complications (bowel/bladder dysfunction, pressure sores, cardiovascular complications), and subsequent risk of injury (falls, impulsivity, impaired judgment, cardiovascular compromise leading to ischemic or hemorrhagic events).

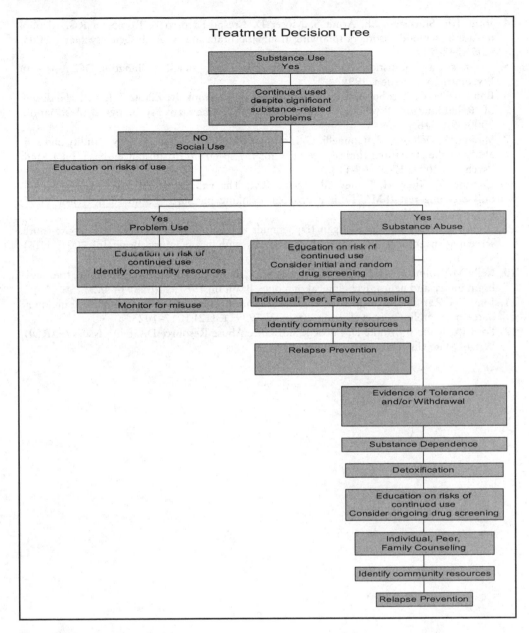

Figure 30.2. Treatment decision tree.

REFERENCES

1. National Association on Alcohol, Drugs and Disability. Access limited substance abuse services for people with disabilities: a national perspective. Report released: January 13, 1999. Washington, DC: National Press Club, 1999.
2. Radnitz CL, Tirch D. Substance misuse in individuals with spinal cord injury. Int J Addict 1995; 30(9):1117–1140.
3. Ray O, Ksir R. Drugs, Society, and Human Behavior. St. Louis: Mosby, 1993.

4. Jorge RE, Starkstein SE, Arndt S, Moser D, Crespo-Facorro B, Robinson RG. Alcohol misuse and mood disorders following traumatic brain injury. Arch Gen Psychiatry 2005; 62(7):742–749.

5. Diagnostic and Statistical Manual of Mental Disorders, 4th ed. Washington, DC: American Psychiatric Association, 1999.

6. Bombardier C. Alcohol and traumatic disability. In Frank R, Elliott T (eds.), Handbook of Rehabilitation Psychology. Washington, DC: American Psychological Association, 2000:399–416.

7. Sbrana, A, Dell'osso, L, Gonnelli, C, Impagnatiello, P, et al. Acceptability, validity and reliablity of the structured clinical interview for the spectrum of substance abuse. Int J Meth Psych Res 2003; 12(2):105-115.

8. Connor JP, Grier M, Feeney GF, Young RM. The validity of the brief Michigan alcohol screening test (bMAST) as a problem drinking measure. J Stud Alchol Drug 2007; 68(5):771.

9. Arenth PM. Bogner JA, Corrigan JD, Schmidt L. The utility of the substance abuse subtle screening inventory-3 for use with individuals with brain injury. Brain Inj 2001; 15(6): 499–510.

10. Kelly MP, Johnson CT, Knoller N, Drubach DA, Winslow MM. Substance abuse, traumatic brain injury and neuropsychological outcome. Brain Inj 1997; 11(6):391–402.

11. Jong CN, Zafonte RD, Millis SR, Yavuzer G. The effect of cocaine on traumatic brain injury outcome: a preliminary evaluation. Brain Inj 1999; 13(12):1017–1023.

12. Ford JA, Rolfe B, Moore D, Lucot J. Substance Abuse Resource Disability Issues (SARDI), Wright State University, Dayton, OH, 1992.

31 | Vision Deficits Following Acquired Brain Injury

Neera Kapoor
Kenneth J. Ciuffreda

Acquired brain injury (ABI) is an umbrella term for an acquired neurologic compromise due to a traumatic brain injury (TBI) or concussion, stroke, aneurysm, tumor, vestibular dysfunction, or postsurgical complications resulting in anoxia or hypoxia (1). In terms of associated deficits following ABI, most of the research has been performed in the area of TBI and stroke, with typical postABI symptoms being related to deficits of cognition, affect, and multimodal sensorimotor abilities, including vision (1–3). In fact, sensorimotor vision symptoms are typically reported in those with ABI in frequencies ranging from 40 to 85%, depending upon the nature of the vision deficit and the criteria used in the study (1,4–6). While the period of natural recovery following ABI varies and, specifically with TBI, is reported to range from a few months to 1–2 years postinjury, it also may remain incomplete (1,3). Therefore, residual deficits evident postinjury ultimately require evaluation, rehabilitation, and monitoring as deemed appropriate.

With respect to vision dysfunctions, most healthcare professionals are familiar with anomalies of ocular health (cataracts, glaucoma, dry eye/blepharitis, pupillary anomalies, optic nerve damage, and retinopathies), the cranial nerves (II, III, IV, V, VI, or VII), and refractive status. However, there are also sensorimotor vision disturbances evident in those with ABI, which, if persistent and disruptive to the individual, may require evaluation and nonsurgical treatment intervention. Since these residual vision anomalies often adversely affect activities of daily living (ADLs; specifically, reading, writing, ambulation, and driving), they are of concern to those with ABI striving to live safely and independently in society.

Vision function impacts the progress of rehabilitation, as well as basic ADLs, because many aspects of rehabilitation are vision-based. For example, with certain reading-related or visual search tasks in cognitive and occupational rehabilitation, patients with visual field defects, blurred vision, or diplopia may have significant difficulty progressing with their rehabilitation. In addition, when performing gaze-stabilization techniques (i.e., techniques that stimulate and normalize the vestibulo-ocular reflex), which underlie a significant portion of vestibular rehabilitation, patients must present without diplopia, strabismus, or nystagmus to perform these vision-based tasks appropriately under binocular (i.e., viewing with both eyes open simultaneously) viewing conditions (1). Therefore, evaluating and treating persistent, residual vision anomalies following ABI may improve the ability to perform the necessary components of rehabilitation, as well as independent ADLs.

While other ocular sequelae may occur with blunt periorbital trauma, including ecchymosis, orbital fracture, hemorrhaging, lid anomaly, corneal and scleral damage, intraorbital damage, pupillary anomalies, and optic nerve damage (4), these conditions will not be discussed in this chapter as they relate more to blunt ocular trauma rather than neurologic damage related to vision function. This chapter provides a cursory review of the basic neurology related to vision, a screening protocol for sensorimotor vision deficits, and an outline of common sensorimotor vision anomalies evident following ABI, in conjunction with their associated symptoms and possible treatment options.

ANATOMY AND PHYSIOLOGY

Primary Visual Pathway

Initially, light passes through the refractive components of the eye, including the cornea, aqueous chamber, crystalline lens, and vitreous, to finally reach the retina, at which point the retinal photoreceptor's signals are transmitted via axons at the level of the optic nerve (cranial nerve II). With two dominant, retinal ganglion cell types (magnocellular and parvocellular), the optic nerve exits the retina and proceeds to the optic chiasm, where a partial decussation occurs separating the visual information into right and left hemi-fields of visual space via corresponding left and right optic tracts of the primary visual pathway, respectively (7). Postchiasmally, the axons travel via the optic tracts to the lateral geniculate body (LGN) for early-stage processing, with the majority of the axons continuing onwards to the occipital cortex (V1). At V1, the neural signals for the primary visual pathway begin the transformation into a high-resolution, neural image with appropriate form, color vision, and contrast, while maintaining peripheral vision integrity (7). After the LGN, and aside from the primary visual pathway, the remaining fibers may travel either to the pretectum to participate in pupillary function and accommodation or the superior colliculus to participate in basic eye movement and visual-motor tasks (7).

Secondary Visual Pathways

Research on the secondary visual pathway of higher-level vision processing suggests evidence for dual, parallel visual processing pathways originating at V1 in the occipital cortex (7). The ventral visual pathway's axons eventually reach the posterior inferior temporal lobe for processing of object identification. The dorsal visual pathway's axons move anteriorly through the middle temporal area and finally reach the parietal lobe for processing related to the performance of visually guided action with appropriate motion control of ocular and limb motility and visual spatial representation.

In addition to the primary and secondary visual pathways, 6 of the 12 cranial nerves (II–VII) as well as numerous cerebral and noncerebral areas of the brain (7–9), are involved in controlling vision function.

Vision Dysfunction and ABI

A compromise of, or anywhere along, the following areas may impair vision function (1,4,5,9): 1) refractive ocular structures, 2) the primary or secondary visual pathways, 3) six of the cranial nerve pathways (or at the level of their respective nuclei) associated with vision function, and 4) cortical and noncortical neurologic substrates involved in ocular motility, including the brainstem, superior colliculus, cerebellum, midbrain, occipital lobe, parietal lobe, and frontal eye fields.

PATIENT ASSESSMENT

Excluding visual perceptual testing, a proposed screening vision protocol (see Table 31.1) for those with ABI commences with an extensive case history, after

Table 31.1

Screening Vision Protocol for Rehabilitation Physicians

Areas of assessment	Components

Case history	• Inquire about:
	  o blur
	  o reading difficulties
	  o diplopia/eyestrain
	  o increased sensitivity to visual motion
	  o increased light sensitivity
	  o bumping into/missing objects on one side of visual space

Refractive status	• Visual acuity

Sensorimotor vision status	• Versional ocular motility(performed monocularly and binocularly), assessing:
	  o fixation: patient should be able to maintain fixation for at least 10 seconds without any drift, gaze instability, or jerk nystagmus of the eyes
	  o pursuit: evaluate the patient's ability to move the eyes smoothly and at the same velocity of the target in all positions of gaze
	  o saccades: evaluate the patient's ability to rapidly move the eyes from the pen cap to the pen horizontally, obliquely, and vertically

Ocular health status	• Color vision using Ishihara color vision plates tested one eye at a time
	• Pupillary responses
	• Visual field testing
	  o confrontation testing
	  o draw a clock test

which the status of at least three major areas is assessed: refractive, sensorimotor vision, and ocular health (10). Equipment required for a vision screening includes a distance visual acuity chart, near visual acuity card, pen (with a pen cap), a 6-inch ruler, Ishihara color vision plates, 8½" by 11" sheet of blank paper, pencil, eye patch, and a penlight or transilluminator. In addition, Table 31.2 provides information for the rehabilitation physician to aid in making appropriate referrals for comprehensive vision evaluations, which are typically performed by neuro-optometrists, ophthalmologists, or neuro-ophthalmologists.

Since many with ABI present with increased sensitivity to light, sound, and visual motion (1,2) as well as word-finding difficulties and slower speed of processing across all sensory modalities (1–3), the following modifications minimize patient discomfort during the vision evaluation:

1. Position hand-held equipment (visual acuity card, occluder/eye patch, penlight, ophthalmoscope, paper, pencil, color vision plates, 6-inch ruler, and pen with pencap) within arm's reach to minimize movement around the patient and reduce the intensity of any response to visual motion.

2. Speak clearly and more slowly than usual, and minimize the use of open-ended questions due to the slower speed of processing and cognitive deficits typically evident (1–3).

Table 31.2

Criteria for Referring for a Comprehensive Vision Evaluation

Case history reports of:
- blur
- reading difficulties
- diplopia/eyestrain
- increased sensitivity to visual motion
- increased light sensitivity
- bumping into/missing objects on one side of visual space

Visual acuities (at near or far viewing distances while the patient is wearing their habitual spectacle correction) that are:
- poorer than 20/20 in one or both eyes
- different between the two eyes

Versional ocular motility observations of:
- nystagmus on fixation assessment
- restriction of eye movements on pursuit testing
- noticeable undershooting or overshooting of the target on saccadic testing

Color vision deficits on monocular testing with the Ishihara color plates

Pupillary anomalies:
- unequal pupil size (anisocoria)
- irregular pupil size
- fixed or minimally reactive pupil(s)
- evidence of relative afferent pupillary defect

Visual field testing revealing:
- hemianopic or quadrantanopic field defects on confrontation testing
- abnormal results with draw-a-clock test

3. Maintain relatively dim room illumination, in conjunction with task illumination, to minimize discomfort from photosensitivity while optimizing contrast and visual acuity. Incandescent, rather than fluorescent, lighting is preferable for room illumination, as the latter with its rapid flickering nature may increase discomfort for those with selective photosensitivity for fluorescent lighting and/or increased sensitivity to visual motion (11).

Vision Screening

The Case History

The case history includes trauma and rehabilitation history, with details of the date and nature of the neurologic insult, including associated past or ongoing rehabilitation. More traditional case history questions follow, such as the review of systems, medical and ocular history for the patient and family, as well as current medications and allergies. Then the individual is asked about current vision symptoms, their impact on ADLs, as well as short- and long-term goals regarding vision and overall rehabilitation. The most typical vision symptoms reported by those with ABI include: 1) blur, 2) difficulty reading, 3) eye fatigue and/or diplopia when reading or regarding objects visually, 4) increased sensitivity to visual motion in association with loss of balance, vertigo, or disequilibrium, 5) increased sensitivity to light, and 6) bumping into/missing objects on one side of usual space.

Refractive Status

Visual acuities may be obtained under monocular (i.e., viewing with one eye at a time) as well as binocular viewing conditions with the patient wearing his or her habitual spectacle correction. Commercially available, portable visual acuity charts are accessible to physicians and take up minimal space.

Sensorimotor Vision Status

Assessing versional ocular motility requires minimal equipment, may be performed under monocular as well as binocular viewing conditions, and provides powerful information regarding neuromotor control of the extraocular muscles. Three dominant components are easily assessed utilizing a pen and pen cap as the physician's tools:

1. Fixation is an eye movement in which the eyes are fixed on a target to maintain the target's image on the fovea. A test for fixation involves instructing the patient to look at a pen tip at a 40-cm viewing distance. The physician evaluates the patient's ability to maintain a steady fixation/gaze on the pen tip for 10 seconds without any ocular drift, gaze instability, or nystagmus (i.e., rapid involuntary oscillation or movement of the eyes).

2. Pursuit is a slow, continuous conjugate eye movement used when the eyes follow a slowly moving object. A test for pursuit involves instructing the patient to look at a target (a pen tip or the physician's forefinger) at a 40-cm viewing distance. The physician evaluates the patient's ability to move his or her eyes smoothly and at the same velocity of the target in all positions of gaze.

3. Saccades are rapid, step-like conjugate eye movements which redirect the line of sight from one position (or object) in space to another. A test for saccades involves instructing the patient to move his or her eyes rapidly from one target to another on command (with the two targets being a pen tip and pen cap separated by 10 cm) at a 40-cm viewing distance. The physician evaluates the patient's ability to rapidly move his or her eyes from the pen cap to the pen tip: horizontally, obliquely, and vertically.

Ocular Health Status

Four techniques serve as strong screening tests: color vision, pupillary assessment, confrontation visual field testing, and draw-a-clock testing. Color vision and pupillary anomalies may accompany optic nerve damage, which frequently occurs with demyelinating diseases and may occur with TBI. Confrontation visual field testing and draw-a-clock testing are particularly helpful in patients with strokes.

1. Color vision testing using the commercially available Ishihara plates should be performed monocularly and may be performed by the rehabilitation physician.

2. Pupillary assessment should be performed in uniformly dim (but bright enough that both the patient and physician are able to see) room illumination using a penlight or transilluminator to stimulate pupillary constriction and 6-inch ruler to aid in estimating pupil size. The physician should measure the size of the pupils and evaluate the pupil shape as round or irregular. Then the pupillary response should be assessed by shining the penlight/transilluminator into the right pupil, which should result in a direct, brisk constriction of the right pupil and a consensual, brisk constriction of the left pupil. Then the physician should assess the pupillary response by shining the penlight/transilluminator into the left pupil, which should result in a direct, brisk constriction of the left pupil and a consensual, brisk constriction of the right pupil. Finally, when moving the penlight/transilluminator from the right eye for 2 seconds to the left eye for 2 seconds and back again to the right eye, there should be no evidence of dilation of the left eye and right eye, respectively, unless a relative afferent pupillary defect is evident.

3. Confrontation visual field testing is typically performed monocularly without any spectacle correction in place so that the frame does not limit the patient's visual field. With physician and patient facing each other and sitting 50 cm from each other, a patch should be placed over the patient's left eye and the physician should close his right eye. The physician should assess the patient's ability to perceive the presence or movement of his or her finger in the following meridians from the patient's perspective, and then this testing should be repeated for the patient's left eye while the physician's left eye is closed: 1) superior, 2) superior temporal, 3) temporal, 4) inferior temporal, 5) inferior, 6) inferior nasal, 7) nasal, and 8) superior nasal visual fields.

4. Draw-a-clock testing is helpful in detecting visual neglect (i.e., visual inattention). The patient should be wearing his or her habitual spectacle correction for near-vision tasks. Using a pencil, the physician draws a moderate-sized circle

centered on a blank 8½" by 11" sheet of paper and writes the number "12" at the top of the circle (as with an analog clock). This paper and pencil are then provided to the patient. The patient is instructed to complete the clock face with the remaining numbers. In those with a left visual inattention (i.e., neglect), the numbers 7–11 will be drawn in positions shifted away from rather than along the left circumferential edge of the clock face, while for those with right inattention, numbers 1–5 would be shifted away from rather than along the right circumferential edge of the clock face.

TREATMENT

Prior to commencing any vision rehabilitation for specific vision anomalies following ABI, an appropriate compensation for refractive error is required. With respect to refractive compensation, multifocal lenses are contraindicated for ambulation in those with gait disturbances, vestibular dysfunction, or cognitive deficits, which are common following ABI (12). Patients should be advised to wear single vision distance spectacles for ambulation and separate single vision near spectacles for prolonged, detailed near-vision tasks. Multifocal lenses may be used for stationary tasks as well as for dynamic tasks performed in familiar environs.

Categories of Ocular and Vision Anomalies

Certain ocular and vision conditions have a greater probability of occurring depending on the nature of neurologic insult. Baker and Epstein (4) referred to five categories of orbital and vision damage related to TBI: soft tissue injuries, orbital fractures, cranial neuropathies, intra-axial brainstem damage, and cerebral lesions (4). The latter three are more likely to contribute to the typical residual vision dysfunctions evident following ABI, which include anomalies of: accommodation, tear film integrity, versional ocular motility (fixation, pursuit, and saccades), vergence (nonstrabismic, as well as strabismic) ocular motility, visual-vestibular integration, photosensitivity, and visual field integrity (1,5,6,12,13–18). Table 31.3 outlines the associated symptoms and possible nonsurgical, neuro-optometric treatment options for these vision anomalies. While anomalies of the tear film integrity may be initially managed by rehabilitation physicians with over-the-counter artificial tears, treatment for the remainder of the conditions described below should be referred to neuro-optometrists specializing in ABI.

Anomalies of Accommodation

Accommodation is the ability to alter focus (i.e., clarity of vision) from a farther object to a closer one and vice versa. While accommodation presents with a physiologic, age-related decline referred to as presbyopia, most individuals do not begin to lose the ability to accommodate at near range until their early to mid-40s. For this reason, accommodative testing is performed on prepresbyopic (i.e., typically those under 45 years of age) individuals only.

Table 31.3

Vision Anomalies Evident Following Acquired Brain Injury with Associated Vision Symptoms and Treatment Options

Category of vision anomaly	Visual symptoms	Treatment options

Accommodation	• Blur
	  ○ constant or intermittent
	  ○ evident when changing viewing distances (i.e., near-far and/or far-near blur)
	• Eyestrain/browaches/eye fatigue evident after brief periods of sustained near vision work
	• Dizziness/nausea/motion sickness during or following a vision-based task
		• Accommodative vision therapy under monocular and binocular viewing conditions
		• Prescription of spectacles for prolonged near vision tasks:
		  ○ instead of, before, in conjunction with, or following accommodative vision therapy

Tear film integrity	• Impaired clarity of vision
	  ○ constant/intermittent
	  ○ fluctuates with blinking
	  ○ at any viewing distance
	  ○ "gritty," foreign body sensation within the eye
		• For mild-to-moderate dry eye:
		  ○ artificial tears three to four times daily in both eyes, in conjunction with lid scrubs
		• For moderate-to-severe dry eye:
		  ○ Systane or Restasis twice daily in both eyes, in conjunction with lid hygiene
		• Possible punctal plug insertion for severe dry eye

Versional ocular motility (fixation, pursuit, and saccades)	• Reading-related difficulty
	  ○ slower reading speed
	  ○ loss of place while reading/skipping lines
	  ○ the print appears to "float"/"swim"
	  ○ avoidance of prolonged vision-related tasks
	• Difficulty shifting to/tracking objects
	• Dizziness/nausea/motion sickness during or following vision-based tasks
		• Versional ocular motor therapy using free space, pencil-paper, and computer-based techniques under monocular and binocular viewing conditions
		• Beneficial compensatory tools:
		  ○ using large-print books for those with best-corrected visual acuity poorer than 20/60
		• Using an aperture-based, typoscopic approach highlighting the text of regard and obscuring irrelevant text on the page to minimize oculomotor-based, reading-related vision symptoms

Table 31.3 (*Continued*)

Vergence ocular motility (strabismic and nonstrabismic)	• Diplopia
	  o eliminated with occlusion
	  o constant or intermittent
	  o at any viewing distance
	  o more evident in one position of gaze than another
	• Eyestrain/eye fatigue/closing or squinting one eye after a brief vision-related task
	• Avoidance of prolonged vision-related tasks
	• Dizziness/nausea/motion sickness during or following vision-based tasks
		• Vergence ocular motor therapy using training devices such as stereograms, vectograms, analyphs, Brock string, and loose prisms

Visual-vestibular interaction	• Same as for vergence and versional oculomotor deficits, with a bias on the vestibular symptoms including:
	  o increased sensitivity to visual motion with difficulty in multiply-visually stimulating circumstances, such as:
	    o supermarkets with high shelving
	    o scrolling on computers
	    o watching television and movies
	    o navigating crowds in busy streets
	    o dizziness, loss of balance, vertigo, nausea
		• Vision therapy for versional and vergence ocular motor deficits
		• Once ocular motility is stabilized, then vestibular rehabilitation is appropriate

Sensitivity to light	• Increased sensitivity to light, which may be:
	  o general: to all types of light
	  o selective: to fluorescent lights which may be
	    o accompanied by increased sensitivity to visual motion
	    o more common in those with vestibular dysfunction
		• Prescription of tinted spectacle lenses:
		  o a 30–40% tint for indoor use
		  o an 80–85% tint for outdoor use
		  o for those with a:
		    o general photosensitivity to all types of lights, use a brown or grey tint
		    o selective photosensitivity to fluorescent lighting, use a light blue or grey tint
		• Recommend wearing a brimmed hat/baseball cap to reduce the illumination directed from the superior visual field

(*Continued*)

Table 31.3 (*Continued*)

Visual field integrity	• Missing a portion of the visual field
	  o with awareness of the defect
	  o without awareness of the defect
	• Difficulty with certain activities of daily living (ADLs):
	  o dressing, eating, shaving/cosmesis, reading, and writing (slower and with reduced accuracy)
	  o ambulation
	    o presenting with an unsteady gait and subjectively feeling off-balance
	    o veering/bumping into objects on one side more so than the other
		• Scanning strategies address the accuracy and speed of small- to large-angle (i.e., 1–40 degrees) saccades and pursuit into the affected visual field
		• Adaptive strategies address the awareness of the affected field by modifying specific aspects of their ADLs
		• Prescription of optical aids, depending upon the nature of the defect and awareness of the defect
		• Treatment options for those with inattention, with or without a visual field defect, include application of yoked prisms in conjunction with scanning and related adaptive strategies
		• Without inattention but with a visual field defect, include application of scanning strategies, often in conjunction with certain optical aids (i.e., sector prisms, spotting prisms, mirrors, and field-expanding lenses)

The study-dependent frequency of occurrence of anomalies of accommodation among prepresbyopic individuals with TBI ranges from 10 to 40% (6,15). While fewer data are available on accommodation in stroke, approximately 12.5% of visually symptomatic individuals with stroke presented with an accommodative anomaly in a recent retrospective study (15). Typical symptoms of anomalies of accommodation include constant or intermittent blur in conjunction with eyestrain or brow aches (12–14). Treatment options for anomalies of accommodation are restorative, compensatory, and adaptive (see Table 31.3) (12,14).

Anomalies of Tear Film Integrity

Dry eye syndrome is an ocular surface anomaly related to the composition and/or uniformity of volume and flow of the tear film. These mechanisms correspond to two predominant categories of dry eye: aqueous deficiency and evaporative loss. With the two types of dry eye co-existing or presenting individually, patients report intermittent lack of clarity of vision, frequent blinking, and a foreign-body sensation (6,17). Standard treatment options for dry eye are compensatory (see Table 31.3) (17).

While dry eye has a reported frequency of occurrence of 10% in the general population greater than 65 years of age (17), a study-dependent frequency of occurrence ranging from 15 to 22% has been reported in those with ABI (6,17). Dry eye, a common ocular side effect of many antidepressant and antihypertensive medications (6,17,19), is an understandable occurrence in the ABI population, since many of these patients are taking these categories of medications. Some antidepressant medications with dry eye as a side effect are fluoxetine hydrochloride, duloxetine hydrochloride, bupropion hydrochloride, venlafaxine hydrochloride, escitalopram oxalate, and citalopram hydrobromide. A few antihypertensive medications with dry eye as a side effect are enalapril maleate, atenolol, and propranalol hydrochloride.

Anomalies of Versional Ocular Motility

Versional ocular motility refers to conjugate (i.e., parallel) changes in eye positions as one regards objects in the visual field. Versional ocular motility, which includes fixation, smooth pursuit, and saccades, has been reported in those with ABI with a study-dependent frequency of occurrence that ranges from 40 to 85% (1,4,15,16). Associated symptoms of anomalies of versional ocular motility include slower speed of reading, loss of place when reading, and dizziness or sensation of motion when reading. The treatment approach for managing versional ocular motor deficits is restorative, compensatory, and adaptive (see Table 31.3).

Vision therapy (i.e., oculomotor learning) (13) for anomalies of versional ocular motility involves stabilizing fixation first (12,14) under monocular and then binocular viewing conditions with the patient viewing a moderately sized target. The duration of fixation should commence at 3–5 seconds and gradually build up to 10 seconds (12).

Once fixation is stabilized, saccades and pursuit are then trained under monocular and then binocular viewing conditions. Small-angle, moderate-angle, and large-angle eye movements (i.e., saccades and pursuit) are trained horizontally and vertically (12,14), with the speed of the eye movement being relatively slow (i.e., ~5 degrees/second or slower, depending upon the individual). Visual scanning and searching techniques may also be performed using pencil-and-paper, as well as computer-based, techniques to improve saccadic and pursuit ability while increasing levels of target complexity, visual discrimination, and speed of processing. Initially, those with ABI should be encouraged to concentrate on the accuracy of versional ocular motor–based tasks, addressing and gradually increasing speed only once accuracy has improved and stabilized (12,14).

Beneficial compensatory tools for those with versional ocular motor anomalies include large-print books and using an aperture-based, typoscopic approach. However, they should be incorporated appropriately. For example, large-print books should only be used in patients with markedly impaired (i.e., poorer than 20/60) best-corrected visual acuity. If the best-corrected visual acuity is better than 20/60, then large-print books make little difference for the patient. However, using an opaque guide (called a typoscope; see Figure 31.1) with a small aperture to highlight or reveal only a few lines of print at a time, while blocking the rest of the printed page, often serves to minimize symptoms of versional ocular motor anomalies and may also be performed with large-print texts. Therefore, a typoscopic approach, in conjunction with the patient's finger to aid in keeping place, should be encouraged as a compensatory tool for those with ABI and symptoms of anomalies of versional ocular motility when reading.

Anomalies of Vergence Ocular Motility

Vergence ocular motility, which refers to disjunctive changes in eye position as one regards objects at varying distances in the visual field, has been reported as being abnormal with varying frequencies, with convergence insufficiency being most commonly reported (6,15,16). Vergence anomalies have been reported with frequencies ranging from 40 (6) to 56% (15) in those with TBI and up to 37% (15) in those with stroke. A common associated symptom with vergence anomalies is constant or intermittent diplopia, which is eliminated with monocular occlusion (i.e., the diplopia is not evident under monocular conditions). It is important to distinguish diplopia evident under monocular versus binocular viewing conditions, as the presence of diplopia only under binocular viewing conditions which is eliminated with monocular occlusion is related to a vergence anomaly. Additional symptoms of vergence dysfunction include eyestrain when reading, vision-related headaches, avoidance of vision-related tasks, and dizziness or sensation of motion when reading (12,14). The treatment paradigm for anomalies of vergence is restorative, compensatory, and adaptive. A few comments are noted below.

Several factors affecting the treatment and prognosis of anomalies of vergence ocular motility include the constancy, direction, magnitude, and comitancy of the ocular misalignment, as well as the patient's ability to fuse under any circumstance (12,14).

If an ocular misalignment is constant and evident under normal binocular viewing conditions, the deviation is referred to as a strabismus. Ocular misalignments evident when binocular viewing is disrupted are referred to as heterophorias. A strabismus is often more challenging to treat than a heterophoria because there is a possibility that the magnitude of the deviation may vary in different positions of gaze. Therefore, if the magnitude of a constantly occurring deviation is the same in all positions of gaze, the strabismus is easier to treat, and its ocular alignment is said to be comitant.

In the presence of constant, comitant ocular deviations with fusion (i.e., ability to perceive a single, cortically integrated image under binocular viewing conditions) evident in conjunction with fusional prism, incorporating this prism in the individual's spectacles is the initial therapeutic step (12,14). Once the individual manifests fusion in primary gaze with or without fusional prism,

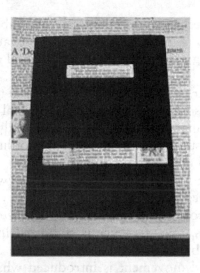

Figure 31.1. (A) Normal view of text on a page. (B) Typoscopic view of a portion of the same text page.

stabilizing fusional vergence in primary gaze using vergence stimuli at varying (i.e., far, intermediate, and near) viewing distances is required (12,14).

Anomalies of Visual-Vestibular Interaction

The purpose of the vestibulo-ocular reflex (VOR) is gaze stabilization—more specifically, stabilization of the retinal images in conjunction with head movement (1,8). While many neural areas contribute to the VOR, the simplest version of the neural arc is for the horizontal VOR, in which the oculomotor nerve communicates with the abducens nerve via the medial longitudinal fasciculus (MLF) and onward to communicate with the acoustic (also known as the vestibulo-cochlear) nerve to stabilize horizontal gaze with horizontal changes in eye/head position (1,8,20). The VOR, referred to as "gaze stabilization" by many vestibular therapists, is also a valuable training tool in the vestibular rehabilitative regimen, which requires stable and accurate extraocular motility (1,8).

Many patients with ABI who have anomalies of visual-vestibular interaction (also referred to as visual vertigo or "supermarket syndrome") may present with symptoms including disequilibrium and increased sensitivity to visual motion in supermarkets, malls, crowds, and multiply visually stimulating environments (1,20). These same patients may also present with difficulty performing "gaze stabilization" tasks in vestibular rehabilitation, which may be related to ocular motor deficits evident during or exacerbated following the ABI, thus resulting in a conflict between the visual and vestibular signals (20). For such individuals, vision therapy for ocular motor anomalies should precede additional VOR training in vestibular rehabilitation (1). Treatment for anomalies of visual-vestibular interactions (see Table 31.3) is compensatory, adaptive, and, to a moderate degree, restorative. The treatment paradigm involves treating anomalies of both versional and vergence ocular motility.

Treating versional ocular motor anomalies with vision therapy in those with visual-vestibular symptoms is similar to treating versional ocular motor conditions in isolation. The primary difference is that, initially, patients should be instructed to perform pursuit and saccadic ocular motility significantly more slowly and gradually build up the speed and rapidity.

With respect to treating vergence anomalies in those with visual-vestibular symptoms, the training regimen commences as with vergence oculomotor anomalies in isolation. Once fusional vergence is stabilized in primary gaze at different viewing distances, then vergence is stabilized in left, right, up, and down gaze (12). After stabilizing vergence in these five cardinal positions of gaze, slow horizontal head movement is introduced while the patient's eyes remain fixed on a target at a given viewing distance to stimulate the slow horizontal VOR (i.e., a frequency of head rotation being 0.5–1.0 Hz). During this slow horizontal VOR training, fusion is monitored using visual feedback cues, including luster, motion blur, and physiological diplopia (14). After stabilizing a slow horizontal VOR, the process of introducing head movement is repeated, but with vertical head movement, after which the patients are ready to commence formal VOR training with vestibular therapists.

Anomalies of Photosensitivity

While photophobia refers to increased light sensitivity with frank ocular pain in the presence of ocular inflammation, photosensitivity refers to increased light sensitivity with discomfort in the absence of ocular inflammation (11,12). More commonly in the ABI population, photosensitivity rather than photophobia is reported, and it may present with increased sensitivity to all lighting or only selectively to fluorescent lighting (11). Selective photosensitivity to fluorescent lighting frequently co-exists with increased sensitivity to visual motion and visual-vestibular disturbances (11). Treatment options (11,12) are delineated in Table 31.3. Since photosensitivity in those with ABI may or may not resolve, the treatment options are compensatory and adaptive, rather than restorative.

Although the precise neurologic substrate responsible for photosensitivity in ABI has not yet been elucidated, anomalies of light (i.e., photopic) and dark (i.e., scotopic) adaptation have been hypothesized for general photosensitivity (11), while anomalous critical flicker fusion frequency thresholds may relate to selective photosensitivity to fluorescent lighting (11). Since it is occasionally suggested that some photosensitive patients presenting with dark sunglasses may be malingering, a complete vision evaluation with a nuero-optometrist, ophthalmologist, or nuero-ophthalmologist is advisable. The evaluation should include the measurement of scotopic and/or critical frequency fusion threshold values for comparison to normative data.

Anomalies of Visual Field Integrity

With respect to lateralized visual field defects, there is a spectrum of four categories of visual field integrity (9): 1) no visual field defect and no unilateral spatial inattention (USI, formerly referred to as visual neglect), 2) no visual field defect, but having USI, 3) a visual field defect in conjunction with USI, or 4) a visual field defect without USI.

Assessment of visual field integrity typically requires visual field testing under monocular viewing conditions while controlling for visual fixation and includes confrontation testing with single presentation, as well as perimetric testing (10). When diagnosing a lateralized (i.e., left or right hemi- or quadrant-inattention) USI, additional pencil and paper diagnostic tests are required, such as drawing of a daisy/clock/person, line bisection, or cancellation (9).

Anomalies of visual field integrity may present as diffuse or lateralized (i.e., a left or right hemianopia or quadrantanopia). Diffuse defects are more common in those with TBI and demyelinating disease, while lateralized defects are more common in those with strokes.

Visual field defects in those with TBI have been reported with a frequency of approximately 35% (5) to 39% (18). A recent retrospective study investigating a sample of visually symptomatic stroke patients found that approximately 67% presented with visual field defects (18). That same retrospective study of visually symptomatic individuals with TBI and stroke found that, out of those with visual field defects, homonymous lateralized defects were found in approximately 23% and 48% of those with TBI and stroke, respectively (18).

Associated symptoms related to anomalies of visual field integrity include bumping into objects on one side of space, difficulty with reading-related eye movements due to the field defect, and lack of awareness that one's visual field is no longer intact. Since lateralized homonymous visual field defects do not typically resolve, the treatment options (see Table 31.3) are compensatory and adaptive, rather than restorative. Further information may be obtained from the literature (9).

Patient Safety

Patients with vision symptoms reported in Table 31.4 are likely to have difficulty living independently and should be advised about specific safety concerns.

Table 31.4

Patient Safety Concerns

Symptom	Safety concern
Blurred vision in both eyes	Delayed recognition of objects (as with identifying signs when driving) Difficulty seeing details, which may affect hygiene in terms of: • washing the face and body • food preparation • cleaning of counters, floors

Frequent (or constant) diplopia	Impaired relative depth perception affecting:
	• driving
	• ambulation:
	  o in busy streets/buildings/environments
	  o up and down stairs/escalators

Hemianopia	Veering toward, bumping into, or missing objects on one side of space poses a safety hazard:
	• for driving:
	  o not seeing cars or pedestrians on one side of visual space
	• for ambulation resulting in bruising, falls, or mild concussions:
	  o bumping into walls, doors, and people
	  o tripping over shoes, children's toys, legs of tables/chairs
	  o potentially being struck by a motor vehicle when crossing the street
	• striking one's head on a cupboard door
	• difficulty with shaving resulting in cuts

Patient Education

Patients and their family members/significant others should be educated about the patient's presenting vision dysfunction(s), associated symptoms, and safety concerns. Educational material should be presented at an appropriate level, taking into account the patient's cognitive limitations.

REFERENCES

1. Suchoff IB, Ciuffreda KJ, Kapoor N (eds.). Visual and Vestibular Consequences of Acquired Brain Injury. Santa Ana, CA: Optometric Extension Program Foundation, 2001.
2. Gillen G, Burkhardt A. Stroke Rehabilitation: A Function-Based Approach, 2nd ed. St. Louis, MO: Mosby Yearbook, 2004.
3. McHugh T, Laforce R Jr, Gallagher P, Quinn S, Diggle P, Buchanan L. Natural history of the long-term cognitive, affective, and physical sequelae of mild traumatic brain injury. Brain Cogn 2006; 60:209–211.

4. Baker RS, Epstein AD. Ocular motor abnormalities from head trauma. Surv Ophthalmol 1991; 35:245–267.
5. Sabates NR, Gonce MA, Farris BK. Neuro-ophthalmological findings in closed head trauma. J Clinical Neuro-ophthalmol 1991; 11:273–277.
6. Suchoff IB, Kapoor N, Waxman R, Ference W. Prevalence of visual and ocular conditions in a non-selected acquired brain-injured patient sample. J Am Optom Assoc 1999; 70:301–308.
7. Miller NR, Newman NJ, Biousse V, Kerrison JB, Walsh FB, Hoyt WF. Walsh and Hoyt's Clinical Neuro-ophthalmology: In Three Volumes, 6th ed. Philadelphia: Lippincott Williams & Wilkins; 2004.
8. Leigh RJ, Zee DS. The Neurology of Eye Movements, 4th ed. New York: Oxford University Press, 2006.
9. Suchoff IB, Ciuffreda KJ. A primer for the optometric management of unilateral spatial inattention. Optometry 2004; 75:305–319.
10. Eskridge JB, Amos J, Bartlett JD (eds.). Clinical Procedures in Optometry. Philadelphia: Lippincott, 1991.
11. Chang TT, Ciuffreda KJ, Kapoor N. Critical flicker frequency and related symptoms in mild traumatic brain injury. Brain Injury 2007; 21:1055–1062.
12. Kapoor N, Ciuffreda KJ. Vision disturbances following traumatic brain injury. Curr Treat Options Neurol 2002; 4:271–280.
13. Ciuffreda KJ. The scientific basis for and efficacy of optometric vision therapy in nonstrabismic accommodative and vergence disorders. Optometry 2002; 73:735–762.
14. Scheiman M, Wick B. Clinical Management of Binocular Vision: Heterophoric, Accommodative, and Eye Movement Disorders, 2nd ed. Philadelphia: Lippincott, 2002.
15. Ciuffreda KJ, Kapoor N, Rutner D, Suchoff IB, Han ME, Craig S. Occurrence of oculomotor dysfunctions in acquired brain injury: a retrospective analysis. Optometry 2007; 78:155–161.
16. Ciuffreda KJ, Rutner D, Kapoor N, Suchoff IB, Craig S, Han ME. Vision therapy for oculomotor dysfunctions in acquired brain injury: a retrospective analysis. Optometry 2008; 79: 18–22.
17. Rutner D, Kapoor N, Ciuffreda KJ, Suchoff IB, Craig S, Han ME. Frequency of occurrence and treatment of ocular disease in symptomatic individuals with acquired brain injury: a clinical management perspective. J Behav Optom 2007; 18:31–36.
18. Suchoff IB, Kapoor N, Ciuffreda KJ, Rutner D, Han ME, Craig S. The frequency of occurrence, types, and characteristics of visual field defects in acquired brain injury: a retrospective analysis. Optometry 2008; 79:259–265.
19. Bartlett JD, Jaanus SD (eds.). Clinical Ocular Pharmacology, 3rd ed. Boston: Butterworth-Heinemann, 1995.
20. Bronstein AM. Vision and vertigo: some visual aspects of vestibular disorders. J Neurol 2004; 251:381–387.

Index